The ROYAL
SOCIETY of
MEDICINE
PRESS Limited

Type 2 Diabetes

in Practice

Andrew J Krentz

Consultant in Diabetes and Endocrinology at
Southampton University Hospitals, UK and
Honorary Senior Lecturer in Medicine at the
University of Southampton, UK

Clifford J Bailey

Head of Diabetes Research at Aston
University, UK

1 Wimpole Street, London W1M 8AE, UK

207 E Westminster Road, Lake Forest, IL 60045, USA

www.rsm.ac.uk

British Library Cataloguing in Publication Data
A catalogue record for this book is available from the British Library

ISBN 1-85315-482-2
ISSN 1473-6845

Typeset by Phoenix Photosetting, Chatham, Kent
Printed in Great Britain by Latimer Trend & Company Ltd, Plymouth

Dedication

To our families

Foreword

Type 2 diabetes is a modern-age epidemic estimated to affect 150 million people worldwide. In most occidental societies, 3–7% of adults develop type 2 diabetes and, in certain ethnic groups, the prevalence is much higher. The complications of type 2 diabetes are formidable: microvascular morbidity is the leading cause of adult blindness, amputations and end-stage renal failure, while premature macrovascular disease reduces average life expectancy by almost 10 years. Management of type 2 diabetes is rarely straightforward. It requires rigorous control of blood glucose and special attention to a syndrome of associated vascular risk factors including hypertension, dyslipidaemia and abdominal obesity. There is no place for mediocrity in the treatment of type 2 diabetes; it must be comprehensive, initiated promptly, delivered as intensively as possible and individually tailored.

This book confronts type 2 diabetes with an analysis of its complex aetiology, pathogenesis and natural history. Against this background, the authors provide a clear practical guide to the early diagnosis, organization and optimization of diabetes care. They show how currently available medications can be used effectively to achieve treatment targets that will minimize the complications. With due diligence, they address the awkward day-to-day problems of type 2 diabetes and suggest a rational framework for good clinical practice and informed decision-making.

We must not flinch from the challenge of type 2 diabetes, and this book provides a valuable resource to assist our endeavours.

Professor Sir George Alberti

President of the Royal College of Physicians, London

President of the International Diabetes Federation

About the authors

Andrew J Krentz is a Consultant in Diabetes and Endocrinology at Southampton University Hospitals and Honorary Senior Lecturer in Medicine at the University of Southampton, UK. He trained in medicine and diabetes in Birmingham, UK and Albuquerque, US. His research interests include insulin action and clinical aspects of type 2 diabetes. Dr Krentz is a member of the European Group for the Study of Insulin Resistance (EGIR) and serves on the editorial boards of several journals.

Clifford J Bailey is Head of Diabetes Research at Aston University, UK. He has served as Secretary of the medical and scientific section of the British Diabetic Association (now Diabetes UK), held editorial positions with several journals and acted as an expert witness to drug licensing authorities. His research involves mainly preclinical development of new antidiabetic therapies.

Preface

The prevalence of type 2 diabetes is growing inordinately, with numbers projected to exceed 300 million by the year 2025. The condition is also emerging earlier in life, magnifying the prospect of long-term complications and the inexorable havoc they bring. Recent research has provided unequivocal evidence that improved control of blood glucose and vascular risk factors will delay the onset and reduce the severity of diabetic complications. Recognized guidelines are now in place which encourage a new philosophy for the management of type 2 diabetes: that of treating to targets. The targets are based on substantial evidence for the reduced risk of complications. Those responsible for the care of patients with type 2 diabetes are strongly urged to adopt an intensive approach to their management programme to achieve these targets whenever possible.

Intensive treatment requires considerable extra commitment, understanding, resources and, above all, the optimal use of those resources. In this book we attempt to lay the foundations and provide the wherewithal to accomplish the task of effective management of type 2 diabetes. We have tried to provide information in a clear and concise format, with easy references, highlighted key facts and practical advice.

We pay tribute to those whose lessons we have heeded carefully: George Bray, Ian Campbell, Michael Fitzgerald, Peter Flatt, Angus MacCuish, Allen Matty, Malcolm Nattrass, Gerry Reaven, David Schade, Ken Taylor, Alex Wright and Tony Zalin. Thank you.

We also acknowledge with grateful thanks those involved in the preparation of this book. Janet Allen in Birmingham, Sandra Messiou in Southampton, and Peter Altman, Tanya Thomas and Sarah Bayer at the RSM.

We hope you enjoy this book, find it useful, and gain something that will improve the management of your patients with type 2 diabetes.

Andrew J Krentz
Clifford J Bailey
March 2001

Contents

1. The burden of type 2 diabetes

Epidemiology
Mortality
Morbidity
Prediction and prevention

The term diabetes mellitus refers to a group of metabolic disorders characterized by chronic hyperglycaemia. These disorders usually result from defects in insulin secretion, insulin action or both. Sustained hyperglycaemia is associated with complications in the macrovasculature, microvasculature and nerves, causing protracted morbidity and premature mortality. Macrovascular complications, particularly coronary artery disease and stroke, are increased two- to four-fold, and diabetic patients have a higher prevalence of peripheral vascular disease. Microvascular complications such as retinopathy and nephropathy, and peripheral and autonomic neuropathy, are also common.

Two main categories of diabetes are distinguished. Type 1 – formerly known as insulin-dependent diabetes mellitus (IDDM) or juvenile-onset diabetes – usually manifests before adulthood and accounts for about 5% of all cases. Type 1 diabetes arises mainly through autoimmune destruction of pancreatic β-cells, which leaves the patient with severe insulinopenia and extreme hyperglycaemia. If untreated, insulin deficiency culminates in fatal ketoacidotic coma. Hence, type 1 diabetic patients are dependent on exogenous insulin administration for survival.

Type 2 diabetes – formerly known as non-insulin dependent diabetes mellitus (NIDDM) or maturity-onset diabetes – usually manifests in later adult life and accounts for about 95% of

all cases. This type of diabetes develops mostly through a combination of insulin resistance and defective β-cell function. This causes less severe hyperglycaemia that is not usually life threatening. However, the catalogue of chronic complications of type 2 diabetes represents a serious clinical burden, eroding quality of life and reducing life expectancy. The progressive and heterogeneous nature of type 2 diabetes adds to the complexity of treatment, which usually requires one or more oral antidiabetic agents and may also necessitate the use of insulin.

In most Western societies, the prevalence of all types of diabetes is 3–7%, and it is the fourth or fifth leading cause of death. Its direct costs are currently estimated at 9% in the UK and 14% in the US of total healthcare budgets. The continuing rise in prevalence of type 2 diabetes makes this condition a major focus for every general medical practice.

Epidemiology

Type 2 diabetes is by far the most common form of diabetes on a global scale, accounting for ~95% of all cases. During the past few decades, type 2 diabetes has reached epidemic proportions in many parts of the world; the increase is closely associated with the development of obesity. The World Health Organization (WHO) has predicted that the global prevalence of type 2 diabetes will more than double from 135 million in 1995 to 300 million in 2025 and that this increase will affect both industrialized and developing countries. The impact on less-developed countries will be disproportionately high. Some of the countries expecting the greatest increases, such as India (up 19 million to 57 million), China (up 16 million to 38 million), Pakistan, Indonesia and Mexico, are also some of the poorest. The public health implications are formidable. In the US, for example, the age-adjusted death rate for diabetes has increased 30% over the past two decades while death rates for other major multifactorial diseases have declined (Figure 1.1).

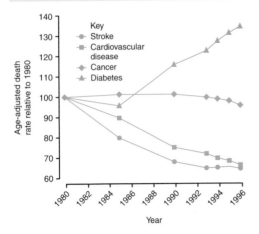

Figure 1.1

Figure 1.1
The increasing mortality associated with diabetes in the US between 1980 and 1996, contrasting with the declining associations with cardiovascular disease and stroke. Sourced from the National Centre for Health Statistics, 1998 and reproduced with permission from McKinaly J, Marceau L. *Lancet* 2000; **356**: 757-61.

Table 1.1
Ethnic variation in type 2 diabetes prevalence in individuals aged 30–64 years. Sourced from the World Health Organization.

	Prevalence (%)	Risk ratio
Pima Indians (Arizona, USA)	50	12
Nauruans (South Pacific)	40	10
Native Australians	25	6
Peninsular Arabs	25	6
South Asians	20	5
West Africans	12	3
Northern Europeans	4	1

The global prevalence of type 2 diabetes is projected to increase to 300 million by 2025

Ethnicity

The prevalence of type 2 diabetes varies more than tenfold between the highest- and lowest-risk populations. The lowest prevalence rates (<3%) have been reported in less-developed countries; by contrast, the highest prevalence (30–50% of adults) is observed in populations such as North American Indians, Pacific Islanders and Australian Aborigines that have experienced radical changes from traditional to 'Westernized' lifestyles during the course of the 20th century (Table 1.1). The Pima Indians of Arizona have the highest reported prevalence of type 2 diabetes: >50% in adults aged 35 years or more. In general, the prevalence of type 2 diabetes is about 3–4% in Europe and about 7% in the US.

Social and behavioural changes are regarded as key factors in the recent global explosion of

type 2 diabetes. Of these, the most important appear to be:

● decreased levels of physical activity
● over-consumption of energy-dense foods.

Ethnicity is an important determinant of susceptibility to insulin resistance, obesity, type 2 diabetes and other cardiovascular risk factors such as dyslipidaemia. Different patterns of plasma lipids (and apoproteins) that exist independently of obesity and insulin resistance may be seen between some of the ethnic groups listed in Table 1.1. For example:

● South Asians tend to have high triglyceride and low HDL-cholesterol concentrations
● Native Americans generally have high triglycerides and low total cholesterol levels
● Peninsular Arabs generally have high triglycerides and high cholesterol levels.

Thus, while South Asians have high rates of insulin resistance and coronary heart disease, Native Americans (with their low total cholesterol concentrations) are relatively protected, despite having a higher prevalence of type 2 diabetes. Similarly, the fact that West Africans tend to have lower triglyceride levels than South Asians and higher HDL-cholesterol levels than Europeans may help to explain the relatively low incidence of coronary heart disease in West Africa compared with North Europe.

Sex ratios

There are reports that type 2 diabetes is more common in men than women (eg in the United Kingdom Prospective Diabetes Study) but other studies have found the converse. The relative prevalences of the sexes vary from population to population and no clear view has emerged. Methodology can have an important influence on measurement of prevalence rates in epidemiological studies.

Genetic and environmental factors

The thrifty genotype hypothesis

In 1962, Neel proposed that certain populations have a high prevalence of genetic traits which once conferred survival advantages during protracted periods of meagre nutrient supply, but which may now be detrimental due to abundant food supplies and reduced habitual levels of physical activity (Table 1.2). During the early 20th century, for example, rates of obesity and type 2 diabetes among the Pima Indians were both very low, corresponding with a physically active lifestyle and limited food availability, but all this has now changed.

The fetal origins hypothesis

Briefly, this hypothesis, formulated by Barker and Hales (Southampton and Cambridge, UK) provides an alternative to the thrifty genotype hypothesis of type 2 diabetes. It proposes that type 2 diabetes results, at least in part, from relative intrauterine malnutrition and that the latter leads to life-long metabolic 'programming'. This includes a reduced complement of islet β-cells combined with insulin resistance in skeletal muscle. Studies in populations in which birth weight has been carefully recorded have consistently demonstrated a correlation between low birth weight and an increased risk of type 2 diabetes in middle age. The risk appears to be particularly high if obesity (a major environmental factor) develops in adulthood. Other cardiovascular risk factors, including hypertension, have also been linked to low birth weight.

Table 1.2
General comparison of traditional and modern lifestyles of aboriginal peoples (the 'thrifty genotype' hypothesis).

	Traditional	Modern
Lifestyle	Hunter-gatherer	Westernized
Food supply	Erratic	Stable
Energy consumption	Low	Excessive
Physical activity levels	High	Low
Obesity	Rare	Common
Type 2 diabetes	Rare	Common

Other genetic factors

A lifetime concordance of approximately 90% for identical twins is strongly suggestive of a genetic component to type 2 diabetes. Commonly, type 2 patients report a family history of the condition: the lifetime risk associated with having a single parent with type 2 diabetes is approximately 40%; it is 50% or more if both parents are affected. However, due to the multiplicity of factors involved, unravelling the genetics of type 2 diabetes has proved highly problematic.

While studies of an uncommon form of diabetes, Maturity-Onset Diabetes of the Young (MODY, page 32), have yielded important evidence for single gene defects, the genetics of most cases of type 2 diabetes involve a polygenic (multigene) inheritance. Many plausible (candidate) genes, such as that for the insulin receptor, have been excluded and, increasingly, attention is being directed to the regulation of:

- genes encoding signalling intermediates within the intracellular pathways of insulin action
- genes involved in the lifecycle of pancreatic β-cells
- genes involved in the insulin secretory function of pancreatic β-cells.

Difficulties in differentiating the insulin resistance attributable to type 2 diabetes *per se* from that associated with obesity may have hampered the identification of causative or predisposing genes. Although the Barker–Hales hypothesis raises the possibility that genetics are not the sole explanation for familial clustering, recent data suggest that diabetogenic MODY genes may also influence birth weight. Thus, it seems that a complex interaction between specific diabetogenic genes, the background genome (as illustrated by ethnic variations), and the intrauterine environment, contributes to the familial aggregation of type 2 diabetes.

Age-related prevalence

The prevalence of type 2 diabetes increases with age; up to 20% of those over 80 years old develop diabetes (Figure 1.2).

The ageing populations of many societies have contributed substantially to the overall increase in the number of patients with diabetes. Glucose tolerance decreases with age, but the extent of the natural deterioration in insulin sensitivity with age remains uncertain. The weight gain that commonly occurs between the fourth and seventh decades of life creates its own state of insulin resistance, particularly if this adiposity is of central (abdominal) distribution.

Recent years have witnessed the emergence of type 2 diabetes in younger groups, including children, adolescents and young adults. This trend is of particular concern, since the clinical course of type 2 diabetes and the development of long-term tissue complications are largely determined by the duration and the degree of hyperglycaemia.

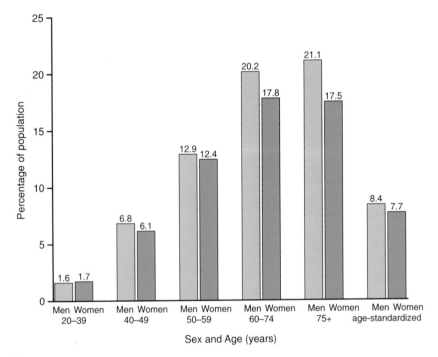

Figure 1.2
Prevalence of diabetes in men and women in the US aged ≥20 years. Included are all diagnosed and previously undiagnosed cases as defined by a fasting plasma glucose ≥7.0 mmol/l (126 mg/dl). Sourced from NHANES III and reproduced with permission from *Diabetes Care* 1998; **21**: 518-24.

Duration x Degree of hyperglycaemia
= Severity of complications

Clinical and metabolic characteristics

Since type 2 diabetes is a heterogeneous disorder, certain features, present in most cases, are regarded as typical (Table 1.3) – but not all will necessarily be present in every affected individual. Factors such as ethnicity, age and stage in the natural history of the disorder will also influence its clinical manifestations.

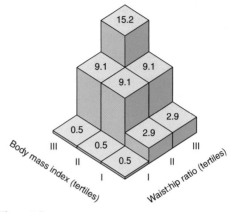

Figure 1.3
Predictive values of tertiles (I is low, III is high) of body mass index and waist:hip ratio for the development of type 2 diabetes in a population of middle-aged Swedish men. The risk of developing type 2 diabetes over a 13-year period is shown for each pillar. Sourced from Larsson B, in Vague J, Björntorp P, Guy-Grand P et al (Eds), *Metabolic complications of the human obesities*. Amsterdam: Elsevier 1985. © 1985. Massachusetts Medical Society.

Table 1.3
Cardinal clinical and metabolic features of type 2 diabetes.

- Presentation usually in middle-age or later life
- Obesity common (present in >75%)
- Symptoms often mild, absent or unrecognized
- Relative rather than absolute insulin deficiency
- Insulin resistance commonly present
- Ketosis-resistant (contrast with type 1 diabetes)
- Progressive hyperglycaemia – even with antidiabetic therapy
- Insulin treatment frequently required to maintain long-term glycaemic control
- Other features of the 'insulin resistance syndrome' – eg hypertension, dyslipidaemia – often present
- High risk of macrovascular complications – which are the main cause of premature mortality
- Hyperglycaemia-related tissue damage may be present at diagnosis

Association with obesity

Associations between obesity and an increased risk of type 2 diabetes have been documented both between and within populations (Table 1.4). The anatomical distribution of adiposity appears to be an important modulator of the clinical impact of obesity. Thus, type 2 diabetes, and other cardiovascular risk factors (chapter 7), are particularly closely associated with visceral (central abdominal, upper body, truncal) obesity, rather than lower body adiposity (Figure 1.3). The waist:hip ratio is a proxy marker for central obesity that is measured easily in clinical practice. Visceral adipocytes

Table 1.4
Age-adjusted relative risk of developing diabetes among US women aged 30–55 and followed for eight years. Sourced from Colditz GA, Willett WC, Stampfer MJ et al. Am J Epidemiol 1990; **132**: 501-13.

Relative risk	Body mass index (kg/m²) at baseline
1.0	<22
5.5	25–26.9
20.0	29–30.1
40.2	33–34.9
60.9	≥35

display several metabolic differences from their subcutaneous counterparts that may partly explain the higher risk of features of the insulin resistance (or metabolic) syndrome (chapter 2). According to some recent studies, low hip circumference may be an independent marker of insulin resistance.

Dietary composition is also important: several studies have shown that an increased proportion of saturated fat in a population's diet is linearly associated with diabetes prevalence. Conversely, the mainly fish diets of the Eskimos and Japanese, rich in omega-3-polyunsaturates, have been reported to improve insulin sensitivity in skeletal muscle.

Other diabetogenic factors

Other factors that may influence the prevalence of abnormal glucose tolerance are presented in Table 1.5. The overall effect of gender is difficult to evaluate and appears to vary between ethnic groups (page 3). The occurrence of diabetes in women increases substantially after the menopause and is positively correlated with parity. Increased circulating concentrations of triglycerides and non-esterified fatty acids are associated with the development of insulin resistance and type 2 diabetes. An accumulation of triglyceride in skeletal muscle, or the increased availability of fatty acids, provides an alternative energy source (to glucose) resulting in decreased cellular glucose use. Chronically raised circulating lipid concentrations also impinge on the intracellular pathways of insulin signalling to reduce insulin sensitivity. A protracted rise in the fatty acid concentration may also impair β-cell function.

Table 1.5
Factors that may influence the prevalence of glucose intolerance and type 2 diabetes.

Age	Diet
Gender	Dyslipidaemia
Ethnicity	History of gestational
Family history of diabetes	diabetes
Obesity	Hyperinsulinaemia
Regional adiposity	Country of residence
Low physical activity	Socio-economic status
Lifestyle	Tobacco use

Mortality

Type 2 diabetes has a major impact on health and survival (Figure 1.1). Patients with type 2 diabetes have a reduced life-expectancy – an average five- to 10-year curtailment if they are diagnosed in middle-age (ie between 40 and 60 years). In developed countries, the age-specific mortality rates are approximately twice those of non-diabetic individuals. The principal cause of premature mortality is cardiovascular disease. Myocardial infarction is the most common cause of death, followed by stroke (Table 1.6).

Table 1.6
Age-specific mortality associated with type 2 diabetes (compared with the non-diabetic population). Sourced from Howlett HCS, Bailey CJ, in Krentz AJ (Ed). *Drug treatment of type 2 diabetes*. Auckland: ADIS International, 2000.

Life expectancy*	Reduced by	~ 5–10 years
Mortality rate	Increased	> 2-fold
Fatal coronary heart disease	Increased	~ 2–4-fold
Fatal stroke	Increased	~ 2–3-fold

*Aged 40–60 years at diagnosis

Insulin resistance and cardiovascular risk

Classic risk factors for cardiovascular disease are often already present when type 2 diabetes is diagnosed. The collective impact of these risk factors has been referred to as a 'ticking clock' for atherosclerosis. The presence of diabetes accelerates these adverse effects. Hypertension and dyslipidaemia are more frequently encountered in patients with type 2 diabetes than in age-matched non-diabetic controls. It has been proposed that insulin resistance – defined as a reduced biological effect of insulin – is a fundamental metabolic defect that links these (and other) risk factors.

Although insulin resistance is widely held to be an important, if not primary, defect in type 2 diabetes, the development of significant glucose intolerance implies an additional defect – impaired insulin secretion. While type 2 diabetes is a metabolically heterogeneous condition, insulin resistance and relative insulin deficiency are prominent defects, and both present in most patients.

> Insulin resistance + β-cell dysfunction
> = Type 2 diabetes

Impaired glucose tolerance

Insulin resistance is also present in subjects with lesser degrees of glucose intolerance. Most patients with type 2 diabetes will have passed from normality through an intermediate stage of impaired glucose tolerance (page 36). The latter state, although not directly associated with a risk of microvascular complications, shares some of the increased risk of atherosclerotic cardiovascular disease that is a feature of type 2 diabetes. In Western societies, more than 5% of younger adults and 20% of those over 65 years of age have impaired glucose tolerance. Since the latter is asymptomatic, most cases remain undiagnosed, but approximately 1–10% of cases will progress to type 2 diabetes each year – the risk is further influenced by factors such as ethnicity, obesity, family history of type 2 diabetes, history of glucose intolerance during pregnancy and the influence of certain drugs with diabetogenic effects (Table 1.5).

The gradual nature of the transition from normal glucose tolerance, through impaired glucose tolerance, finally to type 2 diabetes, may at least partly explain the absence of marked symptoms in many patients. The absence of the typical osmotic symptoms that accompany the onset of type 1 diabetes, for example, would explain the comparative delay in diagnosis in a high proportion of patients. In turn, the delay in diagnosis helps to explain why evidence of diabetes-related tissue damage can be found in up to 50% of newly diagnosed type 2 patients. Backward extrapolations based on the progression of retinopathy have suggested that the onset of pathological hyperglycaemia frequently occurs several (~5–10) years before the diagnosis is made.

The extent of tissue complications at diagnosis reflects the degree and duration of antecedent hyperglycaemia. Thus, the case for earlier identification of individuals with asymptomatic type 2 diabetes, or glucose intolerance, is strengthened. Population screening is one approach, but its cost-effectiveness remains the subject of debate. Factors such as ethnicity and family history of type 2 diabetes will influence the efficacy of screening.

Morbidity

Macrovascular disease

In addition to the high mortality rate associated with atherosclerotic disease (Table 1.6), there is considerable morbidity associated with macro-vascular disease (Table 1.7). For some associated conditions, such as heart failure, the risk is much higher for diabetic patients than matched non-diabetic control subjects. The prevalence of the following atherosclerotic risk factors is increased in patients with type 2 diabetes:

- hypertension is increased approximately 1.5-fold
- dyslipidaemia is increased approximately two-fold.

Table 1.7
Age-specific morbidity from atherosclerotic disease and related disorders in patients with type 2 diabetes. Sourced from Howlett HCS, Bailey CJ, in Krentz AJ (Ed). *Drug treatment of type 2 diabetes*. Auckland: ADIS International, 2000.

Coronary heart disease	Increased ~2–3-fold
Cerebrovascular disease	Increased >2-fold
Peripheral vascular disease	Increased ~2–3-fold
Cardiac failure	Increased ~2–5-fold

Microvascular complications

Patients with type 2 diabetes are also at risk of developing specific long-term microvascular and neuropathic complications:

- retinopathy
- nephropathy
- peripheral and autonomic neuropathy.

Respectively, these may lead ultimately to visual impairment, end-stage renal failure and foot ulceration. In fact, diabetes is now the largest single cause of adult blindness, end-stage renal failure, and non-traumatic amputation in Western societies.

The high, and increasing, prevalence of type 2 diabetes has ensured that microvascular complications make a major contribution to the overall public health burden now associated with diabetes (Table 1.8). Types 1 and 2 diabetes now contribute approximately equal numbers of patients to renal replacement programmes, for example. The relationship between microvascular disease and atherosclerosis is complex and tight. For example, patients who develop diabetic nephropathy are particularly prone to accelerated cardiovascular disease. This explains why most patients with type 2 diabetes who develop proteinuria due to diabetic nephropathy will actually die from coronary heart disease before they reach end-stage renal failure.

Table 1.8
Approximate prevalence of microvascular complications in type 2 diabetes. Sourced from Howlett HCS, Bailey CJ, in Krentz AJ (Ed). *Drug treatment of type 2 diabetes*. Auckland: ADIS International, 2000.

Clinical nephropathy (ie >300 mg/24 hour albuminuria)	~30%
Retinopathy at diagnosis	~20%
Retinopathy (lifetime risk)	~80%
Retinopathy leading to blindness	~2%
Peripheral neuropathy	~60%
Foot ulceration	~5%

Impact of therapeutic interventions

Hyperglycaemia

Results from the 20-year, randomized United Kingdom Prospective Diabetes Study and other prospective studies have confirmed that therapeutic interventions to reduce the level of hyperglycaemia delay the onset, reduce the progression and so reduce the severity of microvascular complications. The beneficial effects of improved glycaemic control on atherosclerosis were less impressive. For this reason, other risk factors for cardiovascular disease must be assessed and treated with lifestyle advice and specific drugs, as necessary (chapters 7 and 8).

Non-pharmacological measures, including dietary management, weight reduction where required, and increased levels of physical exercise, are the cornerstones of diabetes treatment, acting primarily to counter insulin resistance. Several classes of antidiabetic drug are also available. These are required by most patients. Sulphonylureas and other insulin secretagogues raise plasma insulin concentrations; metformin and the thiazolidinediones improve insulin action in certain tissues; α-glucosidase inhibitors reduce the rate of carbohydrate digestion, thus slowing carbohydrate absorption from the gastrointestinal tract. Agents from different classes can often be usefully combined to increase glucose-lowering efficacy.

The United Kingdom Prospective Diabetes Study also demonstrated the difficulties of reinstating near-normal long-term glycaemic control in most patients diagnosed in middle-age. Even insulin treatment was ineffective in maintaining normoglycaemia in the long term. The development of novel oral agents and insulin analogues, combined with a greater understanding of how and when to use these agents, offers the prospect of improved results in the future. It is important to remember that the sulphonylureas, metformin, thiazolidinediones and insulin are also associated with unwanted side-effects and that occasionally these can be serious, even fatal. A careful assessment of the potential risks and benefits of pharmacotherapy must be made for each drug, particularly since diabetic complications such as nephropathy can increase the risks associated with some drugs.

Hypertension

Tight control of blood pressure has been identified as another important therapeutic goal in patients with type 2 diabetes, influencing microvascular complications (notably retinopathy) as well as atheroma. Not only is the prevalence of hypertension increased in type 2 diabetes compared with the non-diabetic population, but the magnitude of overall risk reduction when hypertension is controlled is generally greater in diabetic than non-diabetic individuals. This reflects the higher absolute risk of cardiovascular disease in the diabetic population. Several classes of antihypertensive drug have been shown to confer benefit, but the level of blood pressure attained appears to be more important than the class of agent. The results of a recent clinical trial (MICRO-HOPE; page 102) suggest that the angiotensin converting enzyme (ACE) inhibitors may have cardioprotective effects that are independent of their blood-pressure lowering effects, but this requires confirmation.

Although the results of several large, comparative trials of antihypertensive agents are awaited, it is anticipated that the excess cardiovascular risk attributable to hypertension may not be fully reversible using the current range of drugs. Furthermore, current blood pressure reduction targets present a major therapeutic challenge; combination therapy using several agents from different classes is often required, thus adding to the polypharmaceutical burden faced by patients with type 2 diabetes. The issue of compliance, long-neglected in diabetes, is at last receiving greater attention.

Dyslipidaemia

In the past few years a considerable body of evidence has accumulated from observational studies and randomized intervention trials that have focused attention on the importance of dyslipidaemia and other modifiable risk factors for atherosclerosis. Many middle-aged patients with type 2 diabetes have a 10-year risk of cardiovascular events that equals or exceeds that associated with overt atherosclerotic disease in non-diabetic subjects. In the latter group, the role

of drugs such as statins is well-established as a secondary preventative measure. For patients with type 2 diabetes, the distinction between primary prevention (of cardiovascular disease) and secondary prevention is less clearcut, due to the elevated risk of fatal and non-fatal events. Moreover, those patients with type 2 diabetes who survive a first myocardial infarction have a much poorer prognosis than their non-diabetic counterparts.

For these reasons, patients with type 2 diabetes are regarded as potential candidates for therapeutic interventions such as:

- specific lipid-modifying drugs (statins and fibrates)
- low-dose aspirin (and other antiplatelet drugs, especially following surgical coronary intervention)
- ACE inhibitors (usually as part of antihypertensive therapy or in the treatment of heart failure).

In the UK, the National Service Framework for Coronary Heart Disease (2000) highlighted patients with type 2 diabetes as a group whose absolute 10-year risk will often justify the use of these drugs, in addition to specific antidiabetic and antihypertensive therapy.

Prediction and prevention

It is currently difficult to predict accurately who will develop type 2 diabetes – particularly in populations with a relatively low prevalance of the disorder. Before we improve our predictive skills, major lacunae in our understanding of the aetiology of this heterogeneous disorder need to be filled. However, it is currently possible to define groups at higher-than-average risk. The related factors identified to date include:

- having a first-degree relative (parent or sibling) with type 2 diabetes
- belonging to certain high-risk ethnic groups (page 2)
- being middle-aged or older (earlier rather than later in the high-risk ethnic groups)

- having impaired glucose tolerance (IGT) or impaired fasting glucose (IFG)
- obesity (especially visceral adiposity)
- having certain endocrinopathies (eg Cushing's syndrome or acromegaly)
- receiving treatment with diabetogenic drugs (eg high-dose glucocorticoids)
- a sedentary lifestyle
- having had gestational diabetes
- exhibiting features of the insulin resistance syndrome (page 24)
- small birth weight (Barker–Hales fetal origins hypothesis)
- cigarette smoking.

Clinical studies (eg the Diabetes Prevention Study in Finland) have shown that the risk of progression from a high-risk category such as IGT to type 2 diabetes may be averted, or at least deferred, by measures such as supervised physical training and dietary advice. Large trials evaluating the impact of pharmacological agents (eg the US Diabetes Prevention Program) may clarify the efficacy and safety of drug intervention for IGT, but the latter approach is not currently recommended.

For now, sensible 'lifestyle' advice for higher-risk individuals includes:

- a prudent diet
- avoidance of obesity
- regular aerobic exercise
- avoidance of cigarettes
- avoidance of diabetogenic drugs.

Further reading

Hales CN, Barker DJ. Type 2 (non-insulin dependent) diabetes mellitus: The thrifty phenotype hypothesis. *Diabetologia* 1992; **35**: 595-601.

Harris MI, Flegal KM, Cowie CC *et al*. Prevalence of diabetes, impaired fasting glucose, and impaired glucose tolerance in US adults. The Third National Health and Nutrition Examination Survey, 1988-1994. *Diabetes Care* 1998; **21**: 518-24.

McKeigue PM. Ethnic variation in insulin resistance and risk of type 2 diabetes. In: Reaven G, Laws A (Eds). *Insulin resistance. The metabolic syndrome X*. Totowa, NJ: Humana Press, 1999; 19-33.

Nelson RG, Bennett PH, Tuomilehto J *et al*. Preventing non-insulin dependent diabetes. *Diabetes* 1995; **44**: 483-8.

O'Rahilly S. Non-insulin dependent diabetes mellitus: the gathering storm. *BMJ* 1997; **314**: 955-9.

Reaven GM. Role of insulin resistance in human disease. *Diabetes* 1988; **37**: 1595-607.

Rosenbloom AL, Joe JR, Young RS, Winter WE. Emerging epidemic of type 2 diabetes in youth. *Diabetes Care* 1999; **22**: 345-54.

The Expert Committee on the diagnosis and classification of diabetes mellitus. Report of the Expert Committee on the diagnosis and classification of diabetes mellitus. *Diabetes Care* 1997; **20**: 1183-97.

Zimmet P. The pathogenesis and prevention of diabetes in adults. *Diabetes Care* 1995; **18**: 1050-64.

2. Pathophysiology

Insulin secretion
Insulin action
Insulin resistance

Defects in insulin secretion and insulin action are evident in subjects with type 2 diabetes. Although the temporal sequence of early pathophysiological events has not yet been resolved, the available evidence suggests that a decrease in insulin sensitivity is likely to precede a significant decrease in insulin secretion in most cases. The debate over whether insulin resistance or subtle abnormalities in insulin secretion comes first continues. However, the issue is confused by the fact that defects in secretion can aggravate reduced action, and vice versa. This conundrum is essentially why investigators have shown so much interest in the precursor stage of diabetes, impaired glucose tolerance (pages 28 and 36).

Both islet β-cell function and insulin action are already impaired during the impaired glucose tolerance stage, and while recent insights from uncommon monogenic forms of diabetes have clarified some points, many aspects of the pathophysiology of type 2 diabetes require further elucidation. This chapter outlines the normal physiology of insulin secretion and insulin action before reviewing the main biochemical defects that characterize type 2 diabetes.

Insulin secretion

Insulin (Figure 2.1) is the principal anabolic hormone of the body. It has a multiplicity of acute (within minutes) actions on the regulation of intermediary metabolism. Effects on the cellular transport of nutrients and ions are also prominent and there are many longer-term effects on gene expression (Table 2.1). Insulin is a 51-amino acid peptide composed of two chains, A and B, joined by disulphide bonds and arranged in a complex tertiary structure. Insulin molecules aggregate in pairs (dimers) which then aggregate with zinc to form the hexamers that comprise the insulin granules in the pancreatic β-cells.

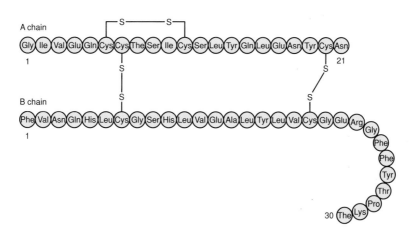

Figure 2.1
Primary structure (amino acid sequence) of human insulin.

Table 2.1
Physiological actions of insulin.

a) Metabolic actions:
   - Suppression of hepatic glucose production
   - Stimulation of glucose uptake by muscle and adipose tissue
   - Promotion of glucose storage as glycogen
   - Suppression of lipolysis and hepatic ketogenesis
   - Regulation of protein turnover
   - Effects on electrolyte balance
b) Other actions (longer-term):
   - Regulation of growth and development (*in utero* and *post-utero*)
   - Regulation of expression of certain genes

Control of insulin secretion

The pre-proinsulin gene is located on the short arm of chromosome 11. Transcription produces pre-proinsulin which is cleaved to proinsulin. Within the Golgi apparatus, proinsulin is then converted via intermediates to the final secretory products, insulin and C(connecting)-peptide (Figure 2.2).

Within the β-cells, insulin molecules associate as hexameric crystals around two zinc ions. When

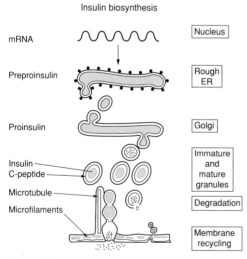

Insulin biosynthesis

mRNA — Nucleus

Preproinsulin — Rough ER

Proinsulin — Golgi

Insulin — Immature and mature granules
C-peptide —

Microtubule — Degradation

Microfilaments —

Membrane recycling

Figure 2.2
Insulin biosynthesis and processing. Insulin and C-peptide are released in equimolar quantities. ER = endoplasmic reticulum.

insulin secretory granules fuse with the cell membrane to release their contents, insulin and C-peptide are released in equimolar quantities.

Insulin secretion is tightly matched to circulating glucose concentrations. While insulin is constantly secreted in regular pulses at a low background (basal) level (this accounts for approximately 50% of daily secretion), it is also secreted in close temporal association to the rise in portal plasma glucose after meals. Glucose is transported into the β-cells by the GLUT-2 glucose transporter protein. Within the cell, it is initially phosphorylated to glucose-6-phosphate by the enzyme glucokinase and subsequently metabolized by the glycolytic pathway and tricarboxylic acid cycle to produce adenosine triphosphate (ATP) (Figure 2.3). ATP generation is proportional to the quantity of glucose entering the cell, which, in turn, is proportional to the extracellular glucose concentration.

ATP serves to close ATP-sensitive potassium channels in the β-cell membrane, leading to depolarization of the cell and an influx of extracellular calcium ions through voltage-gated channels (Figure 2.3). The resulting increase in intracellular calcium concentration activates calcium-sensitive proteins which trigger insulin granule translocation towards the membrane. Finally, fusion of these granules with the cell membrane enables insulin secretion.

Insulin is also secreted in response to other secretagogues such as amino acids. Its secretion is inhibited by certain hormones, notably adrenaline (epinephrine) and somatostatin, and enhanced by others, such as glucagon, glucagon-like peptide 1 (7-36 amide) and gastric inhibitory polypeptide. Insulin is also known to exert autocrine effects, inhibiting its own secretion and, possibly, assisting the growth and division of local islet cells.

The metabolic actions of insulin at tissue level may be antagonized by the classic counter-regulatory hormones: glucagon, the catecholamines, glucocorticoids and growth hormone. These

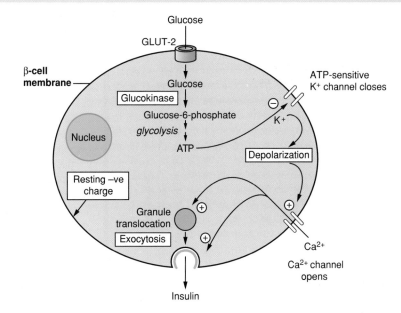

Figure 2.3
Synthesis–secretion coupling model of insulin secretion. GLUT-2 = glucose transporter-2.

hormones exert their anti-insulin actions through direct effects on insulin target tissues.

Defective insulin secretion

Islet β-cells normally adapt to insulin resistance (page 21) in target tissues with a compensatory increase in insulin secretion. In obese people, for example, insulin secretion may be several times higher than normal. As long as insulin secretion is unimpaired, glucose tolerance can be well-maintained – even in rare genetic syndromes of severe insulin resistance such as Leprechaunism. Marked hyperinsulinaemia is the consequence of such resistance to the actions of insulin.

While cross-sectional and prospective studies in animals and humans have shown that insulin secretion increases in line with plasma glucose concentrations, in many individuals the pancreatic β-cells appear to reach their maximum adaptive capability when plasma glucose exceeds approximately 7–8 mmol/l two hours after a 75 g oral glucose challenge. Protracted hyperglycaemia is associated with no further adaptation of β-cell function and, eventually, insulin secretion starts to decline

and the hyperglycaemia escalates. At this stage of impaired glucose tolerance, patients are still generally hyperinsulinaemic, but not sufficiently so to normalize their metabolism. Subsequent progression to type 2 diabetes is associated with progressive failure of β-cell compensation (Figure 2.4a). Absolute insulinopenia becomes apparent with more marked hyperglycaemia; at this stage, the normal phasic responses of insulin secretion have been lost (Figure 2.4b).

Defective insulin secretion kinetics

Advocates for the primacy of β-cell dysfunction in the development of type 2 diabetes point to subtle defects in insulin secretion in 'pre-diabetic' individuals at high-risk of developing the disorder. Some first-degree relatives of subjects with type 2 diabetes have defects in the dynamics of insulin secretion, including loss of the normal pulsatility (usually about every 13 minutes). Impairment of the first phase (two to five minutes) of insulin secretion (probably the release of pre-formed insulin adjacent to the cell membrane) is also an early abnormality in the development of type 2 diabetes.

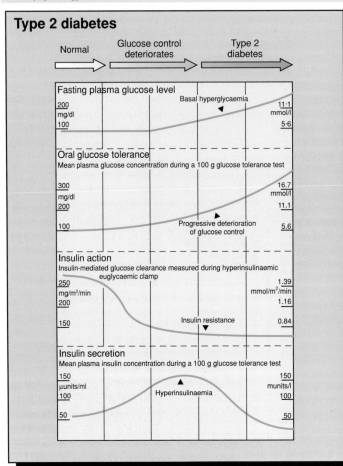

Figure 2.4a
Pathogenesis of type 2 diabetes: changes in glucose and insulin concentration and insulin action during the progression from normal through impaired glucose tolerance (IGT) to type 2 diabetes. To convert munits/l to pmol/l, multiply by 6.
Sourced from DeFronzo RA. *Diabetes* 1988; **37**: 667-87.

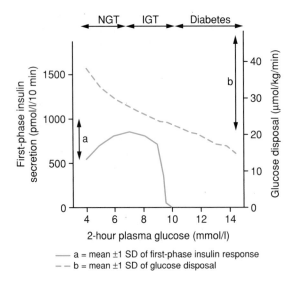

— a = mean ±1 SD of first-phase insulin response
-- b = mean ±1 SD of glucose disposal

Figure 2.4b
Relationship between insulin resistance (insulin-mediated glucose disposal) and first-phase insulin secretion and two-hour post-challenge glucose levels in subjects with normal glucose tolerance (NGT), impaired glucose tolerance (IGT) and type 2 diabetes. Reproduced with permission from Groop LC, Widén E, Ferrannini E. *Diabetologia* 1993; **36**: 1326-31.

Non-diabetic first-degree relatives of people with type 2 diabetes have been shown to have impaired first-phase (and second-phase) insulin release in response to glucose challenge compared with matched healthy controls (Figure 2.5). It is noteworthy that these first-degree relatives are also prone to below-average sensitivity to insulin.

Experimental evidence suggests that defects in the dynamics of insulin secretion may lead to impaired metabolic action in target tissues. Thus, insulin lowers blood glucose more effectively when delivered in pulses rather than as a continuous infusion. Loss of the first phase of insulin secretion has been implicated in the pathogenesis of insulin resistance in target

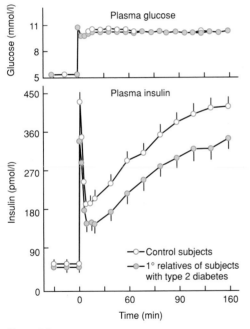

Figure 2.5
Plasma glucose (top) and insulin (bottom) concentrations during hyperglycaemic clamps in 100 non-diabetic first-degree relatives of subjects with type 2 diabetes and a control group of 100 matched healthy volunteers. All were of European ancestry. Note that first- and second-phase insulin secretion in response to hyperglycaemia is impaired in the non-diabetic relatives. Reproduced with permission from Pimenta W *et al. JAMA* 1995; **273**: 1855-61.

tissues; in particular, the suppression of endogenous (mainly hepatic) glucose production is more efficient when the rapid first-phase of insulin secretion is present (or is compensated for by exogenous infusion). This has therapeutic implications because failure to suppress endogenous glucose production sufficiently can lead to early post-prandial hyperglycaemia (endogenous glucose production is normally inhibited by the insulin surge at the beginning of a meal). Impaired post-prandial suppression of circulating glucagon concentrations may help to sustain inappropriately normal to high rates of hepatic glucose production in patients with type 2 diabetes. If the post-prandial plasma glucose concentrations remain elevated, they then continue to stimulate the β-cells, and an extended, later (second-phase) hyperinsulinaemia is produced. In turn, this can lead to down-regulation of tissue insulin receptors.

Defective β-cell proinsulin processing

In the course of synthesis of insulin from proinsulin, partially processed intermediates (mostly 32-33 split proinsulin) are also produced (Figure 2.6a). Since proinsulin and its intermediates cross-react to variable degrees with many of the anti-insulin antibodies used in conventional insulin radioimmuno- and ELISA assays, this can lead to overestimates of the degree of hyperinsulinaemia. Increased circulating concentrations of proinsulin and partially processed proinsulin molecules – all of which have lower biological activity than insulin – have been reported in people with type 2 diabetes or impaired glucose tolerance. Studies using highly specific antibodies and immunoradiometric assays have demonstrated increased proportions of proinsulin and 32-33 split proinsulin in these groups (Figure 2.6b). These abnormalities are detectable even in the absence of the confounding effects of obesity or fasting hyperglycaemia.

Hyperproinsulinaemia in subjects with type 2 diabetes is not corrected by treatment with sulphonylureas, which suggests that

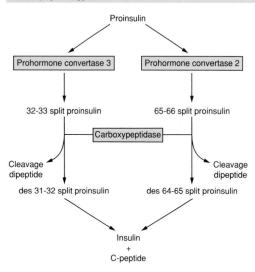

Figure 2.6a
Insulin biosynthesis and intermediates. Proinsulin is processed via prohormone convertase 2 and prohormone convertase 3. The latter is predominant; plasma levels of 65-66 split proinsulin and des 64-65 proinsulin are quantitatively very low.

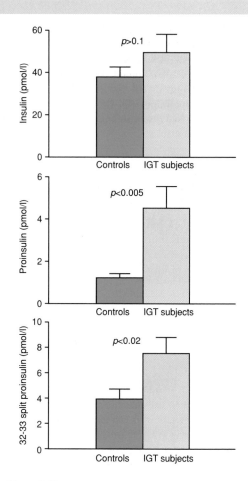

Figure 2.6b
Fasting plasma concentrations of insulin, intact proinsulin and 32-33 split proinsulin (mean + SEM) in eight non-obese men with recently diagnosed impaired glucose tolerance (WHO, 1985; shaded bars) and eight control subjects (all men; solid bars) matched for age and body mass index. p values refer to differences between the groups by unpaired t-test. Reproduced with permission from Krentz AJ et al. Clin Sci 1993; **85**: 97-100. © The Biochemical Society and the Medical Research Society.

ameliorating the detrimental effect of hyperglycaemia *per se* on β-cell function (so-called 'glucose toxicity', page 23) does not normalize β-cell proinsulin processing. Regardless, the reduction of plasma glucose levels through pharmacological or non-pharmacological measures will produce useful secondary improvements in β-cell function.

The molecular mechanisms responsible for impaired insulin secretion in type 2 diabetes are still incompletely delineated. The possibility of defective stimulation of secretion through defective gut-derived factors ('incretins') is given credence by the fact that exogenous glucagon-like peptide 1 (7-36 amide) enhances the endogenous insulin response to meals. The inhibitory effect of chronically raised fatty acid concentrations on β-cell insulin secretion ('lipotoxicity') contrasts with the enhanced glucose-stimulated insulin secretion seen during acute elevations of plasma fatty acids. Further,

fatty acids can induce β-cell apoptosis under experimental conditions. The pathogenic role of fatty acids in type 2 diabetes may not have been fully appreciated and it has been suggested that failure of insulin secretion to suppress lipolysis may be a crucial step in the natural history of this disorder. Since fatty acids provide an energy supply for the process of gluconeogenesis, this could exacerbate fasting hyperglycaemia by accelerating endogenous glucose production. Fatty acids also provide an alternative substrate to glucose for energy production in muscle (page 21). Finally, insulin resistance may be aggravated by progressive β-cell failure in a spiral of metabolic decompensation.

Islet cell amyloid

Histological changes in the islets have long been recognized in subjects with type 2 diabetes. These often include an initial hypertrophy associated with hyperplasia of the β-cells and glucagon-secreting α-cells but, in most cases of established duration, there is a loss of β-cell mass and a relative increase in glucagon-secreting α-cell numbers. Accelerated accumulation of islet amyloid is a prominent histological feature, but the role of amyloid deposition in the deterioration of β-cell function which occurs over time remains uncertain.

β-cell failure

In the United Kingdom Prospective Diabetes Study, mathematical modelling demonstrated a progressive failure of β-cell function, despite treatment with oral antidiabetic agents or insulin. This finding has obvious therapeutic implications, suggesting that, once the process of β-cell failure has become advanced, it proceeds in an apparently unmodifiable or 'programmed' manner – at least with the treatments used in this study.

Susceptibility to subtle abnormalities in β-cell function during the early pathogenesis of type 2 diabetes is believed to reflect the combined effects of genetics and environment. Genetic factors might, for example, include reduced levels of expression of the genes encoding GLUT-2, glucokinase, or the other enzymes of glucose metabolism and energy production. The genes encoding potassium and calcium channels and other signalling components of the insulin secretion pathway may also be subject to limited expression, as may those encoding enzymes involved in the processing of proinsulin to insulin. While the loss of acute

glucose–insulin stimulus-secretion coupling is an early recognized defect of β-cell function, it is not yet clear how this defect occurs. Persistent environmental influences relating to glucotoxicity, lipotoxicity and β-cell overactivity undoubtedly contribute to the early adaptive changes in β-cell function and increased β-cell mass, but the genetic constraints that underlie subsequent failure to maintain either individual β-cell performance or total β-cell population (apoptosis exceeds division and neogenesis) are still unknown.

Summary

Defects in insulin secretion are prominent in subjects with impaired glucose tolerance and type 2 diabetes (Table 2.2); subtle abnormalities in β-cell function can be demonstrated in non-diabetic first-degree relatives of subjects with type 2 diabetes, but the importance of these abnormalities in the aetiology of type 2 diabetes remains unresolved. This may reflect limitations in the techniques available for the assessment of insulin secretion

Table 2.2
Early defects and potential metabolic consequences of islet β-cell dysfunction in impaired glucose tolerance and type 2 diabetes.

Diminished or absent first-phase insulin release
Impaired suppression of hepatic glucose production with resulting post-prandial hyperglycaemia leads to late (second-phase) hyperinsulinaemia

Abnormal pulsatility of insulin secretion
Present in first-degree relatives of subjects with diabetes; diminished glucose-lowering effect of insulin

Increased secretion of proinsulin-like molecules
Marker of early β-cell dysfunction; pathological significance uncertain, but plasma levels correlate with certain metabolic risk markers for atherosclerosis

Progressive β-cell failure
Failure to compensate for insulin resistance in target tissues; defective regulation of lipolysis and glucose metabolism; progressive fasting and post-prandial hyperglycaemia

in humans and the failure of some studies to match for important variables such as obesity and the absolute level of glycaemia. Impaired insulin secretion is a major therapeutic target in type 2 diabetes (chapter 8).

Insulin action

The insulin receptor

The actions of insulin are mediated through the high-affinity binding of insulin to specific receptors located in the membranes of almost all mammalian cells. Certain cells, which show profound acute metabolic responses to insulin, are regarded as classic targets for this hormone. They include:

- hepatocytes
- skeletal muscle cells
- adipocytes.

Other cell types such as erythrocytes do not show matched acute responses to insulin, but this has not deterred investigators from studying insulin–receptor binding in them. Key post-binding events include conformational alterations and autophosphorylation at tyrosines within the β-subunit of the receptor (Figure 2.7). The phosphorylated β-subunit of the insulin receptor acts as a kinase enzyme, initiating several cascades of post-receptor signalling events, the details of which are only partially elucidated. There are at least six intracellular substrates for the insulin receptor, the best characterized of which is insulin receptor substrate-1 (IRS-1). The various pathways of phosphorylation and dephosphorylation reactions leading from these substrates result in the activation or suppression of insulin-sensitive enzymes – the activation of glycogen synthase, for example, which converts glucose-6-phosphate to glycogen. Other pathways result in the genomic effects of insulin – the deinduction (repression) of

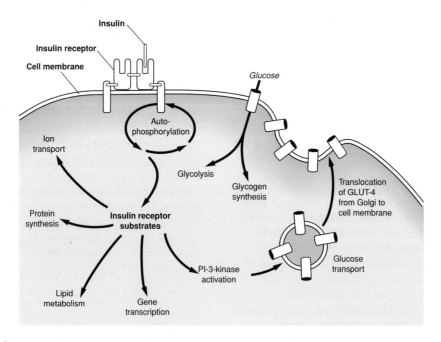

Figure 2.7
Cellular binding of insulin to its receptor and major post-binding events. Sourced from Krentz AJ. *Churchill's Pocketbook of Diabetes*. Edinburgh: Churchill Livingstone, 2000. GLUT-4 = Glucose transporter-4; PI-3-kinase = Phosphatidylinositol-3 kinase.

phosphoenolpyruvate carboxykinase (PEPCK), for example, a key enzyme in the pathway of gluconeogenesis, which converts oxaloacetate to phosphoenolpyruvate.

There are four main mechanisms for impaired insulin action within cells: prereceptor defects, receptor defects, post-receptor defects or effector defects.

Prereceptor defects

Prereceptor defects, such as reduced insulin access to the target cells, may be due to local changes in tissue perfusion, alterations in transcapillary insulin transfer, the presence of insulin antibodies, or a structurally defective insulin molecule. However, these defects have not been identified as making a clinically significant contribution to the common form of type 2 diabetes.

Receptor defects

Receptor defects, such as a reduced number of receptors or a reduced receptor affinity for insulin, may occur in response to chronic hyperinsulinaemia (so-called 'down-regulation'). Although obesity and lesser degrees of glucose intolerance are associated with reduced insulin-receptor binding, mainly by reducing the numbers of receptors, this is largely reversible on treatment. Inherited severe receptor defects (such as those experienced in Leprechaunism) are very rare and do not necessarily result in diabetes.

Post-receptor defects

Defective intracellular events that occur after insulin has bound to its receptor seem to be mainly responsible for insulin resistance in type 2 diabetes. Not only is the maximal response to insulin impaired, but this effect is usually only partially reversible with current treatments. The exact nature of these intracellular defects has not yet been resolved, but reductions in the insulin-stimulated tyrosine phosphorylation of IRS-1 and decreased activity of the subsequent signalling intermediates – such as phosphatidylinositol-3

kinase (PI3K) and protein kinase B (PKB) – have both been noted in the muscle of patients with type 2 diabetes. The known signalling intermediates of insulin action seem to be structurally normal in type 2 diabetes, rather it is the cumulative impact of small changes in the levels of expression and activities of some of these intermediates that seems to impact on insulin sensitivity in obesity and type 2 diabetes.

Effector defects

Effector defects are defects in the final products of the insulin signalling pathways, such as glucose transporters and key glucoregulatory enzymes. The insulin-stimulated translocation of the main insulin-sensitive glucose transporter (GLUT-4) to the plasma membrane of muscle cells is impaired in patients with type 2 diabetes, while the transporters themselves remain structurally normal. Likewise, key insulin-sensitive enzymes remain intact. These facts support the view that the insulin-signalling pathways governing the translocation of glucose transporters to the plasma membrane and the activities of key gluco-regulatory enzymes are the main sites of defective function responsible for insulin resistance.

Glucoregulatory disturbances of insulin resistance

In normal, healthy individuals, venous plasma glucose concentrations are strictly maintained at approximately 5–7 mmol/l. At any time, this concentration reflects a net balance between the rate of appearance of glucose in the circulation and its rate of disappearance from the circulation. The glucose-lowering effects of insulin (Figure 2.8) are primarily:

- suppression of hepatic glucose production (ie reducing the rate of glucose supply into the circulation)
- stimulation of glucose disposal (ie clearance from the circulation, principally by skeletal muscle, but also by adipose tissue).

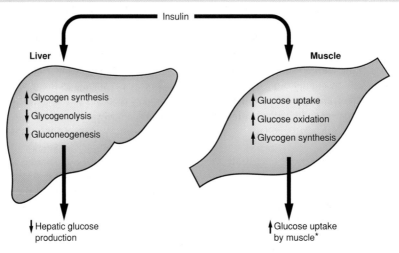

Figure 2.8
Direct actions of insulin on glucose metabolism. Sourced from Krentz AJ. *Churchill's Pocketbook of Diabetes*. Edinburgh: Churchill Livingstone, 2000. *Insulin also stimulates glucose uptake by adipose tissue. However, during a hyperinsulinaemic euglycaemic clamp, ~90% of insulin-mediated glucose disposal occurs in muscle. This is regarded as the 'gold standard' technique for measuring insulin action in humans, but may not accurately reflect normal physiology.

Hepatic glucose production

In the post-absorptive state (ie after an 8–12-hour overnight fast) the rate at which glucose enters the circulation from the liver is the main determinant of the plasma glucose concentration. Initially, this glucose is derived mainly from the breakdown of stored glycogen. As hepatic glycogen stores become depleted (usually after about 24 hours), there is increasing synthesis of *de novo* glucose from 3-carbon precursors such as lactate and various amino acids (gluconeogenesis). Suppression of hepatic glucose production is a major regulatory action of insulin and, in type 2 diabetes, the excessive hepatic glucose production is mainly due to inadequate suppression of gluconeogenesis.

> Hepatic glucose production is the principal determinant of fasting blood glucose concentration

Glucose disposal

Stimulation of glucose uptake (with subsequent entry into the glycolytic pathway or storage as glycogen) requires higher plasma insulin concentrations than are necessary to suppress hepatic glucose production. The stimulation of intracellular translocation of GLUT-4 glucose transporters to the cell membrane for this purpose is a key function of insulin (Figure 2.7). GLUT-4 is strongly expressed in skeletal and heart muscle, and also in adipose tissue. Other isoforms of glucose transporters do not require insulin for translocation to the cell membrane: GLUT-1 is widely distributed and facilitates a continual basal (low) level of glucose uptake; GLUT-2 is found mainly in liver and islet β-cells, where it facilitates a high rate of glucose transport that fluctuates according to changes in extracellular glucose concentration; GLUT-3 provides a steady low rate of glucose transport into tissues that are strongly dependent on glucose, particularly the brain; GLUT-5 is a high-affinity fructose transporter found mainly in the small intestine and testes.

Lipolysis and ketone body metabolism

Another crucial role of insulin is to inhibit the breakdown of adipose tissue stores of triglyceride into non-esterified fatty acids and the gluconeogenic precursor, glycerol. The products of glucose metabolism via glycolysis are lactate (through anaerobic metabolism) and CO_2 (through aerobic metabolism) – the latter is the primary route to energy production. In turn, lactate can be transferred to the liver and there enter the gluconeogenic pathway, leading to glucose formation (the Cori cycle).

Since fatty acids are the principal substrate for ketogenesis within the liver, insulin can suppress ketogenesis by controlling plasma fatty acid levels (Figure 2.9). Both fatty acids and ketones can be used by many tissues as alternative fuels to glucose (eg during starvation and prolonged exercise). The appearance of ketones in the urine of a subject with diabetes indicates severe insulin deficiency. Although ketosis is uncommon in type 2 diabetes, it can develop during severe intercurrent illness and is an indication for prompt insulin treatment.

Insulin resistance

Insulin resistance is a cardinal metabolic feature of type 2 diabetes. It may be defined in generic terms as 'a reduced biological response to a physiological amount of insulin'. The presence of insulin resistance is implied when there is normo- or hyperglycaemia alongside hyperinsulinaemia. For research purposes, insulin action can be quantified using labour-intensive techniques such as the hyperinsulinaemic euglycaemic clamp (also known, more simply, as the glucose clamp), which is widely regarded as the gold standard for quantifying whole-body insulin action. Essentially, it involves simultaneous infusions of insulin and dextrose. The principle is straightforward: the greater the quantity of dextrose that is required to maintain euglycaemia during the sustained hyperinsulinaemia produced by the insulin infusion, the more insulin-sensitive the individual (and *vice versa*).

> Fasting hyperinsulinaemia in the presence of a normal or elevated plasma glucose level implies insulin resistance

In non-diabetic individuals, insulin resistance is usually inferred from the presence of obesity (although there is evidence of heterogeneity within the obese population). It is generally asymptomatic if compensated by hyperinsulinaemia.

> Insulin resistance *per se* is asymptomatic

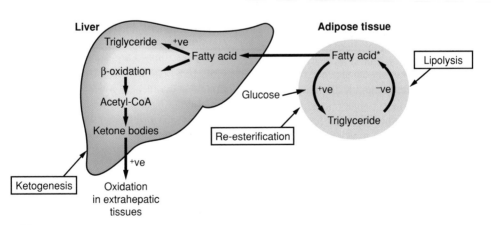

Figure 2.9
Major points of direct regulation of lipolysis and ketone body metabolism by insulin. Sourced from Krentz AJ. *Churchill's Pocketbook of Diabetes*. Edinburgh: Churchill Livingstone, 2000. ⁺ve = Increased by insulin; ¯ve = Decreased by insulin. *The gluconeogenic precursor glycerol is also liberated by lipolysis.

Clinical features

Severe insulin resistance may be accompanied by physical signs such as:

- Acanthosis nigricans – this dermatological feature is found in the axillae, around the nape of the neck, and elsewhere.
- Acrochordons – multiple skin tags.

Other features, present to variable degrees, include:

- Hyperandrogenism – (ie acne, hirsutism) in women of reproductive age.
- Syndrome-specific features – present in some rare congenital syndromes, such as Leprechaunism, Rabson–Mendenhall syndrome, and the lipodystrophic syndromes.
- Acromegaloid features – have also been reported in the absence of elevated growth hormone concentrations.

> Insulin resistance is a prominent feature of type 2 diabetes

Polycystic ovary syndrome

Polycystic ovary syndrome (PCOS) deserves particular mention because it is probably the most common endocrine disorder in young women. It is often associated with obesity and insulin resistance and typically presents with features of hyperandrogenism such as hirsutism, acne, and a history of menstrual and conception problems (oligomenorrhoea). Other biochemical features of the insulin resistance syndrome (page 24) are common in women with PCOS, implying that the risk of cardiovascular disease may be increased in women with PCOS. Retrospective studies also suggest that the risk of developing type 2 diabetes is higher in affected women.

PCOS overlaps with the much less common type A severe insulin resistance syndrome. Hirsutism and cystic ovarian changes are common accompaniments. The insulin resistance of polycystic ovary syndrome is thought to be independent of obesity (although obesity is an important modifier). It is hypothesized that the resulting hyperinsulinaemia stimulates ovarian androgen production.

> Insulin acts as a gonadotrophin in polycystic ovary syndrome

Plasma levels of sex hormone-binding globulin are reduced in the presence of insulin resistance because hyperinsulinaemia inhibits the hepatic production of this carrier protein. This increases target tissue exposure to free (unbound) androgens, mainly testosterone. Weight loss increases plasma levels of sex hormone-binding globulin, reducing free testosterone levels, and may lead to improved insulin action and reduced hirsutism. Reduced levels of sex hormone-binding globulin are regarded as a biochemical marker for subclinical insulin resistance. While recent studies have suggested a potential role for metformin and the thiazolidinediones (chapter 10) in the management of PCOS, their efficacy and safety require further evaluation.

Insulin resistance in healthy populations

Some insulin resistance also seems to exist in apparently healthy populations. In fact, up to 25% of otherwise normal individuals are thought to have unrecognized insulin resistance to degrees similar to those seen in patients with glucose intolerance or type 2 diabetes. While the significance of this insulin resistance is presently uncertain, the prevalence of cardiovascular risk factors is known to increase with increasing plasma insulin concentration.

Reduced insulin sensitivity is observed in certain physiological situations, notably puberty and the second and third trimesters of pregnancy. Insulin resistance may also be induced by drug treatment (eg with glucocorticoids). Compensatory insulin secretion from the pancreatic β-cells (page 13) usually ensures that such episodes of insulin resistance remain subclinical. Other factors that may influence insulin sensitivity include:

- *Gender* – although men and women normally have broadly similar insulin sensitivities if differences in body composition (women have more adipose tissue) and aerobic capacity (lower in women) are taken into account.

- *Ageing* – ageing is reportedly associated with reduced insulin sensitivity. However, this has been disputed, and the contribution of age-related insulin resistance to the decline in glucose tolerance commonly observed in the elderly remains uncertain.

Mechanisms of acquired insulin resistance 1: glucose toxicity

There is evidence that hyperglycaemia *per se* adversely affects insulin action – an effect known as 'glucotoxicity'. The detrimental effect of glucotoxicity on endogenous insulin secretion has been discussed (page 17). The clinical implication is that reducing the level of hyperglycaemia (whether by non-pharmacological measures, oral antidiabetic agents or insulin) may produce secondary improvements in insulin action.

Mechanisms of acquired insulin resistance 2: lipotoxicity

Disturbed fatty acid metabolism is well documented in type 2 diabetes (and lesser degrees of glucose intolerance). Chronically elevated fatty acid concentrations, mainly due to impaired suppression of lipolysis, may be considered to have the following 'toxic' effects:

- impaired insulin-mediated glucose disposal and oxidation (via the glucose–fatty acid or Randle cycle)
- accelerated hepatic glucose production
- suppressed endogenous insulin secretion
- hypertriglyceridaemia (chapter 7).

Increased production of the cytokine tumour necrosis factor-α (TNF-α) by adipocytes may aggravate insulin resistance through inhibitory effects on insulin signalling and GLUT-4 translocation. Elevated circulating fatty acid concentrations have also been implicated in the pathogenesis of hypertension (page 98), but the clinical relevance of the latter observations is uncertain.

Mechanisms of acquired insulin resistance 3: regional adiposity

Insulin action is often reduced in the presence of obesity, but glucose clamp studies have revealed inverse correlations between insulin sensitivity and visceral or abdominal fat deposits, independent of total adiposity (as judged by body mass index). Abdominal obesity is commonly observed in men – although many women also have upper-body obesity with or without lower-body or gynaecoid obesity. Abdominal obesity is strongly associated with an increased risk of type 2 diabetes. The link is believed to result from the increased metabolic activity of visceral adipocytes compared with subcutaneous depots. Visceral adipocytes are not only relatively resistant to the actions of insulin, but exhibit greater sensitivity to the lipolytic effect of the catecholamines. This combination serves to increase the rate of lipolysis resulting in increased portal delivery of non-esterified fatty acids to the liver (page 21). However, some investigators have not confirmed a unique contribution of visceral adiposity to whole-body insulin sensitivity. A recently described hormone, resistin, has been proposed as a link between obesity and insulin resistance.

Hypertension and insulin resistance

Hypertension is very common among patients with type 2 diabetes (page 98). Moreover, many patients with essential hypertension have features of the insulin resistance syndrome. Hypotheses linking insulin resistance with hypertension in patients with type 2 diabetes include:

- Insulin-induced sympathetic activation – which could lead to vasoconstriction and increased peripheral vascular resistance
- Insulin-stimulated renal sodium retention.

Both are speculative and the cause of hypertension in patients with type 2 diabetes – the prevalence of which is also influenced by factors such as age and obesity – remains uncertain. There is intriguing but inconsistent evidence that insulin-sensitizing drugs such as metformin and troglitazone (chapters 9 and 10) can lower blood pressure.

The insulin resistance syndrome

This has a number of synonyms: 'metabolic syndrome', 'syndrome X' and 'Reaven's syndrome'. Insulin resistance has been implicated in a number of pathological states which frequently co-segregate in affected individuals and which are associated with an increased risk of atherosclerotic disease, principally coronary heart disease (Figure 2.10). Key features of the syndrome, originally described by Reaven in 1988 (and refined in 1995) include:

- insulin resistance (defined as decreased insulin-mediated glucose disposal)
- hyperinsulinaemia
- visceral obesity
- glucose intolerance or type 2 diabetes

- dyslipidaemia (hypertriglyceridaemia, low plasma HDL-cholesterol levels and raised small dense LDL-cholesterol levels)
- hypertension
- a pro-coagulant state
- atherosclerosis.

Since there is currently no consensus on the full ramifications of the syndrome, the following may also be included:

- hyperuricaemia
- microalbuminuria
- hyper-homocysteinaemia.

Environmental factors such as high-fat diets and low levels of physical activity may exacerbate insulin resistance. The following criteria have been proposed by the European Group for the study of Insulin Resistance (1999):

A fasting plasma insulin level in the highest 25% of the population in question, together with two of the following:

- a fasting plasma glucose $\geq$6.1 mmol/l
- hypertension (blood pressure $\geq$140/90 mmHg, or treated)

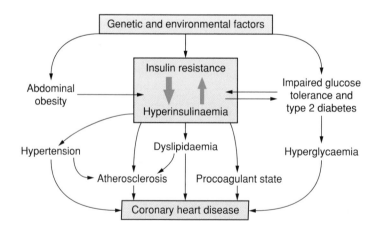

Figure 2.10
Proposed association of key components of the insulin resistance syndrome (metabolic syndrome). Each component is a risk factor for coronary heart disease. Several components are often manifest together in each individual, leading to a substantial increase in the risk of coronary heart disease.

- dyslipidaemia (plasma triglycerides >2.0 mmol/l or HDL-cholesterol <1.0 mmol/l)
- central obesity (waist circumference $\geq$94 cm in men and $\geq$80 cm in women).

There are practical difficulties with such definitions, however, particularly in relation to the lack of population-derived reference ranges for plasma insulin concentration.

Non-alcoholic steatohepatitis

Recently, it has been suggested that fatty infiltration of the liver is associated with other features of the insulin resistance syndrome (such as glucose intolerance and dyslipidaemia) in some patients. An overlap with iron deposition, in turn linked to genes associated with haemochromatosis, complicates the picture.

Clinical implications of insulin resistance

Components of the insulin resistance syndrome are frequently present in combination in subjects with impaired glucose tolerance and type 2 diabetes. Whether tissue insulin resistance is the fundamental metabolic defect which links these abnormalities together is not yet known. However, there is considerable epidemiological and experimental evidence to show that insulin resistance is associated with an increased risk of cardiovascular disease. More importantly, the cumulative effects may be synergistic – ie the magnitude of the risk associated with a combination of factors can be greater than would be expected by simple addition. Finally, there is evidence from longitudinal studies that these metabolic risk factors (a) worsen continuously across the spectrum of glucose intolerance and (b) are present even before diagnosis of type 2 diabetes in high-risk individuals.

> Cardiovascular risk factors magnify the risk of atherosclerosis when present in combination

Taking a different perspective, many patients with essential hypertension have one or more additional components of the insulin resistance syndrome which contribute to their risk of cardiovascular events. Accordingly, it is recommended that management of high-risk patients, such as those presenting with hypertension plus other components of the syndrome, takes account of all vascular risk factors detectable in these individuals. Reduction of cardiovascular risk demands attention to all modifiable risk factors (chapter 7).

> Components of the insulin resistance syndrome should be sought and treated in subjects with diabetes, hypertension or dyslipidaemia

Further reading

Arner P. Not all fat is alike. *Lancet* 1998; **351**: 1301-2.

Barker DJ, Hales CN, Fall CHD *et al.* Type 2 (non-insulin-dependent) diabetes mellitus, hypertension, and hyperlipidaemia (syndrome X): relation to reduced fetal growth. *Diabetologia* 1993; **36**: 62-7.

Davidson MB. Clinical implications of the insulin resistance syndromes. *Am J Med* 1995; **99**: 420-6.

Gerich JE. Insulin resistance is not necessarily an essential component of type 2 diabetes. *J Clin Endocrinol Metab* 2000; **85**: 2113-5.

Iourno MJ, Nestler JE. The polycystic ovary syndrome: treatment with insulin sensitizing agents. *Diabetes Obesity Metab* 1999; **1**: 127-36.

James O, Day C. Non-alcoholic steatohepatitis: another disease of affluence. *Lancet* 1999; **353**: 1634-6.

Kahn SE, Andrikopoulos S, Verchere CB. Islet amyloid. A long-recognized but underappreciated pathological feature of type 2 diabetes. *Diabetes* 1999; **48**: 241-53.

Krentz AJ. *Insulin resistance*. Oxford: Blackwell Science. In press.

Reaven GM. Pathophysiology of insulin resistance in human disease. *Physiol Revs* 1995; **75**: 473-86.

Reaven GM, Laws A. *Insulin resistance: the metabolic syndrome X*. Totowa: Humana Press, 1999.

Shepherd PR, Kahn BB. Glucose transporters and insulin action. *N Engl J Med* 1999; **341**: 248-57.

Shulman GI. Cellular mechanisms of insulin resistance. *J Clin Invest* 2000; **106**: 171-6.

Steppan CM, Bailey ST, Bhat S *et al.* The hormone resistin links obesity to diabetes. *Nature* 2001; **409**: 307-12.

3. Classification

American Diabetes Association and World Health Organization classification systems

Secondary forms of diabetes

Drug induced diabetes

Endocrinopathies

Genetic syndromes

In 1980, the World Health Organization (WHO) proposed a classification of diabetes mellitus based on the recommendations of the US National Diabetes Data Group. This classification (revised in 1985), reflected advances in understanding of the aetiology and pathogenesis of diabetes. Notably, the descriptive terms 'juvenile-onset' and 'maturity-onset' diabetes were replaced with the terms 'insulin-dependent' and 'non-insulin dependent' diabetes respectively. A new category – impaired glucose tolerance (IGT) – was also introduced to describe the intermediate zone of diagnostic uncertainty between normal glucose tolerance and diabetes.

In 1997, the American Diabetes Association (ADA) again reclassified diabetes, revised the diagnostic criteria and introduced another new category – impaired fasting glucose (IFG). This most recent classification attempts to categorize according to disease aetiology rather than treatment. The WHO revised its 1980/1985 classification similarly at about the same time.

> The 1997 American Diabetes Association classification system is based on aetiology, rather than therapy

ADA and WHO classification systems

The 1997 ADA classification of diabetes, subsequently endorsed by the WHO, recognizes four main categories.

Type 1 diabetes

Previously known as 'insulin-dependent' or 'juvenile onset' diabetes – characterized by selective islet β-cell destruction, absolute

Table 3.1

Aetiological classification of diabetes mellitus (American Diabetes Association, 1997).

I. *Type 1 diabetes*
   Islet β-cell destruction usually leading to absolute insulin deficiency:
   A. Immune-mediated
   B. Idiopathic.
II. *Type 2 diabetes*
   Heterogeneous – ranging from predominantly insulin resistance with relative insulin deficiency to predominantly insulin deficiency with insulin resistance.
III. *Other specific forms*
   A. Genetic defects of β-cell function, eg MODY syndromes*
   B. Genetic defects in insulin action, eg Leprechaunism
   C. Diseases of the exocrine pancreas, eg pancreatitis
   D. Secondary to endocrinopathies, eg acromegaly
   E. Drug- or chemical-induced, eg by glucocorticoids
   F. Infections, eg congenital rubella.
   G. Uncommon forms of immune-mediated diabetes, eg anti-insulin receptor antibodies
   H. Other genetic syndromes associated with diabetes, eg Down's syndrome.
IV. *Gestational diabetes*
   Diabetes or impaired glucose tolerance diagnosed in pregnancy – includes pre-existing diabetes.

NB. All patients with type 1 diabetes require life-long insulin treatment. Patients in categories II, III and IV may also require insulin treatment. Thus, use of insulin *per se* can no longer be used to subcategorize diabetes.
*MODY = maturity-onset diabetes of the young due to specific genetic defects of glucokinase, or hepatic nuclear factors.

insulin deficiency and reliance on exogenous insulin to preserve life.

Type 2 diabetes

Previously known as 'non-insulin dependent' or 'maturity-onset' diabetes – occurs mostly in later life, but recent reports of occurrence in children highlight the importance of classifying according to aetiology.

Other specific types

Diabetes may be secondary to a variety of diverse conditions, including specific genetic or acquired syndromes and the use of certain drugs. All are now clearly defined and classified under this subheading.

Gestational diabetes

When diabetes mellitus or IGT is diagnosed during pregnancy, it is referred to as gestational diabetes. Gestational diabetes is pathophysiologically most similar to type 2 diabetes, but insulin is often required for adequate glycaemic control. Gestational diabetes usually resolves post-partum.

Impaired glucose tolerance

The 1980 WHO reclassification introduced the intermediate category of IGT in recognition of the area of diagnostic uncertainty between normality and diabetes. Patients with impaired, but stable, glucose tolerance are not at risk of developing the microvascular complications of diabetes (chapter 6). However, they are at increased risk of developing type 2 diabetes and macrovascular disease (chapter 7). Both IGT and the more recently defined category of IFG are usually asymptomatic, and both are discussed in more detail in chapter 4.

> Impaired glucose tolerance represents an intermediate stage between normality and diabetes

Secondary forms of diabetes

Diabetes mellitus is a feature of various hereditary and acquired diseases and may arise during treatment with certain drugs. Patients with secondary forms of diabetes are just as susceptible to chronic complications as those with primary forms of this disorder.

> Patients with secondary diabetes are also at risk of long-term complications

Pancreatic disease

Acute pancreatitis

Transient hyperglycaemia may require insulin therapy, but permanent diabetes is unlikely to follow a single episode of pancreatitis unless massive pancreatic destruction occurs.

Chronic pancreatitis

Chronic pancreatitis is frequently complicated by glucose intolerance or diabetes and, at least in Western countries, is often attributable to alcoholism. Pancreatic calcification may be evident on radiographs or computerized tomographs. While sulphonylurea treatment may suffice in some patients with an adequate number of functioning β-cells, insulin therapy is often required. Associated intestinal malabsorption and variable degrees of glucagon deficiency (due to α-cell destruction) may predispose to troublesome hypoglycaemia.

Carcinoma of the pancreas

The diagnosis should be suspected in elderly patients presenting with a short history of diabetes including the following features:

- marked and rapid weight loss (especially if disproportionate to the hyperglycaemia)
- upper abdominal pain (especially radiating to the back)
- jaundice with features of biliary obstruction.

Diabetes developing *de novo* alongside pancreatic carcinoma is not, as may be thought, a consequence of insulin deficiency due to islet destruction. Insulin resistance is implicated and glucose tolerance may improve with resection of the tumour. Pancreatic carcinoma may occur more commonly in patients with pre-existing type 2 diabetes.

Pancreatectomy

Pancreatectomy is sometimes required to relieve chronic pancreatitis-associated pain. If more than 80–90% of the pancreas is excised, life-long insulin therapy will be needed – large doses (>30–40 units/day) are rarely necessary in the absence of obesity, because insulin resistance is not usually a feature. Sulphonylureas (chapter 9) are ineffective. Partial distal resection (including that performed on the related donors of segmental pancreatic graft recipients) causes variable degrees of glucose intolerance, including diabetes.

Cystic fibrosis

Diabetes mellitus may complicate cystic fibrosis. Since patients with cystic fibrosis are now living longer, diabetes is emerging as an important complication. Diabetes usually appears in the late teens or early 20s. The recurrent chest infections and intestinal malabsorption associated with cystic fibrosis may complicate diabetes management. Insulin is eventually required in most patients, but sulphonylureas may be useful as an interim measure.

Haemochromatosis

This autosomal dominant inborn error of metabolism is characterized by excessive iron deposition in various organs. Diabetes, for which insulin therapy is often required, also develops in approximately 50% of cases. However, haemochromatosis is an uncommon cause of diabetes. Its alternative name 'bronzed diabetes' describes the associated cutaneous pigmentation (partly due to melanin). Diagnosis should be suspected in patients with hepatomegaly, suspicious pigmentation, pituitary or testicular failure, cardiomyopathy or chondrocalcinosis – a search for the most common mutations causing this disorder is now possible. Hepatocellular carcinoma develops in

approximately 15% of cases. Investigations include measurement of serum iron and ferritin, hepatic imaging and liver biopsy. Family members of a proband should be screened. Treatment is by regular venesection and the prognosis good if adequate treatment is begun before cirrhosis develops.

Malnutrition-related diabetes

Malnutrition-related diabetes encompasses the rare ketosis-resistant subtypes of 'fibrocalculous' or 'protein-deficient pancreatic' diabetes that are encountered in the tropics. Cyanide (derived from the cassava plant) toxicity has been hypothesized, but this has been challenged. Some subjects require high doses of insulin (>200 units/day).

Drug-induced diabetes

Many drugs are associated with the development of glucose intolerance or type 2 diabetes in predisposed individuals. A deterioration in glycaemic control in patients with pre-existing diabetes is also a common clinical problem. Anti-inflammatory doses of corticosteroids, for example, may necessitate the use of insulin in type 2 diabetes previously controlled by oral agents. In fact, major metabolic decompensation, such as hyperosmolar pre-coma or coma can ensue. Post-receptor insulin resistance and activation of the glucose–fatty acid cycle (chapter 2) are implicated.

Individuals with a personal history of glucose intolerance, eg gestational diabetes, are at particular risk from corticosteroid therapy, but the latter may also precipitate diabetes in middle-aged or elderly individuals who have no personal history of glucose intolerance. The typical scenario involves the development of insulin resistance which can progress to diabetes in individuals with a subclinical partial defect in insulin secretory capacity. This is difficult to predict, but a family history of type 2 diabetes should alert the clinician. Whenever high-dose corticosteroids are begun, plasma glucose monitoring is a sensible precaution.

High-dose corticosteroids may precipitate diabetes mellitus in predisposed individuals

For some other drugs, degrees of insulin resistance and/or impairment of endogenous insulin secretion are implicated in the development of glucose intolerance or type 2 diabetes:

Diuretics

Diuretics, particularly high-dose thiazides, have been associated with insulin resistance and hypokalaemia-induced impairment of insulin secretion. Modern prescribing of lower doses of thiazide ($\leq$2.5 mg bendrofluazide, or equivalent) minimizes the adverse metabolic effects. Loop diuretics are held to be less diabetogenic.

β-blockers

Patients with hypertension often have other features of the insulin resistance syndrome (chapter 2). Both β-blockers (non-selective agents, particularly) and thiazide diuretics have been implicated in the development of type 2 diabetes in people with essential hypertension, particularly when used in combination. However, the clinical benefits of lowering elevated blood pressure are likely to outweigh the metabolic disadvantages (chapter 7).

ACE inhibitors

Recent reports indicate that the angiotensin converting enzyme (ACE) inhibitors may actually reduce the risk of type 2 diabetes development in hypertensive subjects. It has been suggested that effective treatment of hypertension *per se* may help to reduce the risk of type 2 diabetes – but this remains speculative.

β-adrenergic agonists

There is evidence that the β-adrenergic agonists, such as ritodrine (used in premature labour), carry a risk of metabolic decompensation in women who have diabetes, or who had gestational diabetes, particularly when given parenterally.

β-blockers and thiazide diuretics can promote the development of type 2 diabetes

Oral contraceptives

Minor metabolic effects have been noted with the use of modern, low-dose oestrogen preparations. Progesterone-only preparations also have very little effect.

Cyclophilin immunosuppressants

Immunosuppression is required for organ transplantation (eg renal transplantation for diabetic nephropathy, chapter 6). Cyclosporin is associated with insulin resistance and β-cell toxicity; similar but greater metabolic derangements have been observed with tacrolimus. Concomitant corticosteroid therapy exacerbates these effects.

Diazoxide

Diazoxide is an infrequently used antihypertensive vasodilator with an inhibitory effect on insulin secretion. It has been exploited in the medical management of insulinoma and severe sulphonylurea-induced hypoglycaemia (chapter 9), but can have potent diabetogenic effects in non-diabetic individuals.

Protease inhibitor-associated lipodystrophy

Recently, a syndrome has been described in patients with human immunodeficiency virus-1 (HIV-1), also receiving treatment with protease inhibitors or nucleoside-analogue reverse transcriptase inhibitors. The cardinal features of this syndrome are:

- peripheral acquired lipoatrophy (face, limbs)
- central adiposity (abdomen and dorsocervical spine)
- hyperlipidaemia

- glucose intolerance
- insulin resistance.

Some suggest that this syndrome represents a programmed adipocyte death (apoptosis) induced by antiretroviral drugs; others suggest mitochondrial toxicity. Type 2 diabetes has been reported in <10% of cases, some in the absence of antiretroviral therapy.

Endocrinopathies

Pathological and chronic hypersecretion of hormones that antagonize insulin action (ie the counter-regulatory hormones, page 12) are frequently associated with glucose intolerance and/or type 2 diabetes mellitus. Deteriorating glycaemic control in a subject with pre-existing diabetes may be the presenting feature of such endocrinopathies.

- *Thyrotoxicosis*: is the most common endocrinopathy encountered in patients with type 2 diabetes. Excess thyroid hormones antagonize the effects of insulin. Increased lipolysis is implicated in the impairment of glycaemic control.
- *Acromegaly*: approximately 30% of patients with acromegaly have IGT and another 30% have diabetes mellitus.
- *Cushing's syndrome*: post-receptor insulin resistance is seen, especially when there are very high cortisol levels secondary to ectopic corticotrophin (ACTH) secretion.
- *Conn's syndrome*: glucose intolerance is reported in about 50% of cases of primary hyperaldosteronism – the effects of hypokalaemia on insulin secretion are implicated.
- *Phaeochromocytoma*: insulin resistance and α-adrenergic inhibition of insulin secretion by adrenaline (epinephrine) (page 12) are associated with this uncommon endocrinopathy.
- *Glucagonoma*: this very rare metabolic syndrome includes a necrolytic migratory erythema rash associated with insulin resistance.
- *Somatostatinoma*: this also very rare

syndrome includes cholelithiasis and is associated with inhibition of endogenous insulin secretion.

- *Hyperparathyroidism*: is associated with subclinical insulin resistance.
- *Prolactinomas*: are the most common functioning pituitary tumours. Hyperprolactinaemia can be associated with hyperinsulinaemia, but glucose tolerance is rarely affected.

In contrast to these endocrinopathies, certain autoimmune disorders are associated with enhanced insulin sensitivity. (These, incidentally, are more frequently encountered in patients with type 1 diabetes as part of a pluriglandular syndrome). There is a tendency to fasting hypoglycaemia in non-diabetic patients with untreated hypoadrenalism.

- *Primary hypothyroidism*: this common autoimmune disorder is associated with a reduced metabolic rate and impaired insulin clearance.
- *Addison's disease*: is rare but requires life-long corticosteroid replacement therapy.
- *Hypopituitarism*: will lead to increased insulin sensitivity (in a sulphonylurea- or insulin-treated patient), thus increasing the risk of hypoglycaemia.

Genetic syndromes

The incidence of diabetes – mainly diabetes with ketosis-resistant, non-insulin dependent phenotypes – is also increased in a number of inherited syndromes. These include:

Chromosomal defects

- *Down's syndrome*: trisomy/translocation of chromosome 21
- *Turner's syndrome*: karyotype 45 XO, mosaics
- *Klinefelter's syndrome*: 47, XXY, mosaics
- *Prader-Willi syndrome*: deletion/ translocation of chromosome 15
- *Bardet-Biedl syndrome*: autosomal recessive disorder – main features are retinitis pigmentosa, polydactyly, central obesity,

mental retardation, diabetes and hypogonadism; genetic loci on chromosome 11 have been described

- *Alström syndrome*: pigmentary retinal degeneration associated with sensorineural deafness, obesity, diabetes, hyperlipidaemia and nephropathy; disease-causing defect mapped to chromosome 2p.

Neurodegenerative disorders

- *Myotonic dystrophy*: this autosomal dominant, multisystem disorder arises as a result of expansion of a trinucleotide repeat on chromosome 19. It is associated with insulin resistance, but overt diabetes is relatively uncommon. The mutation codes for a putative serine–threonine protein kinase.
- *Friedreich's ataxia*: this autosomal recessive disorder is associated with diabetes; insulin resistance and impaired insulin secretion are reported.

Mitochondrial syndromes

Mitochondria are intracellular organelles responsible for the generation of energy by oxidative phosphorylation. Defects in the mitochondrial genome associated with diabetes were first recognized in the 1990s. Mitochondrial DNA is exclusively maternally inherited.

Wolfram syndrome

This is a rare autosomal recessive neurodegenerative syndrome comprising diabetes insipidus, diabetes mellitus (with a tendency to ketosis), optic atrophy and (sensorineural) deafness (hence, also known as DIDMOAD). The deafness may not be clinically evident and many patients also develop hydronephrosis, ataxia and psychiatric disturbances. Death occurs in the third to fifth decades. Although autosomal recessive inheritance has been proposed, mitochondrial defects have been described.

Maternally inherited diabetes

Syndromes associated with mitochondrial DNA mutations account for just a small proportion (<1%) of diabetes in the UK. However, families in which the maternal transmission of non-insulin dependent forms of diabetes (category III diabetes according to the 1997 reclassification) is associated with sensorineural deafness have also been described. A point mutation in mitochondrial DNA at position 3243 in the tRNA$^{LEU(UUR)}$ gene has been identified. While the same mutation is responsible for another rare syndrome – 'myopathy, encephalopathy, lactic acidosis and stroke-like episodes (MELAS)' – diabetes mellitus is not usually a feature of the latter syndrome.

Maturity-Onset Diabetes of the Young (MODY)

This uncommon form of diabetes is a heterogeneous autosomal dominant disorder characterized by hyperglycaemia and relative insulinopenia that presents before the age of 25 years. Offspring with both parents affected by type 2 diabetes have generally been excluded from the molecular genetic studies that have elucidated the aetiology of this heterogeneous syndrome. MODY and the common form of type 2 diabetes differ in several important respects and the main features which distinguish them are presented in Table 3.2.

> There is a 50% risk of diabetes in the offspring of a patient with MODY

Several distinct genetic subtypes have been identified to date, the first having been discovered in 1992:

- *MODY 1* – mutations in the gene encoding hepatic nuclear factor 4α (~5% of cases)
- *MODY 2* – mutations in the gene encoding the 'glucose-sensing' β-cell enzyme glucokinase (~10% of cases)
- *MODY 3* – mutations in the gene encoding hepatic nuclear factor 1α (~65% of cases)
- *MODY 4* – insulin promoter gene mutation
- *MODY 5* – other unidentified mutations.

Table 3.2
A comparison of type 2 diabetes and MODY syndromes.

	Type 2 diabetes	MODY
Age of onset	Predominantly in middle- to old-age, but increasingly recognized in children too*	Childhood to young adulthood
Pathophysiology	Insulin resistance and β-cell dysfunction	β-cell dysfunction
Role of environment	Considerable	Minimal
Associated obesity	Common	Uncommon
Inheritance	Polygenic/heterogeneous	Monogenic/autosomal dominant

*Usually associated with obesity in children, and in those belonging to high-risk ethnic groups. Sourced from Hattersley AT. *Diabetic Med* 1998; **15**: 15-24.

In MODY-2, it seems that mutations in the gene encoding for β-cell (and liver) glucokinase lead to a reduction in insulin secretion involving a shift in the dose–response curve for glucose-stimulated insulin secretion. Thus, at any specified plasma glucose concentration, less insulin is secreted. Fasting plasma glucose concentrations are typically around 7 mmol/l, with post-prandial levels <10 mmol/l; this is a stable defect which is probably present from birth and which shows little progression with time. Patients who are started on insulin at diagnosis appear to be in a chronic 'honeymoon' state, and require less than 0.5 units/kg/day of insulin.

Glycaemic control is good in many individuals without drug therapy; the major exception to this rule is pregnancy where insulin may be required temporarily to ensure optimal control (many cases are, in fact, diagnosed during pregnancy). Use of sulphonylureas in the treatment of MODY has to be undertaken cautiously because of the marked responsiveness of individuals with mutations of the hepatic nuclear factor 1α gene. Short-acting sulphonylureas or meglitinides (chapter 9) may be more suitable. The minor biochemical disturbance associated with MODY is not usually associated with a significant risk of chronic microvascular complications. This relatively stable subtype contrasts with the hepatic nuclear factor mutations which

cause progressive hyperglycaemia. Accordingly, oral agents and even insulin may be necessary and there is a significant risk of long-term complications. The precise molecular mechanisms responsible for diabetes in MODY 1 and MODY 3 remain uncertain. Interference with insulin secretion through altered expression of other genes has been postulated. Since approximately 20% of affected families do not have any of the MODY mutations identified to date, it seems that additional mutations are still to be discovered.

Molecular genetic testing

If genetic testing is negative, no screening will be necessary during childhood. If unaffected offspring are found to have a MODY 2 mutation, then annual testing of fasting plasma glucose is required, and, for females, awareness should be drawn to the importance of excellent glycaemic control before conception. If unaffected offspring are found to have a MODY 1 or MODY 3 genotype, more rigorous regular screening through childhood, adolescence and early adult life is required. It has been suggested that genetic testing should be offered only after appropriate genetic counselling. Whether the knowledge this imparts will ultimately allow intervention to prevent or slow the appearance of diabetes is not yet known.

Further reading

Alberti KGMM, Zimmet P, for the WHO. Definition, diagnosis and classification of diabetes mellitus and its complications. Part 1. Diagnosis and classification of diabetes mellitus. Provisional report of a WHO consultation. *Diabetic Med* 1998; **15**: 539-53.

The Expert Committee on the Diagnosis and Classification of Diabetes Mellitus. Report of the Expert Committee on the Diagnosis and Classification of Diabetes Mellitus. *Diabetes Care* 1997; **20**: 1183-97.

Hattersley AT. Maturity-onset diabetes of the young: clinical heterogeneity explained by genetic heterogeneity. *Diabetic Med* 1998; **15**: 15-24.

Krentz AJ. *Churchill's Pocketbook of diabetes*. Edinburgh: Churchill Livingstone, 2000.

4. Diagnosis and assessment

Clinical presentation
Establishing the diagnosis
Diagnostic criteria
Initial assessment
Initial management
Hyperosmolar, non-ketotic coma
Influence of co-morbidity
Gestational diabetes

Clinical presentation

Most patients with type 2 diabetes are diagnosed in the relatively late stages of a long and complex pathological process. They have often had pathological degrees of hyperglycaemia for several years before the diagnosis is made. The pathogenic process of diabetes has its origins in the patient's genotype, and may be influenced by intrauterine experience, before being moulded throughout life by environmental factors. The condition itself is typically only recognized once symptoms are established or secondary organ damage becomes apparent (Table 4.1).

> Type 2 diabetes is usually diagnosed in the late stages of a complex and progressive pathological process

The presenting clinical features of type 2 diabetes range from surprisingly few symptoms in some patients to the dramatic and life-threatening hyperglycaemic emergency of hyperosmolar non-ketotic coma (page 42). Patients with lesser degrees of hyperglycaemia, whose symptoms may pass unnoticed for many years, may well carry a greater risk of insidious, unnoticed tissue damage.

> Approximately 50% of patients in developed countries with type 2 diabetes are undiagnosed

So, although classic osmotic symptoms are the rule in type 2 diabetes (with the notable exception of significant weight loss compared with type 1 diabetes), a high index of clinical suspicion must be maintained if asymptomatic cases are to be identified (Table 4.1).

Table 4.1
Presenting features of type 2 diabetes.

Minimal	Asymptomatic patients are identified by screening*
Osmotic symptoms	Thirst
	Polyuria
	Nocturia
	Blurred vision
	Fatigue/lassitude
Infection	Recurrent fungal infection (eg genital candidiasis)
	Recurrent bacterial infections (eg urinary tract infection)
Macrovascular complications	Coronary artery disease (angina pectoris, acute myocardial infarction)
	Cerebrovascular disease (transient ischaemic episodes, stroke)
	Peripheral vascular disease (intermittent claudication, rest pain, ischaemic ulceration)
Microvascular and neurological complications	Retinopathy (acute or progressive visual impairment)
	Nephropathy (microalbuminuria/proteinuria, hypertension, nephrotic syndrome)
	Neuropathy (symptomatic sensory polyneuropathy, foot ulceration, amyotrophy, cranial nerve palsies, peripheral mononeuropathies, entrapment neuropathies)
Associated conditions	Glaucoma (disputed association)
	Cataract (occurs earlier in diabetes)

*Usually opportunistic in the UK.

Although its validity has not been confirmed through clinical trials, type 2 diabetes satisfies the accepted criteria for a disorder suitable for screening on a population-wide basis. Screening of individuals with recognized risk factors for type 2 diabetes or the insulin resistance syndrome (page 24) certainly makes sense. The American Diabetes Association (ADA) (1997) recommends that testing (fasting plasma glucose measurements) be performed every three years in all individuals over the age of 45 and in selected high-risk groups of younger people (Table 4.2), but the cost-effectiveness of universal testing is uncertain. Costs would vary according to the demographics of the population screened (chapter 1) and the screening methods used.

The principal determinant of the clinical presentation of diabetes is the degree to which insulin, or insulin action, is deficient (chapter 2). A high renal threshold for glucose, which is particularly common in elderly subjects, may attenuate diabetic symptoms. Glycosuria, and hence osmotic symptoms, are minimal or even absent in the presence of hyperglycaemia in such cases.

> A high renal threshold for glucose may prevent the manifestation of osmotic symptoms, particularly in elderly subjects

The metabolic actions of insulin may be impaired at the cellular level by the direct or indirect actions of counter-regulatory hormones, ie glucagon, the catecholamines, cortisol and growth hormone (chapter 2) – all of which are secreted in response to physical and psychological stresses. The catecholamines are also able to inhibit endogenous insulin secretion and the combination of effects imparted may lead to marked metabolic decompensation in patients with limited insulin reserves. Conditions such as myocardial infarction, acute left ventricular failure or severe sepsis rapidly expose undiagnosed diabetes. Note that patients with type 2 diabetes are predisposed to such complications.

Table 4.2
Criteria for periodic testing for diabetes in asymptomatic individuals aged <45 years. Sourced from the American Diabetes Association, 1997.

- A first-degree relative with diabetes
- Overweight or obesity (especially abdominal obesity)
- Impaired glucose tolerance (on previous testing)
- Impaired fasting glucose
- Previous gestational diabetes or large baby (>4.5 kg)
- Polycystic ovary syndrome
- Essential hypertension
- Hypertriglyceridaemia
- Low HDL-cholesterol levels
- High-risk ethnic origin
- Premature cardiovascular disease
- Corticosteroid, β-blocker, high-dose thiazide therapy
- Primary hyperuricaemia or gout
- Specific endocrinopathies (eg Cushing's syndrome, acromegaly, phaeochromocytoma)
- Certain inherited disorders (eg Turner's syndrome, Down's syndrome)

Impaired glucose tolerance

Since, by definition, plasma glucose levels are not raised to diabetic levels in people with IGT, osmotic symptoms are usually absent. Asymptomatic glycosuria can result (as with type 2 diabetes), but other causes of glycosuria must be excluded (Table 4.3).

> Impaired glucose tolerance is generally asymptomatic

The diagnosis of IGT essentially relies on the performance of a 75 g oral glucose tolerance

Table 4.3
Causes of glycosuria.

- Diabetes mellitus
- Impaired glucose tolerance (IGT)
- Lowered renal threshold for glucose (eg during pregnancy, in children)

NB: fluid intake, urine concentration and certain drugs may all influence results.

test (page 39). The reproducibility of the test has been questioned since a small proportion of individuals seem to revert to 'normal glucose tolerance' on retesting, but it is still the most expedient, in fact only, means of detecting IGT.

Although individuals with stable IGT are not at direct risk of developing chronic microvascular disease, they do seem to suffer an increased incidence of atheromatous disease (chapter 7). Co-segregation of IGT with the classic risk factors for atheroma (eg dyslipidaemia and higher blood pressure) probably accounts for much of this increase. IGT (and even asymptomatic type 2 diabetes) should be considered a potentially co-existent condition in patients presenting with macrovascular disease – ie ischaemic heart disease, cerebrovascular disease and peripheral vascular disease.

Comparative cross-sectional studies currently suggest that IGT and the more recently introduced category of impaired fasting glucose (IFG) (page 38) are not entirely synonymous in terms of their pathophysiology or long-term implications. The contribution of impaired β-cell function, relative to insulin resistance, appears to be greater in subjects with IFG, while insulin resistance seems to be more prominent in individuals with IGT.

Establishing the diagnosis

While a urine test revealing glycosuria is suggestive of diabetes, a positive urine test alone is insufficient evidence on which to base a diagnosis. Glycosuria may occur in the absence of diabetes and *vice versa* (Table 4.3).

Diabetes cannot be diagnosed from glycosuria alone; reliable blood glucose measurement is also necessary

Neither the confirmation nor exclusion of diabetes should rest solely on the measurement of glycated haemoglobin or fructosamine. Although these assays provide highly specific, longer-term indications of blood glucose levels,

they are not yet adequately standardized or sufficiently sensitive. False negative results are particularly likely with less marked degrees of hyperglycaemia and neither IGT nor IFG can be inferred. However, more recently commercially available HbA_{1c} assays – which have been more rigorously standardized – can be useful in confirming suspected cases of diabetes.

Venous plasma glucose

A blood or plasma glucose measurement is the essential investigation in the diagnosis of diabetes. This should be performed by a clinical chemistry laboratory using a specific glucose assay to ensure accuracy. An appropriate sample of venous plasma is collected in fluoride oxalate to inhibit glycolysis.

Reagent test strips for monitoring capillary glucose (most of which give an adjusted reading equivalent to plasma glucose) are convenient and readily available, but the results should be independently confirmed – especially if the result is borderline and the patient asymptomatic. A laboratory-based test *must* be performed to confirm a diagnosis based on a test-strip result. A random or fasting plasma glucose measurement is not only appropriate in such cases, but usually sufficient to establish diagnosis if diabetic symptoms are also present. If the result is borderline, the diagnosis should be confirmed by repeat measurement on a separate day. Repeat testing is particularly important in individuals with no or minimal symptoms of diabetes.

The diagnosis of diabetes should always be confirmed by a repeat plasma glucose measurement in asymptomatic individuals

An oral glucose tolerance test is infrequently required to confirm a diagnosis and should not be regarded as a first-line investigation. Glucose tolerance tests are time-consuming, relatively labour-intensive and less reproducible than fasting plasma glucose measurements.

> A diagnosis of diabetes can usually be established using random or fasting glucose measurements; glucose tolerance testing is not often required

Diagnostic criteria

The revised diagnostic criteria for diabetes (according to the ADA, 1997) are as follows:

- random plasma glucose ≥11.1 mmol/l (200 mg/dl)
- fasting plasma glucose ≥ 7.0 mmol/l (126 mg/dl).

The new diagnostic fasting plasma glucose level is lower than that previously specified by the National Diabetes Data Group (1979) and World Health Organization (WHO) (1980, 1985): ≥7.8 mmol/l (140 mg/dl). The new, lower threshold reflects the results of cross-sectional and prospective studies that focused on the association with microvascular complications, mainly retinopathy. The ADA has accordingly proposed that fasting glucose measurement is the principal means of diagnosis, and now places emphasis on the equivalence of fasting glucose concentrations and at two hours after a 75 g oral glucose challenge. In contrast, the WHO has argued for retention of the oral glucose tolerance test in its reclassification, so the issue is by no means universally agreed. Studies to date suggest that the ADA criteria are more likely to identify patients who are: middle-aged, more obese and relatively more insulin-deficient. Moreover, the overall prevalence of diagnosed diabetes within populations seems to increase when reliance is placed on fasting plasma glucose levels alone.

Impaired fasting glucose

The 1997 ADA criteria introduced a new intermediate category of impaired fasting glucose (IFG), defining it as a fasting venous plasma glucose 6.1–6.9 mmol/l (110–125 mg/dl).

This category denotes an abnormally high fasting glucose concentration, falling just short

of the diagnosis of diabetes. False positive diagnoses of diabetes or IFG may arise if the subject has prepared inadequately (Table 4.4). This is even more relevant now, following the reduction in the diagnostic threshold for diabetes based on fasting plasma glucose to ≥7.0 mmol/l (126 mg/dl). Cross-sectional studies in the US and Europe indicate that there is only ~20–40% concordance between IFG and IGT (diagnosis of the latter is based on 120-minute glucose concentrations >7.8 mmol/l – 140 mg/dl – following a 75 g oral glucose challenge). The situation is complicated further by overlap between these two diagnostic categories – some individuals with IGT will have fasting glucose concentrations that lie within the normal range (ie 6.0 mmol/l or less), others will have values that lie within the IFG range. Finally, US and European studies suggest that post-prandial hyperglycaemia identified using the glucose tolerance test may predict cardiovascular mortality more accurately through identification of patients with IGT. In a recent, large, multinational European study, the Diabetes Epidemiology Collaborative analysis Of Diagnostic criteria in Europe (DECODE) study, IGT (but not IFG) predicted mortality from cardiovascular and non-cardiovascular causes.

Table 4.4
Preparation for a fasting blood test.

- The subject should refrain from consuming any food or drink from midnight before the morning of the test
- Water alone is permitted for thirst
- Regular medication can generally be deferred until the sample has been taken
- The venous blood sample is taken between 0800 hours and 0900 hours the following morning

NB: This preparation is also required for a 75 g oral glucose tolerance test or for measurement of fasting blood lipids. The patient should refrain from smoking before and during the latter test.

Impaired glucose tolerance

A diagnosis of IGT can only be made on the basis of a 75 g oral glucose tolerance test. An equivocal random plasma glucose level (ie <11.1 mmol/l) simply points to the need for a glucose tolerance test.

> Diagnosis of impaired glucose tolerance requires a 75 g oral glucose tolerance test

The oral glucose tolerance test

The oral glucose tolerance test is regarded as the most robust means of establishing a diagnosis of diabetes. Note, however, that the test is contraindicated if there is severe (and, by definition, diagnostic) hyperglycaemia. In individuals (as opposed to epidemiological surveys) the WHO (1998) emphasized that the oral glucose tolerance test was the gold standard, taking both fasting and 120-minute values into consideration.

> The World Health Organization (1998) consultation on the revised diagnostic criteria reaffirmed the importance of the oral glucose tolerance test

Glucose tolerance tests should be carried out under controlled conditions after an overnight fast (page 176). Patient preparation is detailed in Table 4.4. The process is otherwise summarized as follows:

- Subject should be consuming a diet containing adequate amounts of complex carbohydrate (>150g daily)
- Subject can generally defer regular medication on the morning of the test until after the test
- Subject should be encouraged to travel to the clinic by transport (minimal exercise) and to arrive at least 30 minutes before the test to allow time to relax and receive information about the test
- Subject should sit quietly throughout the test
- 75 g anhydrous glucose is dissolved in 250 ml water; flavouring with sugar-free fruit essence and chilling increase palatability and may help reduce associated nausea

- A venous line may be inserted if preferred, and kept patent by flushing with 1.5–2.0 ml sterile isotonic saline. The line should be withdrawn and discarded immediately before subsequent sampling
- Venous blood is sampled before (time 0) and 120 minutes after ingestion of the drink (which should be completed within five minutes)
- Plasma (preferred) or whole-blood glucose samples are taken
- Urinalysis may also be performed every 30 minutes (but is only undertaken if a significant alteration in renal threshold for glucose is suspected).

Interpretation of the results of a 75 g oral glucose tolerance test are presented in Table 4.5. Note that these results apply to venous plasma and that whole blood values are about 15% lower, provided the haematocrit is normal. For capillary whole blood, the diagnostic boundaries for diabetes are ≥6.1 mmol/l (fasting) and 11.1 mmol/l – ie the same as those for venous plasma (Table 4.5). The IFG range (based on capillary whole blood) is 5.6–6.1 mmol/l. Note that marked carbohydrate depletion can impair glucose tolerance; the subject should have received adequate nutrition in the days up to the test.

Table 4.5
Interpretation of 75 g oral glucose tolerance test.

	Venous plasma glucose, mmol/l (mg/dl)	
	Fasting	120 minutes after glucose load
Normal	≤6.0 (108)	<7.8 (140)
Impaired fasting glucose	6.1–6.9 (110–125)	–
Impaired glucose tolerance	–	7.8–11.0 (140–198)
Diabetes mellitus	≥7.0 (126)	≥11.1 (200)

NB: In the absence of symptoms, a diagnosis of diabetes must be confirmed by a second diagnostic test, ie a fasting, random, or repeat glucose tolerance test, on a separate day.

> The type of glucose sample must be known; diagnostic levels vary according to specimen

Impact of acute intercurrent illness

Patients under physical stress (eg surgical trauma, acute myocardial infarction) may experience transient elevations in their plasma glucose, but these often settle rapidly without specific antidiabetic therapy. Such clinical situations are also likely to unmask asymptomatic pre-existing diabetes or to precipitate diabetes in predisposed individuals.

This acute, transient hyperglycaemia should not be dismissed, particularly where it occurs in association with ketonuria in acutely ill patients in whom rigorous treatment is indicated; oral antidiabetic agents (especially metformin) should be avoided. If reassessment six to eight weeks after recovery from the acute illness indicates that glucose tolerance has normalized, it may be that the temporary insulin treatment can be withdrawn (chapter 11). However, patients do appear to benefit from continued treatment after a myocardial infarction and, if appropriate (and in the absence of troublesome hypoglycaemia), insulin should be continued. The management of diabetes during myocardial infarction is described in detail in chapter 7.

Initial assessment

A thorough history and physical examination should be performed:

- Record the mode of diagnosis and presence of symptoms, if any.
- Review the family history of diabetes carefully. Enquire into the obstetric (still births, large babies, gestational diabetes) and menstrual history (oligomenorrhea, especially with features of hyperandrogenism) of women.
- Enquire in detail about drug history, smoking habits and alcohol consumption, and about habitual physical activity and sports interests.

- Measure height and weight and calculate body mass index. Measure waist–hip ratio (>0.95 for men and >0.85 for women are considered undesirable; pages 5 and 181) and note any major weight changes in recent months.
- Identify associated conditions, predisposing and aggravating factors.
- Always investigate occupational, home and family-related factors, and concomitant medical conditions that might influence the prognosis and treatment of type 2 diabetes.
- Remember that features of other endocrinopathies (page 31) may occasionally be evident, that signs of marked insulin resistance are relatively uncommon and that specific diabetic syndromes, such as the lipodystrophies, are rare.
- Measure blood pressure carefully; lying and standing pressures should be recorded if there is any suggestion of postural hypotension arising from autonomic neuropathy.
- Seek evidence of established diabetic complications at diagnosis – examine for retinal, renal, neuropathic, cardiac and peripheral vascular disorders (chapters 6 and 7).
- Investigate symptoms and signs of neuropathy, including autonomic dysfunction where appropriate, and foot disease (chapter 6).
- Examine the fundi (through pharmacologically dilated pupils, unless there are contraindications).
- Consider biochemical testing. A case can be made for routine haematology, blood lipids and hepatic, renal and thyroid function assessment. Abnormal liver and kidney function tests are relatively common and may influence choice of therapy.

Ocular complications

Diabetic retinopathy is discussed in chapter 6. Cataract and possibly glaucoma are more common in patients with diabetes.

Nephropathy

Microalbuminuria (<300 mg/day) or overt (Albustix-positive) proteinuria are hallmarks of diabetic nephropathy. As with the other microvascular complications of diabetes, the development of nephropathy is closely related to the duration and severity of hyperglycaemia. As well as indicating early nephropathy, the presence of microalbuminuria reflects a higher risk of macrovascular disease (chapter 7). Since nephropathy can develop during the asymptomatic phase preceding diagnosis, plasma creatinine should be checked on diagnosis, especially if the new patient is Albustix-positive (has urinary protein loss ≥500 mg/day).

Neuropathy and foot disease

Evidence of these complications should be carefully evaluated at diagnosis (chapter 6).

Macrovascular disease

The close relationship between the components of the insulin resistance syndrome (page 24) should prompt the identification of associated risk factors for atherosclerosis such as:

- hypertension
- dyslipidaemia
- microalbuminuria.

Clinical stigmata of hyperlipidaemia should be sought, pedal pulses palpated and signs of vascular insufficiency noted. Further investigations may be warranted (chapter 7).

Initial management

The pressing clinical consideration is whether or not insulin treatment is required at once. In patients under 35 years with acute symptoms, weight loss and ketonuria, the need to start insulin is clearcut – such cases are likely to have type 1 diabetes. Serious intercurrent illness at diagnosis may also point to insulin being the initial treatment of choice. On the other hand, the overweight or obese middle-aged or elderly patients with typical type 2 diabetes are more likely to be candidates for initial aggressive dietary management. Sulphonylureas or metformin might also be given to the latter group at diagnosis, where the patient is severely hyperglycaemic or symptomatic.

> In newly diagnosed diabetic patients, the first consideration is whether or not insulin treatment is immediately required

Because it is not always possible to assign diagnosed diabetes to a particular subcategory, the choice of initial therapy does not necessarily reflect the aetiology (chapter 3). The problem arises because of unpredictable endogenous insulin deficiency at diagnosis and the rate at which the latter progresses. As already mentioned, patients with type 2 diabetes may need insulin temporarily following diagnosis.

> Initial treatment with insulin does not necessarily confirm a diagnosis of type 1 diabetes

It is sometimes particularly difficult to decide whether a newly presenting, middle-aged, non-obese patient with moderately severe hyperglycaemia has type 1 or type 2 diabetes. Although relatively uncommon in the elderly, type 1 diabetes can present in any age group.

> Type 1 diabetes may present at any age – even in the very old

Even the presence of marked obesity does not guarantee a diagnosis of type 2 diabetes; occasionally obese patients present with marked osmotic symptoms and/or ketonuria indicative of insulin dependence. An insulin trial is probably the most sensible option under these circumstances, with insulin use reviewed after two to three months.

Features of type 1 diabetes sometimes develop in patients with marked obesity; insulin is indicated

Significant ketosis in Caucasian subjects with diabetes means that insulin is required

The situation is complicated as our knowledge of the subtypes of diabetes increases. In many cases, insulin deficiency is the predominant feature but presents less dramatically than in the classic type 1 condition. This has been termed latent autoimmune diabetes in adults (LADA). The diagnosis usually becomes clear retrospectively following the primary failure of treatment with oral antidiabetic agents. However, useful clinical pointers include:

- unintentional weight loss immediately preceding diagnosis
- normal or low body weight for height at diagnosis
- presentation with osmotic symptoms of short duration
- marked fasting hyperglycaemia (eg >15 mmol/l).

Of these, unintentional weight loss is perhaps the most important. Dietary manipulation with or without drug treatment can produce dramatic improvements in this respect. The issue of insulin dependence is particularly vexed in patients of African ancestry, who may present with ketosis, even frank ketoacidosis, yet ultimately prove to have diabetes which is controllable – possibly even with diet alone. Ketonuria (together with hyperglycaemia) is usually indicative of a marked degree of insulin deficiency and requires insulin treatment. However, in patients with otherwise typical features of type 1 diabetes, especially weight loss, the absence of ketonuria at diagnosis should not be taken as unequivocal evidence that insulin therapy is not required. When deciding whether to withdraw insulin, considerable caution is always required (page 173).

Ketonuria in concert with hyperglycaemia suggests marked insulin deficiency

A few young European patients with hyperglycaemia but no ketonuria prove to have relatively uncommon inherited forms of diabetes, such as MODY (page 32). In the past, such patients often received insulin therapy from diagnosis, under the assumption that they had type 1 diabetes.

Hyperosmolar, non-ketotic coma

Hyperosmolar, non-ketotic coma is a life-threatening metabolic complication of type 2 diabetes. Patients presenting with marked hyperglycaemia (>25–30 mmol/l – the upper detection limit of glucose oxidase test strips) should therefore be assessed carefully for a history or evidence of:

- marked osmotic symptoms (such as thirst and polyuria) during preceding days
- dehydration (reduced skin turgor, hypotension)
- impaired consciousness
- acute intercurrent illness (especially sepsis).

This constellation of clinical features should alert the clinician to the possibility of hyperosmolar non-ketosis, a medical emergency requiring prompt hospital admission for iv rehydration and insulin administration (Table 4.6). Patients may be moribund, even comatose, by the time of admission, to the extent that a misdiagnosis of stroke or shock is not uncommon. Hyperosmolar non-ketosis can also develop in patients already receiving treatment for type 2 diabetes. Typical biochemical features include:

- severe hyperglycaemia (plasma glucose often >50 mmol/l)
- hyperosmolarity (see below)
- severe volume depletion with pre-renal uraemia
- electrolyte depletion
- minimal or absent ketosis.

Table 4.6

Guidelines for the management of diabetic hyperosmolar, non-ketotic coma in adults. Sourced from Krentz AJ. Diabetic ketoacidosis, hyperosmolar coma and lactic acidosis. In: Föex P, Garrard C, Westaby S (Eds). *Principles and practice of critical care.* Oxford: Blackwell Science, 1997; 637-48.

a) Fluids and electrolytes

Volumes:	1 l/hour for 2–3 hours, thereafter adjusted according to requirements.
Fluids:	Isotonic ('normal') saline (150 mmol/l) is routine.
	Hypotonic ('half-normal') saline (75 mmol/l) if serum sodium exceeds 150 mmol/l (no more than 1–2 l – consider 5% dextrose with increased insulin if marked hypernatraemia).
	5% dextrose 1l 4–6-hourly when blood glucose has fallen to 10–15 mmol/l (severely dehydrated patients may require simultaneous saline infusion).
Potassium replacement:	No potassium in first 1l, unless initial plasma potassium <3.5 mmol/l.
	Thereafter, add following dosages to each 1l of fluid:
	If plasma potassium is <4.0 mmol/l, add 40 mmol KCl (severe hypokalaemia may require more aggressive KCl replacement)
	If plasma potassium is 3.5–5.5 mmol/l, add 20 mmol KCl
	If plasma potassium is >5.5 mmol/l, add no KCl but repeat measurement of plasma potassium within 1–2 hours.
	Particular care is required in pre-renal uraemia.
	NB: Rhabdomyolysis may cause acute renal failure (rare).

b) Insulin

Using continuous iv infusion:	Give 6 units/hour soluble insulin until blood glucose has fallen to 15 mmol/l.
	Thereafter, adjust rate (usually down to 1–4 units/hour) during dextrose infusion to maintain blood glucose at 5-10 mmol/l until patient is eating again.
	Transfer to subcutaneous insulin.
	Review as outpatient after 1–2 months – withdrawal of insulin may be possible.
	A sulphonylurea or even diet alone may suffice.

c) Other points

Search for and treat precipitating cause (eg sepsis, myocardial infarction).
Hypotension usually responds to adequate fluid replacement.
Monitor for central venous pressure in elderly patients or if cardiac disease present.
If level of consciousness is impaired, pass nasogastric tube to avoid aspiration of gastric contents.
If level of consciousness is impaired, or no urine passed within ~4 hours of start of therapy, insert urinary catheter.
Thromboembolic complications are relatively common. Some clinicians recommend routine anticoagulation; others treat clinically evident thromboses as they arise. Low-dose heparin is a reasonable option, but there are no data from randomized trials.

Consciousness is usually depressed when plasma osmolality has exceeded ~340 mosmol/l. Plasma osmolality may be determined by freezing-point depression or estimated using a formula based on plasma concentrations:

2 x (sodium + potassium) + urea + glucose
(where sodium, potassium, urea and glucose are in mmol/l).

Hyperosmolar non-ketosis is associated with a relatively high case–fatality rate. As many as two-thirds of cases are previously undiagnosed patients and the syndrome tends to be confined to middle-aged and elderly patients – black patients are over-represented in some reports. Precipitating factors are thought to include diabetogenic drugs such as high-dose corticosteroids and infection, both of which antagonize insulin action. The quenching of thirst through carbonated drinks with a high sugar content may also contribute in some cases.

In cases that recover, diabetes can often be controlled by antidiabetic tablets or even dietary measures, which is taken to indicate that patients still have relative rather than absolute insulin deficiency. If insulin is administered for one to two months after recovery, the possibility of successful withdrawal can then be assessed (page 173). Drugs with diabetogenic potential (including high-dose thiazides and non-selective β-blockers) should be used with caution.

While ketonuria is not usually a feature of type 2 diabetes, ketosis, and sometimes ketoacidosis, can be precipitated by acute severe intercurrent illness.

> Patients with type 2 diabetes of African ancestry may present with hyperosmolar non-ketosis or even diabetic ketoacidosis

Influence of co-morbidity

Significant concurrent physical or psychological disease modifies the presentation and management of diabetes. To use an extreme example, alongside a condition such as advanced malignancy (limited life-expectancy), the primary goals of diabetes management would be relief of the osmotic symptoms and prevention of major metabolic decompensation – long-term microvascular complications would not be considered. Insulin may still be the most appropriate therapy in such a case – not only is it likely to provide the quickest relief of osmotic symptoms, but other drugs may be contraindicated, eg because of concomitant renal or hepatic impairment. Use of high doses of potent corticosteroids such as dexamethasone is a relatively common reason for using insulin preferentially in such patients.

> Diabetic patients are frequently affected by significant co-morbidity

Psychological considerations

A diagnosis of diabetes often has a major emotional impact on the patient (and his or her immediate family). Fears about complications such as blindness and amputation are accompanied by significant immediate restrictions on daily life. Factors that may influence the psychological response to diagnosis include: age, the treatment required, the degree and type of self-monitoring required, the presence of complications, co-morbidity, the implications for employment, the impact on recreational activities, and the degree of family and social support.

Furthermore, certain psychosocial characteristics have a bearing both on the initial reaction and on the patient's subsequent success in managing their disease: personality, temperament, health beliefs, cultural or religious conditioning, acute and chronic co-existent psychological states, intelligence, educational achievement, occupation, philosophical leaning. These factors also influence the success of diabetes education. A sympathetic approach, tailored to the individual, is required.

Depression

The overall prevalence of depression in type 2 diabetes is similar to that observed in other chronic diseases. Psychosocial pressures are often cited by patients as reasons for failure to attain or sustain their glycaemic targets, and issues such as compliance are certainly influenced by anxiety and depression. Serious psychiatric disturbance obviously demands expert psychiatric assessment, and chronic psychoses, habitual drug abuse and alcoholism can all place considerable obstacles in the path of successful self-management.

> Depression is more common in patients with diabetes

Gestational diabetes

The 1997 reclassification of diabetes (page 27) recognized gestational diabetes – diabetes first diagnosed in a woman during pregnancy – as a specific sub-category. Diabetes or IGT which is actually precipitated by the pregnancy, and pre-existing diabetes or IGT are now all included in this category. In most women with gestational IGT or diabetes precipitated by their pregnancy, glucose tolerance returns to normal post-partum. The long-term risk of permanent type 2 diabetes is substantially increased, usually in line with the frequency of type 2 diabetes in the relevant population and ethnic group. In the UK, the incidence of gestational diabetes is low (1–2%) in white Europeans and highest (4–5%) in South Asians. Women with MODY are often diagnosed during pregnancy.

> Impaired glucose tolerance in pregnancy is classified as gestational diabetes mellitus

Diagnosis

There is no consensus on the diagnostic criteria for gestational diabetes. In the absence of an unequivocal elevation of blood glucose, diagnosis will rest on the results of a 75 g oral glucose tolerance test. A higher risk of gestational diabetes is conferred by the clinical factors presented in Table 4.7.

Table 4.7
Groups of women associated with a higher risk of gestational diabetes.

- Older women
- Women with a history of glucose intolerance
- Women with a history of large-for-gestational-age babies (birthweight >4.5 kg or >90th centile for gestational age)
- Women from certain high-risk ethnic groups
- Women who have had glycosuria during pregnancy in the past
- Women who are overweight or obese
- Women with a pregnancy complicated by polyhydramnios
- Women with a family history of diabetes in a first-degree relative

Glycosuria is common during pregnancy, but a random blood glucose test or two may be sufficient to allay concerns about diabetes in the absence of other risk factors. In high-risk populations a case can be made for screening for pre-existing diabetes early in pregnancy. Fasting plasma glucose concentrations tend to decline during the first trimester, which renders this test unsuitable. In fact, a complex literature has built up around the issue of gestational diabetes. Expert opinions about the importance of its detection and clinical implications have become polarized. Concerns have been voiced that diagnosis may lead to a higher rate of Caesarian section in the absence of clear clinical indications, but there is an opposing view that some form of screening for glucose intolerance is appropriate. Screening usually takes the form of a blood test between 24 and 28 weeks' gestation. Glycated proteins are not sufficiently sensitive for this purpose. The test described by O'Sullivan is the most widely used in the US.

The O'Sullivan screening test

This test has a cutoff value of ≥ 7.8 mmol/l 60 minutes after an oral 50 g glucose challenge and a high sensitivity and specificity (>80% for each) for glucose intolerance at 20–28 weeks. It may also be applied to high-risk populations in the first trimester, but it is worth bearing in mind that it was designed to determine the risk of subsequent diabetes in the mother, rather than predict the outcome of the index pregnancy.

Management

The detection of gestational diabetes raises important questions about the aims of treatment. It has been argued that there are insufficient data to justify universal screening for gestational diabetes because there is no reliable evidence that subsequent intervention is effective – except perhaps in reducing the proportion of babies with macrosomia (but macrosomia is confounded by maternal obesity). Dietary measures may suffice.

Calorie restriction

A 30% reduction in the daily calorie consumption of obese women will reduce hyperglycaemia. The US National Academy of Science recommends that the total weight gain during pregnancy for obese women should be limited to <6 kg:

Body mass index (kg/m²)	Recommended weight gain (kg)
20–26	11.5–16.0
26–29	7.0–11.5
>29	<6.0

Oral antidiabetic agents

Oral drug treatment is usually avoided, although fears about teratogenicity have not been clearly substantiated. Metformin, for example, has not shown any evidence of teratogenicity *in vitro*. Early experience with the first-generation sulphonylureas, eg chlorpropamide, was marred by reports of profound hypoglycaemia in the neonates of diabetic mothers. However, the role of second-generation sulphonylureas has recently been re-examined. In a US study, glibenclamide (glyburide) was used, apparently safely. This drug does not cross the placenta, but caution must still be exercised and more research is needed before the sulphonylureas can be recommended for gestational diabetes.

Insulin

Insulin is required in approximately 30% of women with gestational diabetes. The merits of attempting to judge control by comparing pre-prandial with post-prandial blood glucose levels have been debated, however no clear answer has emerged with respect to preventing fetal macrosomia. Insulin lispro (rapid-acting insulin analogue, page 156) has been used successfully in gestational diabetes, but in a relatively small number of women. There is a suggestion that the incidence of associated hypoglycaemia may be lower than with conventional short-acting insulin. Lispro is not detectable in cord blood, but further studies are required to establish the safety of insulin analogues during embryogenesis. Ironically, the risk of producing underweight babies as a result of strict maternal glycaemic control has raised theoretical concerns about programming a higher risk of diabetes in the offspring (page 3).

Post-pregnancy follow-up

Follow-up and counselling of mothers with gestational diabetes should include advice about avoiding obesity and the protective effect of regular exercise. Follow-up studies suggest that if body weight is successfully managed during pregnancy, the risk of conversion to type 2 diabetes might be reduced by approximately 50%.

> Maintenance of ideal body weight reduces the risk of future development of type 2 diabetes

In the weeks following delivery, a 75 g oral glucose tolerance test should be performed. Most patients (>90%) will revert to normal glucose tolerance post-partum.

An annual fasting plasma glucose test and instructions to present for additional testing if symptoms of diabetes are experienced are the minimal follow-up requirements. In high-risk populations, such as Hispanic American women, as many as 40% of cases that resolve immediately after the index pregnancy will become re-established as permanent diabetes within six years. In European populations, the rate of progression is much lower, which makes systematic follow-up that much harder. Further, a small proportion of women with gestational diabetes subsequently develop type 1 diabetes. (It is suggested that these patients have slow-onset autoimmune β-cell destruction which is unmasked by the insulin resistance of pregnancy.

Planning pregnancy

Since there is a strong relationship between glycaemic control at conception and the risk of congenital malformations, the importance of planned pregnancy in women with diabetes should be stressed and reminders given whenever the opportunity arises. For the reasons outlined in Table 4.8, diabetic pregnancy is regarded as high risk and should be managed with appropriate specialist diabetic and obstetric supervision. A combined clinic, in which the mother is reviewed at frequent intervals, is favoured by many units.

> Pregnancy should be planned wherever possible in women with diabetes

> Pregnancy in women with diabetes carries additional risks for both mother and child

Table 4.8
Risks associated with diabetic pregnancy.

a) Maternal risks
- Metabolic control deteriorates in the 2nd and 3rd trimesters (insulin may be required)
- Pre-existing complications such as retinopathy and nephropathy may progress
- Risk of pre-eclamptic toxaemia is increased two-fold
- Subclinical coronary heart disease may be unmasked
- Increased risk of urinary tract infection
- Increased rates of Caesarian section

b) Fetal risks
- Risk of congenital malformations is increased
- Rates of stillbirth are increased
- Perinatal mortality is increased
- Incidence of neonatal complications (eg hypoglycaemia, birth trauma) is increased
- Lifetime risk of diabetes in offspring is increased

Certain drugs, eg ACE inhibitors, should be avoided in women at risk of pregnancy. Such drugs are used more frequently in diabetic women. Pre-pregnancy counselling and attainment of excellent glycaemic control (which may necessitate insulin treatment) are aims for all women contemplating conception.

Contraception

Contraception is an important component of planned pregnancy. Selecting appropriate contraception should not present a problem to most pre-menopausal women with type 2 diabetes. Marked obesity, uncontrolled hypertension and the presence of cardiovascular disease may, however, contraindicate the use of combined oestrogen–progestogen oral contraceptives.

The main contraceptive options are as follows; standard contraindications should be observed:

- *Oral combined contraceptive* – metabolic side-effects are usually minimal with the modern, low-dose oestrogen preparations, but there is a reluctance to use the oral combined pill in women with vascular complications of diabetes because of adverse changes in plasma lipid profiles. Hypertriglyceridaemia, in particular, may be aggravated. The progesterone-only pill or other methods are preferred. An associated prothrombotic state is well recognized, and certain progestogens (desogestrel, gestodene) are associated with somewhat higher risks.
- *Progesterone-only pill* – there are no appreciable metabolic side-effects and reports of reduced efficacy may simply reflect non-compliance. These preparations may be used during breast-feeding.
- *Long-acting depot progestogens* – these may be particularly useful if compliance is a problem. There is potential for menstrual irregularity, however, as well as adverse effects on plasma lipids (page 104).
- *Intrauterine contraceptive devices* – effective, without metabolic side-effects, and no specific contraindications in diabetic women.
- *Mechanical barrier methods* – as effective as in non-diabetic patients.
- *Surgical sterilization or vasectomy* – may be preferred by some couples. In the few situations in which pregnancy is

contraindicated, eg severe maternal coronary heart disease, sterilization offers definitive long-term protection.

Further reading

Davies M. New diagnostic criteria for diabetes: are they doing what they should? *Lancet* 1999; **354**: 610-1.

The DECODE study group on behalf of the European Diabetes Epidemiology Group. Glucose tolerance and mortality: Comparison of WHO and American Diabetes Association diagnostic criteria. *Lancet* 1999; **354**: 617-21.

Greene MF. Oral hypoglycaemic drugs for gestational diabetes. *N Engl J Med* 2000; **343**: 1178-9.

Jarrett RJ. Should we screen for gestational diabetes? *Br Med J* 1997; **315**: 736-7.

Metzger BE, Coustan DR (Eds). Proceedings of the fourth international workshop-conference on gestational diabetes. *Diabetes Care* 1998; **21**(2): B1-B167.

O'Sullivan JB, Mahon CM, Charles D, Dandrow RV. Screening criteria for high-risk gestational diabetes patients. *Am J Obstet Gynecol* 1973; **116**: 894-5.

Wareham NJ, O'Rahilly S. The changing classification and diagnosis of diabetes. *Br Med J* 1998; **317**: 359-60.

5. Principles of management

Aims and objectives
Organization of care
Diabetes in primary care
Education
Review schedule
Importance of glycaemic control
Maintaining standards of care
The economics of diabetes care

Aims and objectives

The aims of treatment for type 2 diabetes are focused on optimizing quality of life. They are approached through symptom management, together with measures to both prevent and limit complications and associated disorders. A key aim is to return metabolic control to as near-normal as possible in each individual.

The objectives and priorities of individual care plans will vary with the circumstances of the patient, but a typical list of objectives is given in Table 5.1. It is pertinent to recall that type 2 diabetes is part of the metabolic or insulin resistance syndrome of cardiovascular risk factors detailed in chapter 2 and that the main cause of premature mortality is macrovascular disease. Much of the morbidity is due to microvascular complications and the treatment objectives therefore emphasize the importance of detecting and containing those vascular risk factors that can be modified with proven benefit. Glycaemic control, as a means of improving general metabolic status, must not be compromised, and assiduous attention should be given to atherothrombotic risks including abdominal obesity, hypertension and dyslipidaemia. Helping the patient to understand and contribute fully to the management of their condition ('empowerment') through education and support measures is a valuable means of realizing diabetes control and other objectives. The concept of 'expert patients' has been endorsed by the World Health Organization (WHO) in relation to diabetes.

> Patients should be empowered to self-manage their diabetes wherever possible

Organization of care

Since the treatment of type 2 diabetes can encompass a broad spectrum of disciplines, not just within medicine, but allied professions, it is generally acknowledged that a multidisciplinary team approach offers considerable advantages. A 'diabetes team' will ideally include all the skills and specialisms listed in Table 5.2, but some members may well contribute more than one requirement. The diabetes team will extend links with social workers, community nurses and psychological counselling expertise, and involve substantial administrative commitment.

Table 5.1
Aims and objectives in the management of type 2 diabetes.

General aim	Enhance quality of life through relief and prevention of symptoms
Key objectives	Manage existing symptoms and complications
	Optimize glycaemic control
	Detect and control other risk factors for micro- and macrovascular diseases
	Provide education for healthy living and self-management

Table 5.2
Core members of a type 2 diabetes care team.

Diabetologist	Ophthalmologist
Primary care physician*	Podiatrist
Diabetes nurse specialist/educator	Pharmacist
Dietician	

*Preferably with a special interest in diabetes.

> Diabetes care requires a multidisciplinary team approach

In the UK, for example, the concept of 'shared care' is promoted through close liaison between primary (family general practitioner) and secondary (hospital-based specialist) care. Care teams within a hospital setting are customarily built around specialist physicians, but as the organization of diabetes care moves towards the greater involvement of primary care, geographically adjacent community-based practices are being encouraged to combine resources and build community diabetes teams. Initiatives to bring together appropriate expertise within the primary care setting are usually facilitated by primary care physicians with a particular interest in diabetes. The hospital-based diabetes specialist can serve as a link between a number of teams in primary care, so that overlap is minimal and the best healthcare is delivered. Treatment strategies are usually agreed under the direction of the hospital-based specialist, who also handles all aspects of local diabetes care that cannot be undertaken within the primary care team.

The practicalities of organizing and integrating the breadth of disciplines participating in diabetes care presents a major challenge. Many different structures have been shown to work effectively and there is no single ideal system. Detailed help with setting up a diabetes care team is available from the sources given in Table 5.3. The constraints of healthcare provision (budgets, personnel, other resources and services) and the special needs of different communities (eg the elderly and ethnic groups) means that customization of generalized schemes will best reflect the requirements of the local patients.

Open access (walk-in without appointment) clinics, available on a daily basis and staffed by a diabetes nurse specialist have proved highly successful. These are practicable where large communities are served, provide a valuable opportunity to troubleshoot problems, a forum for patients to help each other and share

Table 5.3
Organization of diabetes care: sources of guidance.

European Diabetes Policy Group 1998-1999. Guidelines for diabetes care. A desktop guide to type 2 diabetes mellitus. *Diabetic Med* 1999; **16**: 716-30.

Kelly DB (Editor-in-chief). *American Diabetes Association Complete Guide to Diabetes*. Alexandria, US: American Diabetes Association, 1996. The American Diabetes Association web address is www.diabetes.org

Delivery and organization of diabetes care. In: Pickup J and Williams G (Eds). *Textbook of Diabetes*, volume 2, 2nd edn. Oxford: Blackwell Science, 1997 (section 19, pages 78.11-81.10).

Diabetes UK (formerly the British Diabetic Association). *Catalogue of information for people with diabetes and healthcare professionals*. London: Diabetes UK, 2000.

Diabetes UK has produced several other helpful documents, including *Recommendations for the management of diabetes in primary care* (2nd edn) and *Recommendations for the structure of specialist diabetes care services*. They can be contacted at 10 Queen Anne Street, London W1M 0BD, and their web address is: www.diabetes.org.uk

difficulties and solutions, and reinforcement of the ethos of diabetes care. A local diabetes telephone helpline can also be very useful for patients, particularly early on in treatment when questions and uncertainties are most common.

Deficiencies and inequalities in the provision of care for people with diabetes in England and Wales were highlighted in a recent Audit Commission report (*Testing Times*, Audit Commission Publications, 2000). This report will inform the first National Service Framework (NSF) for Diabetes. It is hoped that some of the key themes developed in this book will be mirrored in the NSF and that a more equitable and enlightened approach to diabetes care will ensue. It is also hoped that diabetes healthcare professionals in other countries will find this book a sound foundation on which to build (with due recognition of local needs and constraints).

Diabetes in primary care

The long-term management of diabetic patients in the UK is increasingly supervised in part or entirely in primary care – which is particularly appropriate for patients with type 2 diabetes who have satisfactory glycaemic control and no significant diabetic complications. Problems with metabolic control and/or the detection of complications should prompt consideration of specialist advice.

Various models of care have been described:

- *miniclinics* – run in general practice but based on hospital clinics
- *integrated care systems* – patient management is shared between the primary and secondary sectors – but local circumstances will influence the arrangements within a particular health district. Most require close co-operation between hospital-based and primary care, since ready access to the hospital service and diabetes specialist nurses are prerequisites. An effective patient register and recall system are also essential components. Regular audit of process and outcome is required.

> A dynamic and regular process of audit is required to identify deficiencies and ensure improvements in practice

Some studies have shown that specialist-directed management of diabetes in primary care can result in good rates of patient attendance, satisfactory collection of data (blood pressure, retinal examination), and suitable record-keeping. In contrast, unstructured care can lead to losses to follow-up, inferior glycaemic control, inadequate attention to complications and, potentially, increased mortality.

> A specialist-directed recall system is regarded as a prerequisite for successful primary care

In parts of the UK, Local Diabetes Service Advisory Groups have been established with the aim of coordinating general practice, hospital services and other professionals and – crucially – patients involved in diabetes care. Consensus guidelines may help to ensure consistency and minimum standards of care, allowing, for example, a district-wide policy for retinal screening or foot care to be established. The 'annual review' is central to patient care in the UK: this encompasses an assessment of current management, metabolic control and the status of chronic complications, and allows treatment amendments and arrangements for future review to be made.

Information technology

Information technology is increasingly important in data management; paper records may well become obsolete and a district diabetes database should now be regarded as essential. Electronic transfer of clinical and laboratory information between general practice and diabetes centres is becoming more established, but the standardization and complicity of software need further development. Information technology has the potential to:

- review record systems annually using built-in data prompts and risk-assessment programs
- capture digital images thus enabling photographs of retinal and foot lesions to be incorporated into the electronic record
- assist appropriate management by practice nurses and general practitioners (GPs) through decision support
- assist education through interactive computer programs.

> Information technology is an essential component of structured diabetes management

The care plan

Preparing a care plan involves the application of principles and protocols for diabetes management to the local strategy for the provision of care. A checklist of items that need to be covered during the first consultation with a newly diagnosed patient is given in chapter 4, page 40. Based on the first consultation, a care plan can be devised. The care plan should identify the general and specific needs of the individual patient, and set out the treatment programme in a format which is familiar to all

Table 5.4
Example of key components of a care plan for type 2 diabetes.

- Actions required following initial assessment:
  - initial management of existing symptoms and complications
  - immediate referrals, as required
  - further tests, as required
- Antidiabetic treatment
- Monitoring
- Other treatments (new and ongoing)
- Initial advice on living with diabetes
- Initiation of education programme
- Communication with other care team members
- Review schedule

Table 5.5
Agenda for a diabetes education programme.

Initial
- What is diabetes?
- How will diabetes affect my life?
- My diabetes care plan
- Meet the diabetes care team

Ongoing
- Understanding diabetes
- Coping strategies (special counselling if necessary)
- Healthy living (including exercise and stress reduction)
- Dietary management and weight control
- Taking medication (including hypoglycaemia)
- Self-monitoring of blood glucose
- Starting insulin
- Foot care
- Special issues (eg driving, sport, holidays, intercurrent illness)

Occasionally thereafter
- Care update (revision, reinforcement and motivation)
- Dealing with complications

members of the diabetes care team. A sample list of headings for a care plan is given in Table 5.4.

All care plans should be 'negotiated' and agreed with the patient concerned so that the patient is suitably empowered within the limitations of the plan. It is essential that the patient views the plan as a conjoint effort and loose contract, and it is the responsibility of the nurse specialist and/or educator to emphasize this point. Patient involvement will encourage commitment and compliance, and assist self-management.

Education

Education is a key component of every treatment programme for type 2 diabetes, and may be arbitrarily divided into two stages. First, the patient will require an immediate and straightforward explanation of their diagnosis – ie what it is, how it will affect their life, and what will be involved in their care plan. Second, an ongoing programme should be established to provide more details as and when the patient needs them, and to establish a forum for discussion and the trouble-shooting of problems encountered.

A typical agenda of education programme topics is listed in Table 5.5. An initial barrage of information might be quite overwhelming, and care must be taken that facts are metered-out in digestible quantities, at an appropriate pace.

Although the ideal is that all members of the diabetes care team (Table 5.2) are involved in patient education, one figure, usually the specialist nurse, will provide continuity throughout.

Diabetes is inevitably a family affair, affecting all those in close contact with the patient and requiring their understanding, support and encouragement. Including family or friends within a diabetes education programme can enhance a patient's ability to implement the knowledge and experience gained. Meeting with and sharing experiences with other patients is valuable, and patients are often generous and enthusiastic with their time and commitment to helping their peers.

The manner in which an education programme is best delivered is the subject of debate. However, provided it is patient-centred, adaptable and fulfils its objectives, it seems logical to accept that it can take on whatever format best reflects local needs, resources and opportunities. Education must be complemented by motivation and personalization to ensure success and lasting impact. Ideas for the structure, content and delivery of diabetes education can be obtained from the Diabetes Education Study Group in Switzerland, the American Association of Diabetes Educators, the American Diabetes Association and Diabetes UK (details of all these groups are given in Table 5.3 and at the end of the chapter).

Continuing education, possibly linked in with clinic appointments, can be used to maintain rapport between patient and care team, and help to sustain patient motivation, compliance and commitment to the care plan.

Review schedule

The future schedule of appointments will be incorporated into the care plan. Obviously this schedule must be flexible to take account of unforeseen developments.

A checklist for ongoing consultations with the clinician is given in Table 5.6. Since co-morbidity may impact both on choice of therapy and therapeutic targets, a careful general medical assessment should always be made, including a thorough check for vascular risk factors and diabetic complications (chapters 6 and 7). New diagnoses in existing patients should prompt screening of first-degree

---

Table 5.6
Check-list for each consultation with a patient with type 2 diabetes.

I. *Contact frequency*
- Daily for initiation of insulin or change in regimen
- Weekly for initiation of oral glucose-lowering agents or change in regimen
- Routine diabetic visits:
  Quarterly for patients who are not meeting goals
  Biannually for other patients

II. *Medical history*
- Assess treatment regimen
  Frequency/severity of hypo-/hyperglycemia
  SMBG results
  Patient regimen adjustments
  Adherence problems
  Lifestyle changes
  Symptoms of complications
  Other medical illnesses
  Medications
  Psychosocial issues

III. *Physical examination*
- Physical examination annually
- Dilated eye examination annually*
- Evaluate at each visit:
  Weight
  Blood pressure
  Previous abnormalities on physical examination
  Feet

IV. *Laboratory evaluation*
- Glycated haemoglobin or fructosamine assessed every three to six months
- Fasting plasma glucose (optional)
- Fasting lipid profile annually for lipid treatment – follow up profiles as needed and monitor progress towards target
- Urinalysis for protein annually
- Microalbuminuria measurement annually (if urinalysis negative for protein)

V. *Review of management plan*
- Evaluate at each visit:
  Short- and long-term goals
  Glycaemia
  Frequency/severity of hypoglycaemia
  SMBG results
  Complications
  Control of dyslipidaemia
  Blood pressure
  Weight
  Medical nutrition therapy
  Exercise regimen
  Adherence with self-management training
  Follow-up of referrals
  Psychosocial adjustment
- Evaluate annually:
  Knowledge of diabetes
  Self-management skills

*In patients with well-controlled diabetes and blood pressure and little or no background retinopathy, slightly longer intervals may be safe. Extending the intervals between retinal examinations may ease the burden on district-wide screening programmes.
SMBG = self-monitoring of blood glucose.

relatives, where appropriate, especially if they are already known to have one or more of the risk factors.

> Since comorbidity may impact both on choice of therapy and therapeutic targets, a careful general medical assessment should always be made

The annual review

The following checklist is recommended for annual review in primary care; aspects of the review are often shared between a practice nurse and doctor and the date of the review is prompted by the computerized practice register. The checklist should form the basis of practice audit and be supplemented periodically by questionnaire surveys of patient perceptions and satisfaction with care.

> A comprehensive annual review is the cornerstone of structured diabetes management

Interview
- Review general state of health (physical and psychological).
- Review results of self-monitoring.
- Enquire about episodes of hypoglycaemia (where appropriate).
- Reinforce patient commitment to self-management – especially diet, exercise, foot care, and drug compliance.
- Enquire about tobacco and alcohol use.
- Discuss other diabetes-related problems, eg complications, status of co-existing conditions and intercurrent illness.

Physical examination
- Body weight; calculation of body mass index (kg/m^2).
- Waist circumference.
- Blood pressure measurement (sitting).
- Assessment of visual acuity.
- Detailed fundal examination.

- Inspection of feet and footwear.
- Insulin injection sites (where appropriate).

Laboratory investigations
- Glycated haemoglobin (HbA$_{1c}$) concentration (or alternative).
- Urinalysis for protein (or albumin/creatinine ratio) and glucose.
- Serum creatinine and electrolyte concentrations.
- Lipid profile.

Management
- Glycaemic control – review of diet, exercise, weight, lifestyle, and antidiabetic medication.
- Assessment of co-existing conditions.
- Review of ancillary medication.
- Attention to modifiable cardiovascular risk factors – antihypertensive therapy, lipid-lowering therapy, aspirin.
- Management of long-term complications – consider specialist referral where appropriate.
- Agree targets and care plan.
- Arrange review date – patients with complications, suboptimal glycaemic control, uncontrolled hypertension, or other unresolved problems will require earlier review.

Importance of glycaemic control

Glycaemic control is the accepted yardstick for assessing metabolic control in diabetic patients. The justification for optimizing glycaemic control to delay the onset and reduce the severity of microvascular and macrovascular complications is discussed below.

Microvascular complications

All forms of diabetes, be they primary or secondary (chapter 3), are characterized by a risk of the development of long-term microvascular complications (chapter 6). While some patients seem more susceptible than others – perhaps reflecting genetic or other influences – the most important factors determining the risk of development and progression of chronic complications are:

- the duration of the diabetes
- the degree of the hyperglycaemia.

Subclinical (or functional) abnormalities, such as increased retinal blood flow or delayed peripheral nerve conduction velocity, may be present at diagnosis. These usually remain asymptomatic (ie detectable only with specialized techniques) and tend to improve as the hyperglycaemia is controlled. In the longer term, sustained hyperglycaemia will cause tissue damage through a number of postulated mechanisms (chapter 6).

> The risk of chronic microvascular complications is closely related to the degree and duration of the hyperglycaemia

The glucose hypothesis

According to the glucose hypothesis of diabetic complications, permanent – and effectively irreversible – tissue damage is attributable to chronic exposure to pathological degrees of hyperglycaemia. This process usually takes years to become clinically apparent and may be influenced by additional genetic or environmental factors.

> Prognosis of the diabetic patient will be improved not just by treating the hyperglycaemia, but by treating all associated conditions and complications as effectively as possible

Justification for aiming towards the best possible long-term metabolic control derives not just from clinical observation, but builds logically on the results of randomized, controlled clinical trials. The observational Wisconsin Epidemiologic Study of Diabetic Retinopathy supports the view that the basic relationship between degree and duration of hyperglycaemia and the specific microvascular complications of diabetes is similar in both the type 1 and type 2 disease.

Appropriately controlled clinical trials were required to evaluate the risks and benefits of intensified therapy specifically in patients with type 2 diabetes and the results first appeared in the early 1990s. The randomized Kumamoto trial, conducted in 110 lean, insulin-treated Japanese patients with type 2 diabetes, showed that better glycaemic control reduced microvascular complications. The United Kingdom Prospective Diabetes Study was of longer duration and much larger. A summary of the main points of this trial, the largest of its kind, are presented in Table 5.7. The design and results of the Hypertension in Diabetes study – which was embedded within the main trial – are outlined in more detail on page 99.

The key messages to emerge from the United Kingdom Prospective Diabetes Study were:

1. Improved glycaemic control with either sulphonylureas or insulin is associated with beneficial long-term effects, principally in retarding the appearance and progression of microvascular complications. The benefits are continuous until normal glycaemic control is achieved.

2. Very few patients with type 2 diabetes achieve and maintain good metabolic control with dietary modification alone, and most will require drug treatment within three years of diagnosis.

3. Glycaemic control deteriorates with duration of diabetes, even when treated intensively with an oral antidiabetic agent or insulin. Most patients will eventually require a combination of oral antidiabetic agents and/or insulin to maintain glycaemic control (Figure 5.1).

4. Intensive therapy with sulphonylureas or insulin carries a risk of hypoglycaemia and weight gain. The risks and benefits of therapy must be carefully considered for each patient. Initial therapy with metformin may reduce the long-term complications independently of glycaemic control.

Table 5.7
United Kingdom Prospective Diabetes Study details.

Set up to establish:
a) whether intensive therapy using oral antidiabetic agents or insulin reduced the risk of macrovascular or microvascular complications relative to conventional measures (ie diet)
b) whether any particular therapy is advantageous (or disadvantageous).

Study design:
Between 1977 and 1991, 5102 patients (58% male) with newly diagnosed type 2 diabetes were recruited in 26 centres. Patients were stratified according to ideal body weight (<120% or >120%).
- Non-overweight patients. If, after three months' dietary run-in, patients had a fasting plasma glucose 6.1–15 mmol/l and no symptoms of hyperglycaemia, they were randomly assigned to either:
    – conventional policy: dietary therapy aiming for fasting glucose <15 mmol/l
    – intensive policy: aiming for fasting glucose <6 mmol/l using either sulphonylureas (initially chlorpropamide or glibenclamide, and subsequently glipizide) or insulin (commencing with once-daily ultralente or isophane, with short-acting insulin added if pre-meal glucose >7 mmol/l).
- Overweight patients. 753 of 1704 overweight patients with fasting plasma glucose 6.1–15 mmol/l were randomly assigned to receive either metformin as monotherapy (*n*=342), or continued treatment with diet alone (*n*=411). The residual 951 overweight patients were allocated to intensive glycaemic control with chlorpropamide (*n*=265), glibenclamide (*n*=277) or insulin (*n*=409).
- Protocol amendments. During the study, progressive hyperglycaemia was observed in all groups (Figure 5.1). This led to an amendment allowing the early addition of metformin in asymptomatic patients in the intensive group if their fasting glucose remained >6 mmol/l on maximal doses of a sulphonylurea. In this supplementary randomised controlled trial, 537 non-overweight and overweight patients receiving the maximum dose of sulphonylurea were allocated to either continuing sulphonylurea therapy alone (*n*=269), or the addition of metformin (*n*=268). If marked hyperglycaemia recurred, patients were transferred to insulin.

Results:
UKPDS 33: Effects of intensive control with sulphonylureas or insulin.
- Over 10 years the median HbA_{1c} was 7.0% in the intensive policy group vs 7.9% for the conventional (diet) group. There was no difference in HbA_{1c} levels between the different intensive policy subgroups.
- Compared with the conventional (diet) policy group, the intensive policy group showed:
    – 12% risk reduction for any diabetes-related endpoint (*p*=0.029)
    – 25% reduction in microvascular endpoints (*p*=0.0099; Figure 5.2)
    – reduced need for photocoagulation (*p*=0.0031)
    – better preservation of vibration sense at 15 years (*p*=0.0052)
    – 30% reduction in occurrence of microalbuminuria at 15 years (*p*=0.033)
    – 16% reduction in fatal and non-fatal myocardial infarction (*p*=0.052)
    – no significant reductions in either diabetes-related deaths or all-cause mortality
    – no significant difference between the three main intensive agents (chlorpropamide, glibenclamide or insulin) for any of the three aggregate endpoints (any diabetes-related endpoint, diabetes-related death, or all-cause mortality)
    – hypoglycaemia was more common (*p*<0.0001) in the intensive policy groups whether analysed by intention to treat or actual therapy. The highest rate of hypoglycaemia was observed with insulin treatment
    – weight gain was significantly higher in the intensive policy group (mean increase 2.9 kg) than in the conventional group (*p*<0.001). Weight gain was highest for insulin-treated patients.

UKPDS 34: Effects of metformin in non-overweight and overweight patients.
Diet vs metformin in overweight patients:
- Over 10 years, median HbA$_{1c}$ was lower in the metformin-treated group compared with conventional treatment (7.4% vs 8.0%).
- Compared with conventional treatment, patients initially allocated to metformin showed a:
  - 32% risk reduction for any diabetes-related endpoint (*p*=0.002)
  - 42% risk reduction for any diabetes-related death (*p*=0.017)
  - 36% risk reduction for all-cause mortality (*p*=0.011)
  - 30% risk reduction for all macrovascular diseases (*p*=0.02)
  - 39% risk reduction for myocardial infarction (*p*=0.01).

The reduction in diabetes-related endpoints, mortality and stroke was greater for patients initially allocated to metformin (UKPDS 34) than not (UKPDS 33), alongside intensive therapy with sulphonylureas or insulin.

Protocol amendment supplementary study – addition of metformin to maximal dose sulphonylurea:
- In the substudy, continued therapy with a sulphonylurea alone was associated with a much lower mortality (about one-third) than in the main study, whereas addition of metformin lowered mortality to a lesser extent (about two-thirds of the mortality rate of the main study).

Combined analysis of the metformin studies:
- Combined analysis of these two metformin studies showed that addition of metformin had an effect comparable to that observed with intensive therapy (sulphonylurea or insulin) in UKPDS 33 with a 19% net reduction in any diabetes-related endpoint (*p*=0.033). However, the beneficial effect on cardiovascular outcomes observed after initial randomization to metformin was not substantiated after secondary addition of metformin to sulphonylurea in the supplementary study.
- Metformin improved glycaemic control without inducing weight gain and was associated with fewer reported episodes of hypoglycaemia than the other intensive therapies.

An additional substudy showed minor benefits of acarbose when added to other therapies.

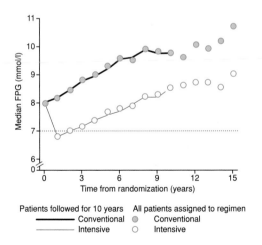

Patients followed for 10 years　　All patients assigned to regimen
——— Conventional　　⚫ Conventional
——— Intensive　　○ Intensive

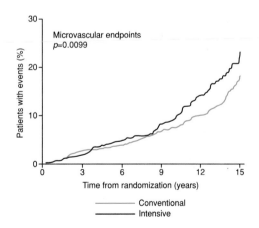

——— Conventional
——— Intensive

Figure 5.1
Cross-sectional and 10-year cohort data for fasting plasma glucose (FPG) for patients on intensive (sulphonylureas or insulin) or conventional (dietary) therapy in the United Kingdom Prospective Diabetes Study. Reproduced with permission from the *Lancet* 1998; **352**: 837-53.

Figure 5.2
Kaplan-Meier plots of aggregate microvascular endpoints for intensive and conventional treatment groups.
Reproduced with permission from the *Lancet* 1998; **352**: 837-53.

The results of this complex and lengthy study point to the potential for major health benefits from improved glycaemic control in patients with type 2 diabetes (alongside vigorous treatment of hypertension; chapter 7); and suggest that a combined approach targeting hyperglycaemia and hypertension is particularly advantageous. During the study all antidiabetic therapies had to be titrated up, or additional therapy introduced, to keep up with the progressive nature of the disorder – on average, a major adjustment such as an additional therapeutic agent, was required every four to five years. The small but sustained difference in glycaemic control between the conventional (diet) and intensive policy groups was associated with clinically relevant reductions in microvascular endpoints. Both sulphonylureas and insulin treatment were associated with increases in plasma insulin concentrations and weight gain, but insulin was eventually required in a substantial proportion of patients. The risks and benefits of insulin, including the risk of a higher rate of hypoglycaemia (~2% of patients suffered a major episode each year), require that the circumstances of the individual patient are considered thoroughly before insulin treatment is started. Insulin treatment is customarily reserved for type 2 patients who fail to respond adequately to diet and oral antidiabetic agents alone (in contrast to its use in this study).

Macrovascular disease

Although evidence from observational studies also suggests a link between the magnitude of the hyperglycaemia and the risk of atherosclerotic vascular disease, the United Kingdom Prospective Diabetes Study was unable to demonstrate a statistically significant reduction in macrovascular events through improved glycaemic control alone by lowering HbA_{1c} 0.9% over 10 years. To some extent, this may reflect the design, size and patient selection of the trial. A reduction in the incidence of myocardial infarction was noted, but this fell just short of conventional statistical significance ($p=0.052$). However, a subsequent analysis of the data (UKPDS 35) showed that a 1% reduction in HbA_{1c} would result in an average 14% reduction in myocardial infarction ($p<0.0001$). Thus, the data support the notion that glycaemia is a modifiable risk factor for myocardial infarction, and it is possible that the benefits of glycaemic control on coronary heart disease were underestimated in the United Kingdom Prospective Diabetes Study.

There is additional evidence suggesting that good metabolic control is also important immediately after a myocardial infarction, but it is generally accepted that reducing macrovascular disease – the principal cause of mortality in type 2 diabetes – will also require attention to other major modifiable cardiovascular risk factors such as dyslipidaemia, hypertension and smoking (UKPDS 23). Contrary to theoretical concerns, no adverse cardiovascular effects were observed with either sulphonylurea or insulin use in the United Kingdom Prospective Diabetes Study.

Metformin

The results of this study provided evidence for a beneficial effect on macrovascular complications where metformin was used as initial therapy in overweight patients. However, improved glycaemic control did not explain the more favourable outcome with metformin, and this led to speculation that other actions, such as improved fibrinolysis, might be involved. Further, metformin's benefits were not sustained when the drug was added-in to the treatment of a more heterogeneous (and relatively small) subgroup of patients already receiving the maximal dose of a sulphonylurea. The reason for this remains uncertain but it is now widely regarded as a statistical aberration rather than a real effect, particularly since the sulphonylurea subgroup exhibited much lower mortality than the main randomization. Sulphonylureas are considered in more detail in chapter 9 and metformin in chapter 10.

Assessment of glycaemic control: urinalysis (glycosuria)

Semi-quantitative testing for the presence of glucose using reagent-impregnated test strips is of limited value. Urinalysis provides retrospective information about glucose levels over a limited period of time. Other limitations include the effects of renal threshold, urinary concentration, neuropathic bladder and inability to detect hypoglycaemia.

Renal threshold

The renal threshold for the reabsorption of glucose in the proximal convoluted tubule – 10 mmol/l (180 mg/dl) on average – varies between individuals. Thus, patients with a low renal threshold will tend to show glycosuria more readily than patients with a high threshold. In fact, some individuals with a low renal threshold may have glycosuria but normal glucose tolerance ('renal glycosuria') – children are particularly likely to test positive for glucose. Conversely, a high threshold, which is common among the elderly, may give the misleading impression of apparently satisfactory control. The renal threshold of a particular individual will also change with time according to circumstances – it is usually lowered in pregnancy, for example.

Urinary concentration

Recent fluid intake and urine concentration also affect glycosuria. Renal impairment may elevate the threshold for glucose reabsorption.

Neuropathic bladder

Delayed bladder emptying, due to diabetic autonomic neuropathy (page 75), will reduce accuracy of measurements through dilution.

Hypoglycaemia

Hypoglycaemia cannot be detected by urinalysis.

Good, long-term metabolic control requires more accurate information about blood glucose in the range generally below that reflected in urinary glucose measurements. In elderly patients with type 2 diabetes, urinalysis may mislead completely (see above) and pathological degrees of hyperglycaemia go undetected. Urinalysis must be supplemented by tests for glycaemia in all patients in whom the therapeutic objectives extend beyond simply the avoidance of osmotic symptoms.

> Urinalysis alone is an inadequate means of assessing metabolic control in most diabetic patients

Assessment of glycaemic control: glycated haemoglobin

Glycated haemoglobin (HbA$_{1c}$) is formed by the post-translational non-enzymatic glycation of the N-terminal valine residue of the β-chain of red cell haemoglobin. The process of non-enzymatic glycation (which in other tissues is implicated in the pathogenesis of the long-term complications of diabetes) is considered in more detail in chapter 6, but the proportion of HbA$_{1c}$ to total haemoglobin (normal non-diabetic reference range approximately 4–6%) provides a clinically useful index of average glycaemia over the preceding six to eight weeks. Average HbA$_{1c}$ levels collected over a longer period (ie years) provide an estimate of the risk of microvascular complications. Sustained high concentrations identify patients in whom efforts should be made to improve long-term glycaemic control.

Glycaemic targets

Clearly, targets must be adjusted to suit the circumstances of the individual. As discussed above, a patient with advanced complications might not be expected to gain tangible benefits from tight glycaemic control; indeed, such an approach might carry unacceptable risks of severe hypoglycaemia.

Frequency of measurement

It is generally recommended that HbA$_{1c}$ should be measured every six months. Monitoring should be more frequent if indicated. Pregnancy, for example, requires monthly monitoring.

Previous sample collection

Blood can be collected by venesection before the clinic visit, in primary care, by the hospital phlebotomy service or even by the district nurse. Alternatives include rapid assays for clinic use, and self-collection of a fingerprick sample (into a capillary tube or onto filter paper) which is then mailed to the laboratory.

Limitations of HbA$_{1c}$ measurement

Although HbA$_{1c}$ levels are a reliable indicator of recent average glycaemic control, they do not provide information about the daily pattern of blood glucose fluctuation, which is required for logical fine-tuning of insulin dosing. Fortunately, this complementary information can be obtained from the patient's self-test results. More recent changes in glycaemia (within the preceding four weeks or so) will influence current HbA$_{1c}$ level more than current glucose level. Spurious HbA$_{1c}$ levels may arise in states of:

- blood loss/haemolysis/reduced red cell survival (low HbA$_{1c}$)
- haemoglobinopathy – elevated levels of HbS (low HbA$_{1c}$) or elevated levels of HbF (high HbA$_{1c}$)
- uraemia due to advanced diabetic nephropathy (page 81) is associated with anaemia and reduced erythrocyte survival , and this may also falsely lower HbA$_{1c}$ level.

Fructosamine assay

The generic term 'fructosamine' refers to the protein-ketoamine products that result from the glycation of plasma proteins. The fructosamine assay measures these glycated plasma proteins (mainly albumin) to reflect average glycaemia over the preceding two to three weeks. This shorter period may be particularly useful when rapid changes in control need to be assessed, eg during pregnancy, and fructosamine assessment is also less expensive than an HbA$_{1c}$ assay (an important consideration in some laboratories).

The methodology is suitable for automation and rapid results can be obtained for use in the clinic or office, which obviates the need for a prior blood test. Albumin levels can be misleading in certain hypoalbuminaemic states such as nephrotic syndrome, however, and some fructosamine assays are subject to interference by hyperuricaemia or hyperlipidaemia.

Patient self-testing

Patient self-monitoring of capillary blood glucose obtained by fingerprick has become an established method for monitoring glycaemic control. Enzyme-impregnated dry strip methods are available, which give an approximate visual indication of blood glucose. Ideally, these should be used in conjunction with a portable meter for a more accurate measurement. Most colorimetric strips are based on the glucose oxidase reaction:

$$\text{Glucose} + O_2 \xrightarrow[\text{oxidase}]{\text{Glucose}} \text{Gluconic acid} + H_2O_2$$

The hydrogen peroxide generated by this reaction then reacts with a reduced dye in the test strip and produces an oxidized colour proportional to the amount of H_2O_2 formed. This, in turn, reflects the amount of glucose oxidized. In most test strips, there is a separating layer which excludes cells and allows penetration by plasma. Thus, the reading obtained from the blood sample is actually a *plasma* glucose value.

Alternatively, glucose oxidation by glucose oxidase can be linked to the conversion of ferricinium to ferrocene. Ionization of ferrocene back to ferricinium liberates electrons which alter the current passed along a platinum wire, to give an accurate glucose measurement on a portable meter.

Practical considerations

Many different strips and dedicated meters are available. More expensive options include the storage and retrieval of multiple test results within a memory facility and the ability to download these results into a personal computer. Meters with large digital displays or audio output are available to aid the visually impaired and guidance from trained personnel with up-to-date knowledge of testing systems ensures that patients acquire the most appropriate device for their particular requirements. Supervised instruction of patients (or their carers) in the use of the chosen system should be provided and the manufacturers' instructions must be followed meticulously if reliable measurements are to be obtained.

> Guidance from the diabetes care team is helpful in the selection of an appropriate test system for self-blood glucose monitoring

Some systems use light reflectance to provide readings accurate to 0.1 mmol/l. Factors such as the adequacy of the capillary sample and calibration of the meter require attention. Test strip containers may carry a barcode strip or number which needs to be programmed into the meter. Control solutions of specified concentration are available from manufacturers – their telephone helplines are also useful sources of customer support. Sub-optimal storage of test strips is a potential source of error. It should be emphasized that quality control is essential.

Elderly patients often cope remarkably well with self-testing and many gain reassurance from it, but practical, patient-related limitations to self-testing include:

- inadequate manual dexterity, eg through deforming rheumatoid arthritis or advanced neuropathy or post-stroke
- intellectual inability or incapacity
- visual handicap.

Initiation of self-testing is an important preliminary step in patients who will eventually require insulin, but frequent self-testing has not been clearly demonstrated to improve control in others; testing every few days before breakfast and occasionally at other times (including 1–2 hours post-prandially) will usually suffice.

Efficacy

Self-testing remains a controversial issue. While, intuitively, it would seem that any additional information about glycaemic control would be advantageous, there is little firm evidence to support the assumption that routine self-monitoring improves glycaemic control. The evidence-base for this activity is small though, all the more surprising in view of the data suggesting that glycaemic control is suboptimal in a large proportion of patients (Figure 5.3). There is a need for good randomized trials of self-testing in type 2 diabetes patients.

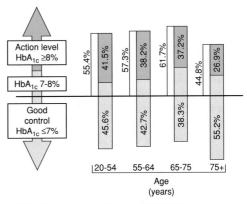

Figure 5.3
Glucose control (to ADA criteria) in type 2 diabetes patients in the US (NHANES III). Reproduced with permission from *J Am Geriatr Soc* 2000; **48**: 264-7.

Maintaining standards of care

Initiatives at local, national and international level are necessary to improve standards of care for patients with diabetes. At national level the interests of patients with diabetes are served by organizations such as Diabetes UK and the American Diabetes Association. These bodies act as advocates for people with diabetes. Generation of funds for research is another important aspect of their activities; both the UK and US national diabetes organizations publish peer-reviewed clinical and scientific papers in their respective journals. Annual scientific meetings under the auspices of these bodies bring together doctors, nurses, other healthcare professionals and scientists to share and evaluate progress in areas ranging from basic science to clinical care. These national meetings are amplified by international gatherings such as that of the European Association for the Study of Diabetes. The International Diabetes Federation, founded in 1950, holds triennial international meetings.

The Saint Vincent Declaration

Inevitably, there is a political dimension to the provision of diabetes care. International collaborations such as the Saint Vincent Declaration in Europe in 1989 represent another facet to the quest for improved patient outcome. This declaration resulted from a meeting between various representatives of European government health departments and patient organizations under the aegis of the regional offices of the World Health Organization and the International Diabetes Federation. The meeting produced a unanimous agreement on a series of recommendations of general goals and five-year targets. A demand for formal recognition by policy-makers of the public health problems presented by diabetes was accompanied by recommendations for research and the setting of laudable, if ambitious, targets for improvements in care:

- to reduce new blindness due to diabetes by one-third or more
- to reduce the numbers of diabetic patients entering end-stage renal failure by at least one-third
- to reduce diabetic morbidity and mortality from coronary heart disease
- to improve pregnancy outcome in women with diabetes so that it approximates to that in non-diabetic women.

The 1997 Lisbon Statement acknowledged the initiation of diabetes action programmes in most of the countries that were signatories to the Saint Vincent Declaration. The latter was coupled with a resolution to continue collaborative efforts to improve the healthcare of diabetic patients in Europe.

The economics of diabetes care

Since diabetes is a common and chronic disorder, it consumes a considerable proportion of the healthcare budgets of developed countries. In 2000, data suggested that diabetes was responsible for an estimated 9% of the total direct healthcare costs of the UK and 14% of the total direct healthcare costs of the US. The estimated annual costs of foot ulceration alone have been put at £13m in the UK and $500m in the US. Indirect costs are very difficult to estimate because they include those costs attributable to acute and chronic morbidity and premature mortality leading to loss of occupational productivity.

Diabetes consumes a disproportionately large part of national healthcare budgets and also incurs an extensive burden in terms of indirect and intangible costs such as social factors and reduced quality of life

The cost-effectiveness of new treatments using relatively expensive therapies is an increasingly important dimension of care. Vigorous treatment of hyperglycaemia, hypertension and the many associated complications of type 2 diabetes (chapters 6 and 7), demands investment in drugs and effective healthcare delivery systems. This outlay can reasonably be expected to be recouped through a reduced requirement for later interventions against complications such as retinal photocoagulation or renal replacement therapy. However, analyses of the cost-effectiveness of treatment pose considerable difficulties for health economists and this is still a relatively imprecise and speculative discipline. The projected massive global increase in the number of patients with diabetes (page 2) points to a need for even greater expenditure in the future and this will undoubtedly present major challenges, particularly for less economically developed countries.

Further reading

American Diabetes Association. Clinical practice recommendations 2000. *Diabetes Care* 2000; **23**: S32-42.

Coster S, Gulliford MC, Seed PT *et al*. Self-monitoring in type 2 diabetes mellitus: a meta-analysis. *Diabetic Med* 2000; **17**: 755-61.

Coutinho M, Wang Y, Gerstein HC, Yusuf S. The relationship between glucose and incident cardiovascular events. *Diabetes Care* 1999; **22**: 233-40.

European Diabetes Policy Group. A desktop guide to type 2 diabetes mellitus. *Diabetic Med* 1999; **16**: 716-30.

Goldstein DE, Little RR, Lorenz RA *et al*. Tests of glycaemia in diabetes (technical review). *Diabetes Care* 1995; **18**: 896-909.

Klein R. Hyperglycemia and microvascular and macrovascular disease in diabetes. *Diabetes Care* 1995; **18**: 258-68.

Stratton IM, Adler AI, Neil AW *et al*. Association of glycaemia with macrovascular and microvascular complications of type 2 diabetes (UKPDS 35): prospective observational study. *Br Med J* 2000; **321**: 405-12.

St Vincent Declaration. Diabetes care and research in Europe. *Diabetic Med* 1990; **7**: 370.

Testing times: a review of diabetes services in England and Wales. London: Audit Commission Publications, 2000. (www.diabetes.audit-commission.gov.uk)

Tuomilehto J. Controlling glucose and blood pressure in type 2 diabetes. *Br Med J* 2000; **321**: 394-5.

UK Prospective Diabetes Study Group. Effect of intensive blood-glucose control with metformin on complications in overweight patients with type 2 diabetes (UKPDS 34). *Lancet* 1998; **352**: 854-65.

UK Prospective Diabetes Study Group. Intensive blood-glucose control with sulphonylureas or insulin compared with conventional treatment and risk of complications in patients with type 2 diabetes (UKPDS 33). *Lancet* 1998; **352**: 837-53.

UK Prospective Diabetes Study Group. Risk factors for coronary heart disease in non-insulin dependent diabetes (UKPDS 23). *Br Med J* 1998; **316**: 823-8.

Contact information

Diabetes Education Study Group. Division of Therapeutic Education for Chronic Diseases, 3HL, University Hospital, 1211 Geneva 14, Switzerland.

American Association of Diabetes Educators, 444 North Michigan Avenue, Suite 1240, Chicago, IL80611, USA

American Diabetes Association at www.diabetes.org/ and www.news@diabetes.org/.

Diabetes UK at www.diabetes.org.uk.

Medscape at www.medscape.com (endocrinology).

6. Microvascular complications

Biochemistry of diabetic complications
Ocular complications of diabetes
Diabetic neuropathy
Diabetic foot disease
Diabetic nephropathy

Although the acute symptoms of diabetes can usually be controlled with appropriate therapy, all forms of diabetes are also associated with the insidious development of specific damage to the small vessels of certain organs. The small vessel (microvascular) complications of diabetes primarily affect the retina, the renal glomerulus and the peripheral nervous system. All three tissues are freely permeable to glucose and are closely linked to glycaemic control. The ultimate clinical consequences of diabetic microvascular disease are failure of the related major systems and visual impairment, chronic renal failure and neuropathic foot ulceration, respectively. Type 2 diabetes is also associated with an increased mortality from atherosclerotic (macrovascular) complications, particularly coronary heart disease, but these will be discussed in the next chapter. Together, the micro- and macrovascular complications of diabetes are major (and growing) causes of diabetic morbidity and mortality on a global scale.

Biochemistry of diabetic complications

Studies in animal models have provided insight into the biochemical mechanisms responsible for the chronic microvascular complications of diabetes. The principal hypotheses which link tissue damage to long-term exposure to high glucose concentrations include the polyol pathway, protein kinase C activity, and non-enzymatic glycation.

The polyol pathway

Increased activity of this ubiquitous biochemical pathway leads to intracellular accumulation of osmotically active sorbitol and fructose through the action of the enzyme aldose reductase. Depletion of myo-inositol and impairment of Na^+-K^+-ATPase activity are associated disturbances that have been implicated, particularly in the pathogenesis of diabetic neuropathy. Alterations in cellular redox state, leading to a state of 'pseudo-hypoxia' through the following reactions, may also be relevant:

$$Glucose + NADPH + H^+ \longrightarrow Sorbitol + NADP^+$$
Aldose reductase

$$Sorbitol + NAD^+ \longrightarrow Fructose + H^+$$
Sorbitol dehydrogenase

Protein kinase C activity

Accumulation of diacylglycerol as a result of high intracellular glucose concentrations activates protein kinase C-β in endothelial cells. This alters vascular permeability and increases basement membrane synthesis – an important early histological feature of the microvascular complications of diabetes. Pathological changes result:

↑ Glucose → ↑ Diacylglycerol → ↑ Protein kinase C-β

Secondary increases in the expression of growth factors with effects on vascular permeability may contribute to neovascularization in the retina.

Non-enzymatic glycation

The long-term modification of proteins such as collagen and nucleic acids by non-enzymatic glycation (ie attachment of glucose to the amino groups of proteins at a rate proportional to the mean glucose concentration) also contributes to tissue damage. Physical cross-linking of biochemically altered proteins modifies their structure and function – in the vascular wall, for example. While the earliest biochemical changes are reversible with restoration of good glycaemic control, the reversibility falters with time, and advanced glycation endproducts (AGEs) are eventually formed.

Glucose + Protein → Schiff base → Amadori product → AGEs

This process is the basis of glycated haemoglobin assays for the determination of medium-term glycaemic control.

Drug treatment

Drugs such as aldose reductase inhibitors, protein kinase C inhibitors and aminoguanidine block these metabolic pathways independently of glycaemia, and may prevent the development of certain complications in animal models of diabetes. In 2000, phase II clinical trials with a novel therapeutic agent, ALT-711 were announced. This drug cleaves the protein–glucose cross-links of AGEs. Since clinical trials of promising drugs such as the aldose reductase inhibitors have proved disappointing to date, excellent metabolic control remains fundamental to the prevention of microvascular complications. The results of the United Kingdom Prospective Diabetes Study (page 56) reinforced the relationship between glycaemic control and microvascular complications of type 2 diabetes, demonstrating that each 1% reduction in HbA_{1c} for 10 years was associated with a 37% reduction in microvascular complications and a 21% reduction in diabetes-related endpoints and deaths. Four important observations were made during analysis of the results (UKPDS 35):

- The lower the glycaemia, the lower the risk of complications
- Any rise in HbA_{1c} above the normal range carries an increased risk of glycaemic complications (no threshold was identified)

- Any improvement in glycaemia is likely to be beneficial
- Near-normoglycaemia should be the aim for as many patients as possible.

> The microvascular complications of type 2 diabetes increase in line with the extent and duration of the accompanying hyperglycaemia

Ocular complications

Clinical ocular complications associated with type 2 diabetes include:

- transient visual disturbances secondary to osmotic changes
- retinopathy – responsible for >80% of blindness in diabetic patients
- cataracts – these develop earlier in diabetic patients
- glaucoma – which may be primary or secondary to diabetic retinopathy.

Key points about diabetic retinopathy

- Diabetes is the principal cause of partial sight and blind registration in adults in westernized countries.
- Diabetic retinopathy is asymptomatic until well advanced.
- Effective treatment is available.
- Laser photocoagulation must be applied before the retinopathy becomes too advanced.
- Patients must be screened thoroughly and regularly.

> Retinal screening must be undertaken regularly in patients with type 2 diabetes

Population-based studies show that the prevalence of any degree of retinopathy is highest in younger, insulin-treated patients than in non-insulin treated older patients with type 2 diabetes. Severe retinopathy may develop in both major types of diabetes, but with some important differences. Factors other than hyperglycaemia, notably hypertension, have an important influence, particularly in patients with type 2 diabetes, as demonstrated in the Hypertension in Diabetes study (page 99).

> Hypertension has a major influence on the progression of retinopathy in type 2 diabetes

Moreover, studies in the US have shown that the risk of retinopathy is higher among certain ethnic groups, namely Native Americans, Mexican Americans and African Americans. The higher risk in these groups does not appear to be attributable to differences in glycaemic control or other recognized risk factors.

Approximately 20% of patients may have some evidence of retinopathy at diagnosis of their diabetes, but the prevalence increases with age. Careful fundoscopy is therefore mandatory in newly presenting patients. Maculopathy is the major cause of visual loss in those with retinopathy at diagnosis, but cataract (page 72) is also relatively common. Control of blood pressure is important in the prevention of visual impairment due to maculopathy. The benefits of long-term tight glycaemic control are well established and this should be carefully explained to the patient. However, several studies (mainly in patients with type 1 diabetes) have shown that pre-existing retinopathy can deteriorate transiently shortly after rapid improvements in glycaemic control and careful expert surveillance – with timely laser photocoagulation if necessary – is therefore required when glycaemic control is improved acutely. Acute reduction in retinal blood flow leading to retinal hypoxia is a postulated mechanism.

> Pre-existing retinopathy may deteriorate transiently when glycaemic control is improved

Ocular symptoms

Until it is very advanced, diabetic eye disease is largely asymptomatic. However, ocular symptoms attributable to diabetes include:

- Transient disturbance of refraction, usually myopia. This may be a presenting symptom of diabetes or may occur with the institution of antidiabetic therapy. Patients are advised to defer eye tests until diabetic control has been stabilized. Osmotic changes within the ocular lens are thought to be responsible.

Other less commonly encountered symptoms include:

- Gradual loss of vision, suggestive of the development of maculopathy or cataract.
- Sudden, painless, loss of vision due to vitreous haemorrhage. Retinal arterial and venous thrombosis may also occur in patients with diabetes.
- Appearance of 'floaters', possibly due to small or recurrent vitreous haemorrhages.
- Chronic pain and redness, due to rubeosis and secondary glaucoma.
- Field defects and impaired night vision, which are sequelae of extensive laser photocoagulation.

In addition, extraocular cranial nerve palsies may cause diplopia.

> Diabetic retinopathy and its sequelae are usually asymptomatic until well-advanced

Screening for diabetic retinopathy

Early recognition of diabetic retinopathy is essential if laser therapy is to be administered early enough for useful vision to be preserved. Annual checks of corrected visual acuity combined with expert evaluation of the fundus are required. In the UK, diabetologists, trained general practitioners or optometrists have generally performed direct fundoscopy in the clinic or surgery. Elsewhere, an ophthalmologist or optometrist might provide this service.

Visual acuity

Corrected best visual acuity is measured at 6 m using a well illuminated Snellen chart. Patients should wear their long-distance glasses, if required. A pinhole will correct refractive errors to approximately 6/9. Each eye should be tested separately. Visual acuity should be tested before mydriatic eye drops are applied. Impaired visual acuity that does not improve with pinhole testing is suggestive of maculopathy or cataract.

Retinal examination

If direct ophthalmoscopy is employed, the pupils must first be pharmacologically dilated by applying 1% tropicamide 10–15 minutes before the examination. Transient local discomfort is common and the effect of tropicamide may take several hours to wear off. Additionally, the pupils of elderly patients, and particularly patients with overt diabetic neuropathy, may not dilate well; autonomic imbalance is postulated. Cautions and contraindications to mydriasis (pupil dilation) are few:

- *Driving* – which should be avoided, if possible. Dazzle from headlights and impaired visual acuity (which may fall transiently below legal requirements) carry obvious risks after tropicamide; alternative transport should preferably be arranged in advance. Although pilocarpine is sometimes used to reverse the effect of tropicamide the effect may only be partial, with the pupil becoming fixed in mid-dilatation. Reading may also be temporarily impaired.

- *A history of intraocular surgery* – although this is rarely a problem, the advice of the ophthalmologist should be sought. Some types of intraocular lens implant may dislocate with pupillary dilatation.

- *Precipitation of acute glaucoma* – has long been feared in susceptible patients, but a recent re-evaluation suggests that the risk may have been overplayed.

Non-mydriatic retinal photography

Non-mydriatic retinal cameras can provide colour photographs of the optic disc and macula and these have been extensively used in screening programmes in the UK. The photographs obtained require expert evaluation but studies suggest that cameras may improve the detection rate for maculopathy. High-resolution video cameras with digital data capture are a more recent development; digital data have the additional advantage of being suitable for electronic transfer and incorporation into computer-based record systems. Retinal photography is emerging as the screening method of choice in the UK.

Frequency of screening

The possibility that retinopathy may have developed before diagnosis of diabetes and the tendency for maculopathy to develop within a few years of diagnosis means that all patients need to be examined both at diagnosis and annually thereafter. More frequent examination should be considered if retinopathy is detected and patients who default from follow-up should always have their eyes examined when the opportunity presents.

> Patients who have defaulted should always have a detailed eye examination on reattendance

Classification of diabetic retinopathy

For clinical purposes, diabetic retinopathy is classified into several well defined stages (Table 6.1). It is not inevitable that the retinopathy will pass from one stage to the next. The clinical importance of the classification derives from the likelihood of treatment success in the earlier stages. The benefits of photocoagulation have been proven in randomized, controlled studies initially using the xenon arc and later the argon laser.

Table 6.1
Classification of diabetic retinopathy.

- Background retinopathy
- Pre-proliferative retinopathy
- Proliferative retinopathy
- Advanced diabetic eye disease
- Maculopathy

Note that these categories are not necessarily mutually exclusive, nor are they as distinct as the classification suggests.

Maculopathy denotes retinopathy concentrated at the macula, ie within the temporal vessels, approaching the fovea. Maculopathy may threaten central vision, particularly in patients with type 2 diabetes. Advanced diabetic eye disease includes the sequelae of vitreous haemorrhage and secondary rubeotic glaucoma – visual impairment is always present to some degree, and often blindness.

> Proliferative retinopathy and maculopathy are potentially sight-threatening forms of diabetic retinopathy

a) Background retinopathy

Background retinopathy (Figure 6.1) is characterized ophthalmoscopically by microaneurysms, intraretinal blot or (less frequently) flame haemorrhages, and hard exudates (waxy-looking lipid deposits from damaged vessels). In isolation, venous dilatation is not regarded as evidence of retinopathy. All of these features are asymptomatic, and each may fluctuate, with microaneurysms and haemorrhages, for example, sometimes disappearing on re-examination.

- *Surveillance* – careful periodic review is essential and usually recommended about every six months for all but the most minimal or slowly progressive cases.
- *Explanation* – it is usually appropriate to inform the patient of the discovery of retinopathy, at which stage the importance of regular review can be stressed. Accurate prognosis may be difficult (although risk of serious visual impairment is likely to be greatly reduced by therapy) but a reassuring approach is best.
- *Search for other complications* – carefully, and notably for hypertension and nephropathy (page 81). The latter may, in turn, influence progression of retinopathy.
- *Review glycaemic control* – the importance of glycaemic control should be discussed in terms appropriate to the patient, but the setting of unrealistic glycaemic targets is likely to generate anxiety and frustration.

b) Pre-proliferative retinopathy

Pre-proliferative retinopathy (Figure 6.2) is characterized by venous loops, beading or reduplication, arterial sheathing, intraretinal microvascular abnormalities (arteriovenous shunts), cotton wool spots (retinal infarcts), and multiple, extensive haemorrhages. These features denote increasing retinal ischaemia, the extent and degree of which tend to be underestimated by the ophthalmological appearance. Specialist investigations such as fluorescein angiography may be indicated. Pre-proliferative retinopathy, by definition, carries a relatively high risk of progression to new vessel formation within 12 months.

- Ophthalmic referral – a specialist opinion is indicated within a few weeks.

c) Proliferative retinopathy

Proliferative retinopathy (Figure 6.3) is characterized by new vessel growth on the optic disc or in the periphery of the retina in response to growth factors released by areas of ischaemic retina. These new vessels are friable and likely to cause pre-retinal or vitreous haemorrhage. Those on the optic disc are the most-feared in this respect. The vessels are asymptomatic in the absence of haemorrhage. When a large haemorrhage occurs, the patient will present with sudden, painless, monocular vision loss. Following a large haemorrhage, there is loss of the normal red reflex on ophthalmoscopic examination. Smaller bleeds may cause the patient to notice 'floaters' in the visual field. On examination, the new vessels appear frond-like, and extend into the subhyaloid space from their origin at the retinal surface. Widespread retinopathy elsewhere is usual, but it may be impossible to discern any retinal features on fundoscopy because of blood in the vitreous humour.

- *Urgent ophthalmic referral* – immediate expert assessment is indicated for suspected acute vitreous haemorrhage or sudden vision loss.
- *Laser photocoagulation* – timely argon laser therapy can reduce the risk of severe visual

loss by >50% over five years in patients with proliferative retinopathy. Laser therapy must be given before visual loss is too advanced. Panretinal photocoagulation, which may involve thousands of retinal burns, is associated with potential complications including: impaired night vision, visual field constriction, impaired colour vision and progression of macular oedema. New vessels regress in response to photocoagulation and the stimulus to further new vessel formation is removed by destruction of the ischaemic retina. Successful photocoagulation may induce permanent quiescence of proliferative retinopathy, but this treatment is more appropriately regarded as a palliative procedure. Intraocular haemorrhages must be absorbed before laser treatment can be applied, which may take several weeks.

Sudden loss of vision necessitates immediate referral to an ophthalmologist

---

d) Advanced diabetic eye disease

Advanced diabetic eye disease includes retinal detachment due to fibrous traction and rubeosis iridis (new vessels on the iris). Severe panretinal ischaemia may lead to new vessel formation on the iris. Obstruction of the drainage angle by new vessels may then cause painful secondary rubeotic glaucoma. Retinal detachment – a grey elevation of the retina – may be obscured by vitreous haemorrhage. Painless sudden loss of vision is the presenting symptom in both cases. Action:

- *Urgent ophthalmic referral* – immediate expert assessment is indicated for retinal detachment.
- *Panretinal photocoagulation*.
- *Surgical vitrectomy* – this highly specialized procedure may restore useful vision in selected patients with advanced diabetic eye disease. Intraocular microsurgical techniques permit removal of fibrous

plaques and re-attachment of areas of retina; direct intraocular laser procedures are also feasible.

- *Enucleation* – this is the last resort for a painful, blind, rubeotic eye.

e) Maculopathy

Maculopathy (Figure 6.4) mainly affects patients with type 2 diabetes. Three types are recognized:

- exudative (may develop into circinate plaques)
- oedematous (cystic or diffuse; may be difficult to visualize with direct ophthalmoscopy or photography) and
- ischaemic (the least amenable to laser treatment).

Maculopathy should be suspected if a significant reduction in visual acuity (ie by two lines on the Snellen chart) occurs in the absence of an obvious cause, such as cataract. Expert slit-lamp examination may be needed to confirm diagnosis. Leaking capillaries may be more easily identified by fluorescein angiography.

- *Ophthalmic referral* – this is recommended for hard exudates (well defined waxy lesions) within two disc diameters of visual fixation. Unexplained deterioration in visual acuity also merits referral, whether or not retinopathy is apparent – it may be due to treatable macular oedema. If in doubt, always obtain an expert opinion.
- *Photocoagulation* – the focal type is recommended for microaneurysms and the grid type for diffuse macular oedema.
- *Control of hypertension* – hypertension should be sought and treated vigorously.

Visual handicap

Patients with severe visual impairment should be registered as partially sighted (best corrected acuity 6/60) or blind (3/60 or worse), as appropriate. This will trigger financial benefits and social service support. Low vision aids and

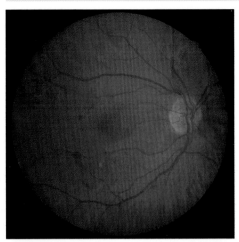

Figure 6.1
Background retinopathy

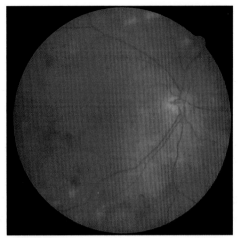

Figure 6.2
Pre-proliferative retinopathy

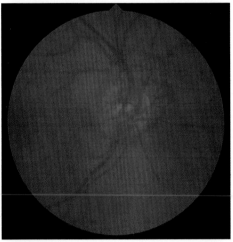

Figure 6.3
Proliferative retinopathy

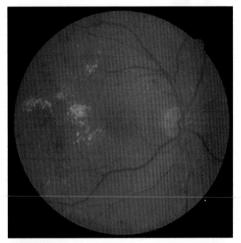

Figure 6.4
Maculopathy

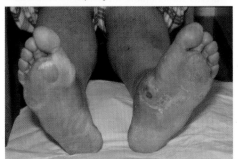

Figure 6.5
Charcot neuroarthropathy: bilateral changes with ulcerating deformity on medial aspect of left foot.

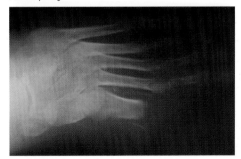

Figure 6.6
Charcot neuroarthropathy: extensive degenerative changes in mid-foot. Note partial surgical removal of first metatarsal and arterial calcification.

Figures 6.1–6.4 reproduced with permission from Krentz AJ. *Churchill's Pocketbook of Diabetes*. Edinburgh: Churchill Livingstone, 2000.

adapted household appliances are available. Pen injectors and other devices may be useful for patients requiring insulin. Self-monitoring of capillary glucose is possible, with glucose meters modified to give an audible result. Other support might include: braille instruction, large print and audio books, and guide-dog provision. Depression is understandably common, but peer-support, generally arranged through patient organizations, can be helpful.

Cataract

Opacities of the crystalline lens are usually asymptomatic in the early stages of development, but a common cause of treatable visual impairment. Cataracts are features of conditions such as myotonic dystrophy and chronic corticosteroid therapy, which can be associated with diabetes. Type 2 diabetes is a risk factor for cataract formation and the lesions may also progress more rapidly in diabetic patients.

> Cataracts are more common in diabetic patients and appear earlier than in non-diabetic individuals

Treatment is indicated if the cataract is interfering significantly with daily activities or the assessment of retinopathy. Surgical extraction with implantation of an intraocular lens is a routine procedure once the cataract has matured.

Glaucoma

In diabetic patients, glaucoma may be:

- *Primary* – chronic, open-angle glaucoma may be more common in diabetic patients; there is a suggestion that its presence may protect to a degree against retinopathy
- *Secondary* – due to advanced diabetic eye disease (such as rubeosis iridis).

Diabetic neuropathy

Neuropathy is the most common chronic complication of diabetes. It is a cause of considerable morbidity and its contribution to premature mortality may be underestimated. Diagnosis is essentially clinical; specialized techniques are usually unnecessary. Electrophysiological measurements are often abnormal at diagnosis of diabetes but tend to improve with control of glycaemia; overactivity of the intraneural polyol pathway (page 65) has been implicated. In chronic cases of diabetic neuropathy, however, there appears to be a major contribution from microangiopathy of the vasa nervorum. Only a minority of diabetic patients will go on to develop clinical neuropathy. Several stages are recognized, the earliest of which are usually asymptomatic:

- Intraneural biochemical abnormalities – sorbitol accumulation and associated myoinositol depletion.
- Impairment of electrophysiological measurements – decreased nerve conduction velocity.
- Clinical neuropathy – may be symptomatic or asymptomatic. Histological changes evident (research tool only).
- End-stage complications – foot ulceration and Charcot neuroarthropathy (page 81) are major and effectively irreversible derangements of neural structure and function.

Classification of established diabetic neuropathy is also essentially clinical, reflecting the differing manifestations and natural histories of the various forms (Table 6.2).

Table 6.2
Classification of diabetic neuropathies.

- Focal neuropathies – eg cranial nerve palsies, carpal tunnel syndrome
- Distal symmetrical polyneuropathy – glove and stocking; may be asymptomatic
- Acute painful sensory neuropathy – uncommon; may follow initiation of insulin treatment
- Motor neuropathies – uncommon; usually resolve
- Autonomic neuropathy – erectile dysfunction is the most common manifestation; other forms are rare

Clinical syndromes

a) Focal neuropathies

Focal neuropathy can affect the cranial nerves, eg the third, fourth or sixth. While oculomotor nerve palsies are usually incomplete, diplopia is prominent. However, the pupil is often spared and ptosis is uncommon. It can also affect the peripheral nerves, eg median, ulnar, common peroneal. Localized vascular lesions are thought to be responsible. Mononeuritis multiplex denotes the involvement of several peripheral nerves; distinguishing it from generalized peripheral neuropathy may be difficult. Transient focal neuropathies may also occur occasionally in hyperosmolar non-ketotic coma (page 42).

Spontaneous recovery of cranial nerve lesions within three months is the rule; in the absence of features such as ptosis, the patient can usually be reassured about the likely cause of a third cranial nerve palsy without resort to computed tomographic imaging. Recurrence is recognized. Persistent carpal tunnel syndrome merits investigation with nerve conduction studies; local injection therapy or decompression may help. Foot drop may benefit from an orthopaedic support. Ulnar nerve lesions may cause wasting of the dorsal interossei and hypothenar eminence.

b) Chronic symmetrical distal polyneuropathy

Chronic symmetrical distal polyneuropathy is common but often remarkably asymptomatic. Symptoms, if present, are usually confined to the legs and feet and start distally. Advanced neuropathy may also affect the hands and limit daily activities, such as insulin administration. Symptoms may include:

- *Paraesthesiae* – unpleasant sensations, akin to walking on pebbles, are characteristic.
- *Numbness* – loss of sensation may not be noticed by the patient. Instead, the patient may complain of subjectively cold feet, particularly in bed. The presence of pedal pulses on palpation together with signs of neuropathy will confirm the correct diagnosis.
- *Pain* – unremitting, burning, or lancinating pain.
- *Allodynia* – unpleasant sensations resulting from contact with bedclothes, trousers, etc, are reported.
- *Muscular leg cramps* – again especially in bed.
- *Impaired sense of position* – this may result in unsteadiness of gait and a tendency to trip. This can be a prominent but sometimes underrecognized symptom.

Classic signs of diabetic peripheral neuropathy are, however, easily detected on clinical examination:

- *Absent ankle jerks* – an early feature, but age-related loss is also common in the elderly.
- *Diminished vibration sense* – a 128 Hz tuning fork is applied to a distal prominence, such as the dorsum of the terminal phalanx of the hallux (big toe). If sensation is absent, the fork should be moved progressively proximal to the medial malleolus, then along the upper tibia (avoiding soft or oedematous tissue). Vibration sense may also diminish with age. More quantitative devices, eg the biothesiometer, are available, but are expensive and so usually confined to research studies. Age-related reference ranges are available.
- *Reduction in other sensory modalities* – position, light touch, pain and temperature – may accompany or follow loss of vibration sensation. Insensitivity to the application of a 10 g (5.07) Semmes-Weinstein monofilament will identify patients at high risk of neuropathic ulceration (page 78). This simple and reproducible test involves the perpendicular application of a nylon filament to a callus-free surface of the sole until it buckles under the gentle pressure.
- *Warm, dry skin* – with fissuring due to local sympathetic denervation.

- *Dilated superficial veins* – and sometimes bounding pedal pulses due to vascular shunting.
- *Clawed toes* – denervation of intrinsic foot muscles produces 'clawing' of the toes, exposing the metatarsal heads; this predisposes to ulceration.

Management should involve the following:

- *Education* – insensitive feet may be scalded by hot bathwater or in front of a heater or open fire. Injuries by unperceived foreign bodies in footwear may occur; prevention is paramount. Non-diabetic anatomical abnormalities such as hallux valgus predispose to ulceration. Basic elements of foot care are presented in Table 6.7; these should be reinforced at regular intervals.
- *Exclusion of other causes of neuropathy* – alternative causes of neuropathy, notably chronic excessive alcohol consumption, should be identified. A detailed history and simple biochemistry and haematology tests will identify most alternatives. Discontinuation or avoidance of drugs with neurotoxic potential is important. Uraemia due to advanced nephropathy may exacerbate diabetic neuropathy.
- *Glycaemic control* – should be optimized; the United Kingdom Prospective Diabetes Study (UKPDS 33) also showed that better glycaemic control was associated with less deterioration in vibration sense at 15 years. However, the effects of improving glycaemic control have not been substantiated in controlled trials in symptomatic patients. Studies of the effect of hyperglycaemia on pain thresholds have produced conflicting results.
- *Analgesia* – therapeutic options are limited for painful neuropathic syndromes. Analgesia appropriate to the degree of pain must be provided; paracetamol is usually inadequate; opiates may be required. Start with codeine or dihydrocodeine. Beware the nephrotoxic potential of non-steroidal anti-inflammatory drugs in patients with renal impairment (in fact these drugs are often not very effective for neuropathic symptoms). The centrally acting opioid-like non-narcotic agent tramadol may be useful for short-term therapy.
- *Antidepressants* – tricyclic antidepressants (imipramine 25–50 mg before bed or, as a second choice with a higher risk of side-effects, amitryptiline) may be useful adjuncts to simple analgesics; their antidepressant effects may also be useful, but these drugs block noradrenaline (norepinephrine) reuptake thereby reducing pain. Their hypnotic effect may also aid sleep, but response is variable.
- *Anticonvulsants* – carbamazepine (starting at 100 mg/day) or phenytoin (100 mg/day) can sometimes alleviate shooting pains. Gabapentin has recently been licensed for painful neuropathic syndromes and may be effective when other approaches have failed. Its safety profile appears to be superior to that of the tricyclics, but transient dizziness and somnolence are reported in up to 25% of patients.
- *Other therapies* – reported benefits for aldose reductase inhibitors (page 66) have been unimpressive to date and these drugs are not licensed in the UK. Capsaicin (0.075% cream), a recently introduced topical alkaloid derived from capsicum peppers, depletes levels of a peptide neurotransmitter, substance P, in nociceptive C fibre nerve terminals. Clinical experience to date is limited; transient stinging pain and erythema have been reported; the cream must be applied three to four times daily. Sheathing painful limbs with surgical adhesive may help to alleviate allodynia, but a bed-cradle to avoid contact with bedclothes is more practical. Implantable spinal cord stimulators are occasionally of reported benefit in patients with severe, intractable pain. Quinine has long been used for night cramps. The role of complementary therapies, such as acupuncture, is uncertain.
- *Psychological support* – its importance should not be underestimated and it should always

be underpinned by explanation of the prospect of improvement in acute neuropathies.

c) Acute painful sensory neuropathy

This uncommon syndrome presents as acute severe distal neuropathy, usually following the institution of insulin therapy. Recovery can be expected, but may be incomplete. Histological studies have shown regenerating nerve fibres; these are thought to be the origin of the symptoms. Treatment is symptomatic – good long-term glycaemic control should be maintained.

d) Motor neuropathies

Motor neuropathies include classic diabetic amyotrophy which may cause constitutional disturbance and weight loss (neuropathic cachexia of Ellenberg). The patient is typically a middle-aged male with type 2 diabetes in whom recent antecedent glycaemic control may have been surprisingly satisfactory. The presentation – pain (possibly severe) and weakness in the quadriceps – is abrupt. Muscle wasting follows rapidly. The weakness may be profound, leading to falls and immobility and painful hypersensitivity of the skin over the anterior aspect of the thigh is also characteristic. The symptoms lead to insomnia, anorexia, weight loss and depression. The knee jerk is characteristically absent and the plantar response may be extensor. While the nature of the responsible lesion remains uncertain, some features point to spinal cord or nerve root damage. An acute vasculopathy of the vasa nervorum is a popular explanation, but the predilection for the femoral nerve roots is unexplained. Other motor neuropathies are recognized (usually painful with hyperaesthesia; localized muscle weakness may occur), but truncal neuropathies affecting the abdomen are rare.

In classic amyotrophy few, if any, investigations are required. The major differential diagnoses are a nerve root or cauda equina lesion. Radiographs of the lumbar spine are usually unhelpful; magnetic resonance imaging may sometimes be indicated. Cerebrospinal fluid protein concentrations can be elevated and nerve conduction studies may show a localized femoral neuropathy – although evidence of spinal lesions is also recognized. Treatment is symptomatic and supportive with adequate analgesia and physiotherapy. Maintenance of good glycaemic control is recommended (although there is no clear relationship to recovery). Recovery (sometimes incomplete) usually occurs within a few months. Ipsilateral recurrence is uncommon.

e) Autonomic neuropathy

Diabetes-associated autonomic dysfunction usually remains asymptomatic. The most common clinical manifestation in men is probably erectile dysfunction (estimated to affect around 30%), although factors other than diabetic neuropathy are often contributory. Subclinical abnormalities of autonomic function are also relatively common and can be detected by simple bedside tests of cardiovascular reflex integrity, including:

- *Heart rate variability* – mainly assesses parasympathetic (vagal) function during deep breathing over 1 minute. The mean ratio of the electrocardiographic R-R interval in expiration to inspiration is calculated; less than 1.20 is considered abnormal (ie heart rate shows reduced variability).

- *Orthostatic blood pressure response* – this is a test of sympathetic integrity. Many variations, including the heart rate response to standing (the ratio at 30 and 15 seconds), or the Valsalva manoeuvre, for example, have been described. More sophisticated computer-aided systems are now available to provide comprehensive assessments of autonomic function.

- *Other specialized techniques* – such as the acetylcholine sweat spot test and measurement of pupillary adaptation to dark are chiefly used for research purposes.

Studies of spectral analysis of heart rate variability and baroreceptor reflex sensitivity may reveal even more subtle abnormalities of autonomic function, the long-term clinical implications of which are uncertain.

Patients with clinically overt autonomic neuropathy have been found to have a relatively high mortality rate in some follow-up studies. Autonomic dysfunction has been implicated in the sudden perioperative death of some diabetic patients. The electrocardiographic QT interval may be prolonged in diabetic patients; another measure, QTc dispersion, predicted death in a recent prospective study of patients with newly diagnosed type 2 diabetes. Improvements in glycaemic control have little beneficial effect on symptomatic autonomic neuropathy since advanced histological changes within nerves (axonal loss, demyelination, obliteration of vasa nervorum) are only partially, if at all, reversible. The United Kingdom Prospective Diabetes Study (page 56) was unable to demonstrate any benefits of improved glycaemic control, but the multifactorial Steno type 2 diabetes intervention study showed a 62% reduction in the risk of progression of measurements of autonomic neuropathy.

Erectile dysfunction is the most common manifestation of diabetic autonomic neuropathy in men, particularly with advancing age and use of antihypertensive drugs – notably the β-blockers and thiazide diuretics. Psychological factors are often present, making the distinction between primary organic and psychogenic impotence difficult. Devices enabling detection of nocturnal tumescence may sometimes be helpful, but many clinicians adopt a more pragmatic approach. Physical examination concentrates on genital anatomy (phimosis, Peyronie's disease) and evidence of peripheral neuropathy or peripheral vascular disease. Hormonal investigations (plasma testosterone, prolactin, gonadotrophins) are indicated if there is loss of libido or other features suggesting hypogonadism. The therapeutic options include:

- Counselling – by a clinician or specialist nurse. Should include demonstration of therapeutic options.
- Mechanical devices – vacuum tumescence devices, very occasionally surgical penile implants.
- Vasoactive drugs – prostaglandin E_1 administered intracorporeally or intraurethrally by the patient before intercourse; also α-blockers such as phenoxybenzamine.
- Sildenafil – this recently introduced oral agent is a popular option and appears to improve sexual function in 50–60% of diabetic men. The drug is administered at a starting dose of 50 mg approximately one hour before intercourse, although studies to date suggest that diabetic patients generally require a higher dose than non-diabetic individuals. Sildenafil inhibits the breakdown of cyclic guanosine monophosphate (cGMP) by a specific type 5 phosphodiesterase. It does not induce an erection; appropriate visual, psychological or physical stimuli are necessary. It is generally well-tolerated and no major problems such as priapism (which occasionally complicates injection therapy) have been reported. One major contraindication has emerged: concomitant use of nitrate drugs may cause a precipitous fall in blood pressure which has been implicated in some deaths. The drug may be contraindicated in approximately 10% of men.

In general, care should be exercised by men with cardiovascular disease – particularly severe angina or major impairment of left ventricular function – for whom sexual activity may be hazardous.

> Sildenafil is contraindicated in patients taking nitrate drugs

Orthostatic hypotension is defined arbitrarily as an otherwise unexplained fall in systolic blood pressure of 25–30 mmHg or more in a volume-replete patient on standing for two minutes. In fact, blood pressure may continue to fall for up to 15 minutes. This rare complication can be very disabling and difficult to manage. The differential diagnoses include other causes of autonomic failure in middle-aged or elderly patients (eg Shy-Drager syndrome), Addison's disease (uncommon) and hypopituitarism (uncommon). Antihypertensive agents and tricyclics may aggravate orthostatic hypotension and should be avoided. Support stockings may help to prevent venous pooling. Careful use of fluorocortisone may be beneficial but higher doses carry a risk of supine hypertension, oedema and hypokalaemia. Another alternative is midodrine, an α-adrenergic agonist.

Gastroparesis and diabetic diarrhoea rarely affect patients with type 2 diabetes. The motility agent cisapride, which had been used for gastroparesis, was withdrawn in 2000 following reports of serious cardiac arrhythmias, mainly in patients on concomitant therapy or with contraindications. Recent animal research suggests a pathophysiological role for diminished nitric oxide generation raising the possibility of novel forms of therapy. However, metformin (chapter 10) and acarbose (chapter 9) are much more common iatrogenic causes of gastrointestinal symptoms in patients with type 2 diabetes. On rare occasions, bladder paresis may produce hesitancy and retention and predispose to urinary infection. Prostatic disease should be excluded, but self-catheterization may be necessary in a few patients.

Also rarely, patients with diabetic autonomic neuropathy may suffer drenching sweats of the head and upper torso while eating. This is known as gustatory sweating and is unrelated to hypoglycaemia. Anticholinergic drugs have been tried, but their side-effects are often intolerable. Peripheral oedema is another rare consequence of autonomic neuropathy. Ephedrine may be helpful and exacerbation of lower limb oedema avoided through use of drugs such as nifedipine, amlodipine and the thiazolidinediones.

Diabetic foot disease

Diabetic patients have an approximately 15-fold increased risk of non-traumatic lower-limb amputation compared with the non-diabetic population. In elderly patients with type 2 diabetes, there is a significant mortality rate associated with such major amputation; this largely reflects serious co-morbidity in this group. In the UK, foot complications remain the most common reason for the hospitalization of diabetic patients. All health districts should establish a specialist foot clinic to which patients can be referred, or self-refer, for urgent assessment of serious lesions. Combined foot clinics with input from a podiatrist, vascular surgeon and diabetologist have been shown to reduce amputation rates.

> Diabetic patients with foot disease are at greatly increased risk of surgical amputation

The syndrome of diabetic foot disease includes elements of:

- *Peripheral neuropathy* – this is the major factor, manifest as insensitivity, motor imbalance with abnormal pressure distribution, and the consequences of local sympathetic denervation.
- *Peripheral arterial disease* – this leads to impaired tissue perfusion and is present in more than half of all cases; in combination with peripheral neuropathy, this comprises the neuro-ischaemic foot.
- *Tissue infection* – this occurs secondary to trauma or neuropathic ulceration.

The neuropathic foot

The neuropathic foot is insensitive (due to sensory neuropathy), dry (due to sympathetic denervation) and warm (well perfused in the absence of co-existing peripheral vascular disease; page 95). Note that peripheral arterial disease may modify these features. Areas of high pressure develop with weight bearing due to alterations in foot anatomy. The latter, in turn, is a consequence of denervation of intrinsic foot muscles and tearing of the plantar fascia at the distal insertions. The resulting 'clawing' of toes exposes the metatarsal heads to abnormally high local pressures during normal gait. Calluses develop over these areas in response to the high pressure. Neuropathic toes may be compressed (painlessly) by ill-fitting or inappropriate footwear. Patients with 'at-risk' feet should receive verbal instruction about foot care, supplemented, where appropriate, by a written leaflet (Table 6.3); advice should be reinforced by regular contact with a podiatrist.

Table 6.3

Basic rules for care of the neuropathic foot.

- Inspect feet daily (or have someone else inspect them)
- Check footwear for foreign objects before use
- Have feet measured carefully when purchasing shoes
- Buy lace-up shoes with plenty of toe-room
- Attend for regular podiatry
- Keep feet away from heaters, hot water bottles, and other hot objects
- Check temperature of bath water before entry
- Avoid walking barefoot, especially outdoors
- Use moisturizing cream for dry, fissured skin
- Avoid unaccustomed lengthy walks, eg on holiday

> Callus formation indicates chronic local high pressure with risk of ulceration

Shearing forces during normal walking can disrupt the tissues under a callus which may lead to local haemorrhage. In fact, haemorrhage under a callus is a sign of imminent ulceration, secondary infection and, ultimately, gangrene due to septic arterial thrombosis. The major risk factors for ulceration are listed in Table 6.4. Previous ulceration is particularly important, as recurrence is common. The elderly, socially isolated patient who cannot inspect or perhaps even reach his or her feet is also a high-risk case. Oedema from congestive cardiac failure,

---

Table 6.4

Indicators of feet at increased risk of ulceration.

- Neuropathy – especially with callus, blisters or fissures
- Ischaemia
- Previous ulceration
- Previous amputation
- Anatomical abnormalities, eg hallux valgus
- Impaired mobility due to age or co-morbidity
- Social isolation or low socioeconomic status

---

nephropathy or immobility renders feet vulnerable as does the chronic deformity associated with Charcot neuropathy (page 81).

> Haemorrhage within a plantar callus is a warning sign of impending ulceration

Referral

Patients should be referred to the podiatry service if they have any of the indications presented in Table 6.5. Regular callus debridement is required to reduce the risk of ulceration. Amateur treatment by the patient directed against lesions such as corns or deformed toenails should be discouraged. For established ulcers, particularly indolent or recurrent ulcers, three innovative therapies have recently become available:

- *Platelet-derived growth factor* – alongside good wound care, becaplermin (0.01% gel) has been shown to improve healing of chronic, uninfected ulcers compared with placebo. Further studies are required.

Table 6.5

Indications for referral to a podiatrist.

- Patients with peripheral neuropathy
- Patients with significant ischaemia
- Patients with other foot lesions (eg callus, corns, ingrowing toenails)
- Patients requiring detailed foot assessments for other indications

---

- *Cultured dermis* – this preparation is akin to a skin graft constructed from neonatal fibroblasts embedded in a synthetic matrix (supplied deep frozen). Studies to date suggest that more ulcers can be healed if this treatment is applied, but, again, infection must be controlled before application.
- *Fibrinogen adsorption* – this represents a major departure from conventional topical treatments. The process requires extracorporeal passage of plasma through a sepharose matrix. Evidence of efficacy and safety is presently inadequate.

Healthcare professionals such as district and general practice nurses and appropriately trained community podiatrists should be able to refer urgently to the local (hospital) specialist foot clinic. Patients should also be able to self-refer, if necessary. Indications for referral are listed in Table 6.6.

Table 6.6
Criteria for referral to a specialist diabetes foot clinic.

- Patients with neuropathic ulceration which has not responded to treatment within four weeks
- Patients with a foot infection not responding to antibiotics
- Acute or chronic Charcot neuroarthropathy
- Patients requiring special shoes or insoles
- Patients requiring weight-relieving casts

Infection

Infection with spreading cellulitis and/or deep infection represents an immediate threat to the viability of the foot, and sometimes even to the patient's life. Unless there is a prompt and convincing response to initial outpatient treatment the following actions are required:

- *Hospital admission* – bed rest to facilitate ulcer healing. An ulcer will not heal if the patient continues to walk and pressure-relief is essential; failure to rest is usually responsible for recurrence. Provided the infection is controlled, a removable or lightweight plaster cast can be applied to allow healing; a window is left in the plaster to enable inspection. Simultaneous care must be taken to avoid the consequences of immobility, notably decubitus neuro-ischaemic heel ulcers in debilitated patients. Action should also be directed towards relevant co-morbidity such as peripheral oedema, which is common in diabetic patients with multiple complications and co-morbidities.
- *Assessment of the extent of the infection and state of the peripheral vasculature.* Radiographs will exclude chronic osteomyelitis in deep infections. They may, however, appear normal in the earliest stages of osteomyelitis. Neuropathy in the absence of bone infection may produce translucency of the metatarsal heads. Arterial calcification is asymptomatic but may also be visible on radiographs of feet exhibiting extensive diabetic neuropathy. Vascular calcification needs to be documented, because the results of Doppler studies of the peripheral vasculature may be misleading. Chronic, deep-seated infection has a general debilitating effect and hypoalbuminaemia (a negative acute-phase reactant), a mild normochromic normocytic anaemia, is common. Additionally, erythrocyte sedimentation rate and C-reactive peptide concentrations are usually elevated during active infection and tissue repair.

Radiographs of feet with deep or chronic infection should be taken to exclude osteomyelitis

---

- *Bacterial treatment.* A mixed bacterial growth is common, usually containing *Streptococcus pyogenes, Staphylococcus aureus* and anaerobic species, such as the bacteroides (notable for their odour). Radiographs should be checked for tissue gas formation; gram-negative bacilli may contribute to deep infections. Deep wound swabs will guide the choice of antibiotic, but action against all the organisms listed above will be required in cases of serious infection. Initially, antibiotic therapy may be required, particularly if peripheral arterial supply is impaired. Subsequently, oral treatment may need to be continued for several weeks in cases of deep tissue infection or osteomyelitis. Examples of commonly used antibiotic regimens are presented in Table 6.7. If, after 12 weeks of appropriate therapy, an ulcer can be probed down to underlying bone, surgical resection of the osteomyelitic bone may be indicated.

Table 6.7
Examples of antibiotic regimens for diabetic foot infections.

Superficial infections
- Oral ampicillin + flucloxacillin
- Oral amoxicillin/clavulanate
- Azithromycin (if penicillin allergy)

Deep-tissue infections
- Intravenous ampicillin + flucloxacillin + oral metronidazole
- Intravenous amoxycillin–clavulanate
- Intravenous ciprofloxacin + clindamycin

Osteomyelitis
- Fusidic acid
- Trimethoprim
- Clindamycin
- Rifampicin

Methicillin-resistant Staphylococcus aureus
- Fusidic acid
- Trimethoprim
- Rifampicin
- Vancomycin (requires monitoring of blood levels)
- Teicoplanin

Notes: Liaison with the local microbiology service is recommended. Appropriate safety monitoring is required with some agents. Complications (eg pseudomembranous colitis) may develop during or after antibiotic therapy. Infection with methicillin-resistant *S. aureus* (MRSA) is an increasing problem in many units. Debridement and local antiseptic measures may be useful.

Radiographs should be taken to exclude gas formation by *Clostridium* spp

---

- *Surgery.* Judicious debridement, digit amputation and deep abscess drainage (beware the patient with neuropathy who has severe foot discomfort) can all be performed by a trained podiatrist or surgeon. The aim is always to preserve the limb but life-threatening infection may demand major intervention such as mid-foot or, as a last resort, below-knee amputation.

Severe discomfort in an infected neuropathic foot raises the possibility of abscess formation

---

- *Amputation* may be required for non-healing lesions (eg through an inadequate peripheral blood supply), gangrene, osteomyelitis, or recurrent lesions at a single site. 'Ray' amputation of the second, third or fourth toes, taking the associated metatarsal, can result in a highly satisfactory outcome (although healing will take some weeks), but major amputation is usually a devastating event. The prospects for successful rehabilitation are often remote. Walking using a below-knee prosthesis increases energy expenditure by 50%, which is an impossible target for many elderly or debilitated patients. Further, the risk of ulceration in the contralateral foot tends to increase due to compensatory weight-bearing. Confinement to a wheelchair may be the unfortunate consequence.
- *Prevention of recurrence.* Education of patient and carer, provision of special footwear, home help, and careful follow-up in the foot clinic will all help to prevent recurrence. Orthotist assessment is essential in patients with severe deformity. Ready-to-wear boots may be helpful in the short term, but are unaesthetic, so compliance is poor. Shoes may need to be made to order to accommodate special

insoles. Technology can now be used to identify local high-pressure sites, aiding insole and shoe design. Sports training shoes are worn by some patients, being a relatively inexpensive and acceptable alternative.

Charcot neuroarthropathy

Increased blood flow through the foot, secondary to local autonomic denervation together with abnormal pressure loading, may lead to unsuspected fractures resulting from minimal normal daily trauma. Patients often present acutely with a foot that is warm, tender and oedematous – palpable pedal pulses are characteristic. While these features strongly suggest an acute Charcot neuroarthropathy, (Figures 6.5 and 6.6), erroneous diagnoses of infection, inflammatory arthritis or even deep venous thrombosis are not uncommon. A penetrating ulcer that can be probed down to bone is probably the most reliable single sign of osteomyelitis; if there is doubt, antibiotics should be given. Contrary to common belief, some degree of discomfort is often present in the acute Charcot foot.

Radiographs will usually confirm the diagnosis, except in the earliest phases, when they may appear normal. Initially fractures (of a metatarsal, for example) may be apparent, but these progress rapidly to extensive subluxation, fragmentation and disorganization with remodelling. Isotope bone scans are often unhelpful in distinguishing acute neuroarthropathy from infection, since local uptake of tracer occurs in both circumstances. Magnetic resonance imaging and computed tomography are more helpful. Plasma levels of bone-specific alkaline phosphatase are often elevated. Once remodelling is complete, the patient is left with a deformed neuroarthropathic foot at high risk of ulceration (Figure 6.5). A 'rocker bottom' deformity is characteristic and bilateral changes are often evident on radiographs (Figure 6.6), even in the absence of clinical evidence of bone destruction.

> Radiographs must be taken if a patient with neuropathy presents with an acutely swollen hot foot

Management

Treatment during the acute stages of Charcot neuroarthropathy is controversial; no adequate randomized controlled trials have been performed. The ultimate aim is to minimize the degree of deformity in the quiescent phase:

- *Immobilization* – a walking plaster or removable cast is usually favoured, taking care to avoid trauma and ulceration from the cast itself. It is recommended that weight-bearing be recommenced very gradually over a period of weeks.
- *Intravenous bisphosphonates* – these drugs inhibit osteoblast activity and have been used in the hope of suppressing bone remodelling.
- *Custom-made footwear* – will help to prevent subsequent ulceration – if worn! (Ask the patient and inspect footwear.)
- *Reconstructive orthopaedic techniques* – realignment techniques have recently been described, especially to help patients with unstable hind feet, but surgical intervention should only be considered as a last resort.

> Charcot neuroarthropathy is associated with high risk of recurrent foot ulceration

Diabetic nephropathy

It is estimated that approximately 25–30% of patients with type 2 diabetes develop some degree of nephropathy. Certain ethnic groups, eg African–Americans, South Asians and Native Americans, appear to be at higher risk. Diabetic nephropathy is currently the single largest cause of end-stage renal failure in Westernized countries and the rapidly increasing global incidence of type 2 diabetes seems set to ensure that it continues to be a major consumer of healthcare resources. Diabetes is now responsible for more than one-third of all patients starting renal replacement therapy.

> Diabetes is the single largest cause of end-stage renal failure in developed countries

Diabetic nephropathy does not only result in progressive renal failure; it is also closely associated with increased morbidity and mortality from coronary heart disease, cerebrovascular disease and peripheral arterial disease. In fact, most patients with type 2 diabetes will die from atherosclerotic disease before they develop end-stage renal failure. Renal replacement therapy does not diminish this risk. Thus, diabetic nephropathy, in common with other causes of chronic renal failure, may be regarded as a state of greatly accelerated atherosclerosis.

> Diabetic nephropathy is associated with a greatly increased incidence of atherosclerosis

Natural history

Several distinct (if somewhat arbitrary) phases are recognized in the natural history of nephropathy. The earliest are asymptomatic. The important prognostic implications of this condition necessitate regular (annual) testing of urine for albumin – its presence being the earliest clinical indicator of nephropathy. While distinct stages in the development of nephropathy are recognized, the pathogenic process is actually a continuum (Table 6.8).

> Proteinuria is the clinical hallmark of diabetic nephropathy

Considerable emphasis has been placed on pharmacological intervention in the early stages of nephropathy, particularly with angiotensin converting enzyme (ACE) inhibitors. These are advocated even in the

Table 6.8
Natural history of diabetic nephropathy.

- *Stage 1: Functional changes*
  These include an increased glomerular filtration rate and filtration fraction at diagnosis; such subclinical changes are fairly common in type 2 diabetes, demonstrable in approximately 30% of patients. Glycaemic control reduces glomerular filtration rate, but the abnormalities persist in some patients.

- *Stage 2: Renal structural lesions*
  Early structural (subclinical) changes may be present even at diagnosis in some patients with type 2 diabetes.

- *Stage 3: Microalbuminuria*
  Blood pressure starts to rise (although remaining within the normotensive range); otherwise asymptomatic. Glomerular filtration rate tends to be stable up to this point.

- *Stage 4: Overt clinical nephropathy*
  Dipstick tests for protein become positive, initially intermittently then persistently. Nephrotic syndrome may develop. Glomerular filtration rate starts to decline and plasma creatinine starts to rise. Hypertension is usually well established by this stage (if not present at an earlier stage).

- *Stage 5: Progression to end-stage renal failure*
  Plasma creatinine rises above 500 µmol/l, usually at a constant rate for individuals who have had clinical nephropathy for seven to 10 years, but with considerable inter-individual variation. Once plasma creatinine has exceeded 200 µmol/l, the point at which dialysis will be required can be predicted using a plot of the reciprocal of the plasma creatinine concentration. Blood pressure is usually difficult to control by this time. The rate of decline in glomerular filtration rate is closely associated with elevated systolic blood pressure in patients with type 2 diabetes. Intercurrent illnesses, eg urinary tract infection or pharmacological over-diuresis, may cause a temporarily rapid decline in renal function. Fluid retention may result in pulmonary or peripheral oedema, which may be misinterpreted as cardiac decompensation. The incidence of macrovascular events (myocardial infarction, stroke, peripheral vascular disease) is dramatically increased by this stage.

Note: these stages have been identified mainly through studies in patients with type 1 diabetes.

absence of overt hypertension, reflecting an apparent renoprotective effect that is held to be independent of changes in systemic blood pressure. However, the methodology used for screening for early nephropathy and the timing and type of pharmacological intervention are all areas of controversy; the debate reflects the absence of long-term outcome data, but studies are seriously hampered by the long natural history of this complication. Most interventional studies to date have been relatively small and short-term. Moreover, they have tended to rely on surrogate endpoints such as transition from microalbuminuria to clinical grade proteinuria. Finally, they have mostly been performed in patients with type 1 diabetes. To complicate the picture further, microalbuminuria is recognized as a less specific predictor of nephropathy in type 2 diabetes – progression in only about 25% of cases compared to 50–70% of those in patients with type 1 diabetes. Thus, although progression, defined as the crossing of arbitrary proteinuria thresholds, may suggest renoprotection, extrapolation to the long-term outcome is fraught with difficulties. Despite all this, evidence has accumulated to suggest that it may be possible to delay the progression of diabetic nephropathy, at least in some patients.

> Annual testing for proteinuria is recommended in order to detect the development of diabetic nephropathy

Diagnosis

Microalbuminuria

The concept of 'microalbuminuria' was introduced in the 1960s. In the earliest clinically detectable stage, urinary albumin excretion is increased to 30–300 mg/day. Sensitive assays are required to measure albuminuria accurately, and these are best performed as a timed overnight collection. An albumin concentration <20 mg/l is regarded as normal. A urinary albumin:creatinine ratio, measured in the first-voided sample of the morning is a more practical alternative:

2.5 mg/mmol in adult men and 3.5 mg/mmol in adult women are diagnostic of microalbuminuria (assuming exclusion of confounding factors and alternative possibilities). Cross-sectional studies in patients with type 2 diabetes have suggested a prevalence of microalbuminuria ranging from 15% to >50%, depending on ethnicity. Microalbuminuria is also a marker for cardiovascular risk and overall mortality. It is typically associated with a constellation of risk factors for cardiovascular disease: insulin resistance, poor glycaemic control, dyslipidaemia, left ventricular hypertrophy, endothelial dysfunction and abnormalities of blood pressure regulation (impaired nocturnal 'dipping').

> Microalbuminuria: 30–300 mg/day
> Proteinuria: >300 mg/day

Proteinuria

When albumin excretion exceeds 300 mg/day, the Albustix (or equivalent) dipstick test becomes positive, marking the development of clinical nephropathy. Nephrotic syndrome may occasionally develop, with distinctive symptoms including urinary protein excretion >5 g/day, hypoalbuminaemia and peripheral oedema. However, urinary protein excretion may be influenced by several factors, including:

- *Hyperglycaemia* – tests for microalbuminuria at diagnosis and during periods of poor glycaemic control may be misleading because of transient increases in urinary protein excretion.
- *Intercurrent illness* – especially urinary tract infection, is common. It may be asymptomatic and therefore must be excluded.
- *Posture* – an upright posture increases protein excretion. Testing the first-voided sample of the day avoids this effect.
- *Exercise* – also increases urinary protein excretion.
- *Congestive cardiac failure* – is a prominent cause of proteinuria.

- *Other renal pathology* – such as glomerulonephritis and drug-induced renal disease (eg penicillamine). Renal vein thrombosis is closely associated with the nephrotic syndrome.

Thus, care must be exercised before concluding that proteinuria is attributable to diabetic nephropathy. Rather, microalbuminuria or a positive Albustix test result should prompt exclusion of these alternatives. Albuminuria should be confirmed with at least one additional sample, especially if treatment is being considered and for levels within the microalbuminuria range. The following screening strategy has been suggested by expert groups:

- Once diabetes has been stabilized, the albumin:creatinine ratio should be checked at least annually up to the age of 70 years.
- A positive result should prompt re-testing and exclusion of alternative possibilities.
- Timed overnight urine samples are regarded as the gold standard test, but repeat early morning albumin:creatinine ratios are also acceptable and far more practical.
- Persistently positive results should lead to careful assessment of glycaemic control, blood pressure, plasma lipids, plasma creatinine and to a careful search for other micro- and macrovascular complications.

Further investigations

Renal biopsy is usually unnecessary unless there are atypical features, such as rapid (and otherwise unexplained) deterioration in renal function, absence of significant diabetic retinopathy, development of nephrotic syndrome, and features suggesting alternative pathology such as haematuria, or evidence of autoimmune disease. Once diabetic nephropathy is well advanced, microscopic haematuria may be detectable on dipstick testing, but alternative renal tract pathology should be excluded. Macroscopic haematuria is not a feature of diabetic nephropathy.

Co-morbidity

By the time dialysis is required, most patients will have significant multiple diabetic complications. In particular, retinopathy will have resulted in severe visual impairment in some patients. Indeed, the association between retinopathy and nephropathy is so strong that the absence of the former should prompt consideration of alternative reasons for renal failure. Patients are also likely to have advanced neuropathy, not infrequently with features of autonomic dysfunction (page 75). The risk of neuropathic ulceration is high and may be exacerbated by pedal oedema. Postural hypotension may occasionally pose management difficulties, particularly in relation to haemodialysis (page 86). The incidence of major ischaemia of the peripheries is greatly increased with chronic renal failure – with concomitant risk of gangrene in the upper and lower limbs.

Management

Glycaemic control

The United Kingdom Prospective Diabetes Study (page 56) showed a 30% reduction in the risk of microalbuminuria at 15 years' follow-up with intensive therapy. Care should be taken to avoid oral antidiabetic agents that may be hazardous in the presence of renal impairment, notably long-acting sulphonylureas such as glibenclamide (glyburide) (page 129) and metformin (page 141). Insulin is often the treatment of choice, but doses may have to be reduced in patients with renal impairment since a proportion of insulin is cleared via the kidney. Anorexia may also require a reduction in insulin dose. On the other hand, insulin resistance associated with microalbuminuria and renal failure and intercurrent illnesses may make glycaemic control difficult to attain. The key points of the Steno type 2 diabetes study, in which multiple risk factors including hyperglycaemia were targeted in high-risk patients with microalbuminuria, are presented in Table 6.9.

Table 6.9
The Steno-2 study. Intensified multifactorial intervention in patients with type 2 diabetes and microalbuminuria. Sourced from the *Lancet* 1999; **353**: 617-22.

Study design
Randomized, unblinded trial comparing intensive multifactorial therapy (low-fat diet and exercise, smoking cessation, ACE inhibitors, vitamins C and E, aspirin and stepwise therapy directed against hyperglycaemia, dyslipidaemia and hypertension) in a specialized hospital diabetes centre (*n*=80) with standard treatment by general practitioners (*n*=80). Mean age of patients 55 years; mean follow-up 3.8 years.

Results
Compared with patients in the standard treatment group, those in the intensive group had reduced risks for clinical nephropathy (56% relative risk reduction; *p*=0.01), progression of retinopathy (40%; *p*=0.04), blindness in one eye (85%; *p*=0.03), progression of autonomic neuropathy (62%; *p*=0.01) and the combined endpoint of death and macrovascular events (37%; *p*=0.03).

Interpretation
Multifactorial intervention reduced the development of nephropathy and other complications. However, the relative contribution of each intervention to outcomes was unclear.

Control of hypertension

Blood pressure gradually rises as urinary albumin excretion increases. It may remain within the normotensive range in the initial stages, but will still be elevated for the individual patient concerned. Glomerular filtration declines with progression to end-stage renal failure (over about a decade but with considerable inter-individual variation). Polymorphisms of the ACE gene may have prognostic and therapeutic implications for patients with diabetic nephropathy. Patients with the DD genotype are homozygous for deletion of a 287 base-pair repeat sequence within intron 16 of the gene. Patients with type 2 diabetes and the DD genotype reportedly have higher circulating levels of ACE and more rapid loss of renal function – they may require higher doses of ACE inhibitors. Further studies are required.

> Genetic factors that may increase susceptibility to nephropathy in diabetic patients have been identified

Control of hypertension is essential. Tight blood pressure targets have been proposed by expert groups. The US Joint National Committee on Detection, Evaluation and Treatment of Hypertension, for example, recommends targets of <130/85 for all diabetic patients and <125/75 for diabetic patients with nephropathy. Such targets have been derived from studies showing that tight control of blood pressure is associated with a slower decline in glomerular filtration rate. While blood pressure control may be more important than the type of drug used to achieve it, differences between classes of antihypertensive agent have been noted, particularly in terms of reducing proteinuria. Although a firm evidence-base for the use of ACE inhibitors has been amassed, their superiority in this specific subgroup remains uncertain – in animal models, they have been shown to have renoprotective effects independent of their effects on systemic blood pressure. Combination therapy will usually be required in the pursuit of target blood pressures (page 104). There is some evidence that non-dihydropyridine calcium antagonists (eg diltiazem) have greater antiproteinuric effects than dihydropyridines (eg nifedipine). Recent short-term data suggest that combining an ACE inhibitor with an angiotensin II receptor antagonist may be advantageous in providing superior blood pressure control. Further studies are required. Care is required to avoid the development of hyperkalaemia in patients with overt nephropathy. Care must also be taken with ACE inhibitors in women of childbearing age.

> Hyperkalaemia is a hazard with potassium-retaining drugs in patients with nephropathy

The potential dangers posed by bilateral renal artery stenosis in patients with type 2 diabetes are discussed in chapter 7. A combination of antihypertensive drugs is often required, particularly in patients with type 2 diabetes and clinical nephropathy. Use of loop diuretics, β-blockers, long-acting calcium antagonists and centrally acting drugs may all be necessary. In particular, the early addition of a loop diuretic such as frusemide is helpful; as plasma creatinine concentrations rise, large doses of the latter agent may be required.

> Combinations of antihypertensive agents are usually required for patients with clinical nephropathy

Blood pressure and renal function should be assessed at least every three months, more frequently in some patients.

Treatment of dyslipidaemia

The high toll from accelerated macrovascular disease suggests that routine use of statins is indicated in nephropathy, but there are presently no data from randomized controlled trials to confirm the benefits. Unfavourable alterations in lipid profiles – increased low-density lipoprotein (LDL)-cholesterol, increased triglycerides, reduced high-density lipoprotein (HDL)-cholesterol – can be detected before creatinine levels rise; increases in plasma levels of atherogenic lipoprotein(a) may also contribute. The risk of myositis is increased when statins are co-prescribed with cyclosporin following renal transplantation and fibrates are contraindicated in patients with renal impairment because of the high risk of myositis.

Cigarette smoking

Cigarette smoking should be avoided completely.

Protein restriction

A modest restriction in diet to 0.6–0.7 g/kg/day is often recommended for patients with clinical nephropathy, but the benefits remain controversial.

Dialysis

Survival rates have improved for patients with diabetic nephropathy on dialysis. If a patient is considered unsuitable for renal transplantation, dialysis is used as the sole long-term therapy. Because of a greater tendency to fluid retention, dialysis may have to be introduced at an earlier stage in some diabetic patients. By the time that plasma creatinine level has reached 500 μmol/l, dialysis should be a serious consideration.

> Dialysis should be considered once plasma creatinine levels have reached 500 μmol/l

Continuous ambulatory peritoneal dialysis is now the favoured form of therapy: it is relatively inexpensive compared with haemodialysis, avoids rapid fluctuations in intravascular volume and is therefore better suited to patients with cardiovascular disease or autonomic neuropathy. No vascular access is required and insulin may be delivered into the peritoneal cavity by injection into the dialysate; its pharmacokinetics are altered by factors including the volume of dialysate and the tonicity (ie isotonic vs hypertonic), approximately 50% is systemically absorbed. Reported survival rates remain less favourable for diabetic patients but also similar to those achieved on haemodialysis. Peritonitis is the principal complication.

Haemodialysis requires the construction of vascular access, either an arteriovenous fistula or an artificial graft. These not only tend to fail more rapidly in diabetic patients, but distal necrosis of digits may occur. Autonomic neuropathy-related hypotension may make removal of excess fluid problematic and blood glucose concentrations may be erratic. Survival is generally worse in elderly patients. There is some evidence that high-dose antioxidant therapy (vitamin E 800 units/day) can reduce cardiovascular event rates in patients with a history of cardiovascular disease undergoing haemodialysis.

Renal transplantation

Renal transplantation is usually cadaveric but sometimes from a living related donor and the treatment of choice in patients with end-stage diabetic nephropathy. Patient and graft survival rates remain slightly inferior to those of non-diabetic recipients but, otherwise, rehabilitation is usually satisfactory. Several key selection criteria must usually be fulfilled for renal transplantation in the UK (Table 6.10).

Table 6.10
Criteria for renal transplantation in diabetic patients.

- Age <65 years
- Absence of severe cardiovascular or cerebrovascular disease
- Absence of significant sepsis
- Absence of life-limiting co-morbidity

Assessment of the coronary vasculature is routine; coronary angiography is required by most centres. The diabetogenic effects of immunosuppressive agents (corticosteroids, cyclosporin and tacrolimus) may necessitate increased insulin doses post-transplantation. Dyslipidaemia may also be exacerbated by immunosuppressive therapy. The main causes of death post-transplantation are atheromatous cardiovascular disease and sepsis, but autonomic neuropathy (page 75) may also be a factor. There is an increase in the risk of neoplastic disease with long-term immunosuppressive therapy.

Further reading

Aiello LP, Gardner TW, King GL *et al*. Diabetic retinopathy (technical review). *Diabetes Care* 1998; **21**: 143-56.

Anon. Drug treatment of neuropathic pain. *Drug Ther Bull* 2000; **12**: 89-93.

Backonja M, Beydoun A, Edwards KR *et al*. Gabapentin for the symptomatic treatment of painful neuropathy in patients with diabetes mellitus. *JAMA* 1998; **280**: 1831-6.

Clark CM Jr, Lee DA. Prevention and treatment of the complications of diabetes mellitus. *N Engl J Med* 1995; **332**: 1210-7.

Cooper ME. Pathogenesis, prevention and treatment of diabetic nephropathy. *Lancet* 1998; **352**: 213-9.

Edmonds ME. Progress in the care of the diabetic foot. *Lancet* 1999; **354**: 270-2.

Embil JM. The management of diabetic foot osteomyelitis. *Diabetic Foot* 2000; **3**: 76-84.

Ferris FL III, Davis MD, Aiello LM. Treatment of diabetic retinopathy. *N Engl J Med* 1999; **341**: 667-78.

Gaede P, Vedel P, Parving H-H, Pedersen O. Intensified multifactorial intervention in patients with type 2 diabetes mellitus and microalbuminuria: the Steno type 2 randomized study. *Lancet* 1999; **353**: 617-22.

Kohner E, Allwinkle J, Andrews J *et al*. Saint Vincent and improving diabetes care. Report of the visual handicap group. *Diabetic Med* 1996; **13**: S13-26.

Mason J, O'Keeffe C, McIntosh A *et al*. A systematic review of foot ulcer in patients with type 2 diabetes mellitus. 1: prevention. *Diabetic Med* 1999; **16**: 801-12.

Mayfield JA, Reiber GE, Sanders LJ *et al*. Preventive foot care in people with diabetes (technical review). *Diabetes Care* 1998; **21**: 2161-77.

Stratton IM, Adler AI, Neil HAW *et al*. Association of glycaemia with macrovascular and microvascular complications of type 2 diabetes (UKPDS 35): prospective observational study. *Br Med J* 2000; **321**: 405-12.

Thomas S, Viberti G-C. Proteinuria in diabetes. *J R Col Physicians Lond* 2000; **34**: 336-9.

Tuomilheto J. Controlling glucose and blood pressure in type 2 diabetes. *Br Med J* 2000; **321**: 394-5.

UK Prospective Diabetes Study Group. Tight blood pressure control and risk of macrovascular and microvascular complications in type 2 diabetes (UKPDS 38). *Br Med J* 1998; **317**: 703-13.

UK Prospective Diabetes Study Group. Efficacy of atenolol and captopril in reducing risk of macrovascular and microvascular complications in type 2 diabetes (UKPDS 39). *Br Med J* 1998; **317**: 713-20.

Viberti G-C, Marshall S, Beech R *et al*. Saint Vincent and improving diabetes care. Report on renal disease in diabetes. *Diabetic Med* 1996; **13**: S6-12.

Wieman TJ, Smiell JM, Su Y. Efficacy and safety of a topical gel formulation of recombinant human platelet-derived growth factor-BB (becaplermin) in patients with chronic neuropathic diabetic ulcers. *Diabetes Care* 1998; **21**: 822-7.

7. Macrovascular disease

Risk factors for atherosclerosis
Coronary heart disease
Acute myocardial infarction
Peripheral arterial disease
Cerebrovascular disease
Hypertension
Dyslipidaemia

Type 2 diabetes is a strong risk factor for cardiovascular disease in both men and women. Longitudinal studies indicate that the risk of atherosclerotic cardiovascular disease is two to four times higher in patients with type 2 diabetes than in non-diabetic individuals. The annual rate of fatal and non-fatal cardiovascular disease among people with type 2 diabetes is 2–5%. This risk is largely independent of the classic risk factors for atherosclerosis. Further, it is operative in many different populations with dissimilar background rates of cardiovascular disease. The prevalence of cardiovascular risk factors, including glucose intolerance, however, does differ between ethnic groups (page 2).

> Coronary heart disease is the principal cause of premature mortality in patients with diabetes

Patients with proteinuria (microalbuminuria or clinical proteinuria) are at significantly increased risk of atheromatous cardiovascular disease; the reasons remain only partially understood. Cardiovascular event risk is increased nearly two-fold by the presence of microalbuminuria and it has been hypothesized that microalbuminuria reflects generalized endothelial dysfunction which predisposes to

atheroma. The vascular endothelium has a complex structure and disturbances of endothelial function have been reported in patients with type 2 diabetes. However, this should not detract from the fact that type 2 diabetes *per se* is a major risk factor for coronary heart disease, amply demonstrated by the observation that the normal protection from coronary heart disease afforded to pre-menopausal women is negated by diabetes. In fact, some studies indicate that rates of atherosclerotic cardiovascular disease are higher in diabetic women than diabetic men, relative to their non-diabetic counterparts.

> The normal protection from cardiovascular disease afforded to pre-menopausal women is negated by diabetes

Risk factors for atherosclerosis

Both longitudinal and interventional studies have indicated that glycaemia is an independent risk factor for atherosclerotic cardiovascular disease. Current evidence suggests that there is a linear association between glycated haemoglobin (HbA_{1c}) levels and cardiovascular risk in patients with type 2 diabetes. This was demonstrated by prospective population-based studies in Finland (Figure 7.1) and Sweden in which cardiovascular mortality was linearly associated with glycaemia, independent of mode of treatment. In a second Finnish study, elevated HbA_{1c} was significantly associated with coronary heart disease mortality after adjustment for other cardiovascular risk factors. In the United Kingdom Prospective Diabetes Study (UKPDS 23), increased baseline HbA_{1c} and fasting plasma glucose concentrations were associated with coronary heart disease. Other predictive risk factors included an increased LDL-cholesterol concentration, a decreased HDL-cholesterol concentration and an increased fasting triglyceride concentration (but triglycerides were no longer independently predictive when other risk factors were included in the analysis). The estimated hazard ratio for smokers compared with non-smokers was 1.41. The multicentre European DECODE Study showed that elevated two-hour plasma glucose concentrations correlated more strongly with cardiovascular mortality than fasting hyperglycaemia.

> Elevated fasting plasma glucose concentrations and elevated HbA$_{1c}$ levels are associated with an increased risk of coronary heart disease

The main modifiable risk factors for atherosclerosis in diabetic patients are identical to those in non-diabetic individuals, ie:

- hypertension
- dyslipidaemia
- cigarette smoking.

The adverse effects of hypertension and

dyslipidaemia also seem to be amplified by the presence of diabetes. Lipid levels and blood pressures that might be regarded as acceptable in non-diabetic subjects are not acceptable in diabetic patients.

When a multiplicity of risk factors is present, the risk of macrovascular disease is greatly enhanced (Figure 7.2). The impact of other cardiovascular risk factors, such as fibrinogen, plasminogen activator inhibitor-1, lipoprotein(a) and homocysteine, has yet to be fully elucidated.

> The coronary risk associated with dyslipidaemia, hypertension or cigarette smoking is amplified by the presence of diabetes

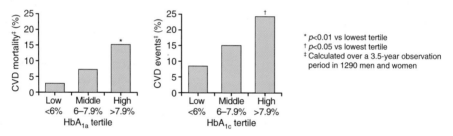

* $p<0.01$ vs lowest tertile
† $p<0.05$ vs lowest tertile
‡ Calculated over a 3.5-year observation period in 1290 men and women

Figure 7.1
Glycated haemoglobin (HbA$_{1c}$) at baseline as a predictor of cardiovascular disease in nearly 1300 Finnish men and women (aged 65–74 years). Reproduced with permission from Kuusisto *et al. Diabetes* 1994; **43**: 960-7.

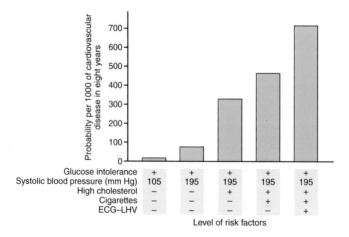

Figure 7.2
Effect of multiple risk factors for coronary heart disease. Reproduced with permission from Kannel WB, McGee DL. *Diabetes Care* 1979; **2**: 120-6.

Coronary heart disease

Coronary heart disease is the most common cause of mortality among patients with type 2 diabetes. The magnitude of the increased risk in diabetic patients was forcefully demonstrated in a population-based study. During a seven-year follow-up, Finnish patients with type 2 diabetes who had no overt coronary heart disease at entry were found to be at as high a risk of myocardial infarction and cardiovascular death as non-diabetic individuals who had already sustained a myocardial infarction (Figure 7.3). While this study can be criticized, patients with type 2 diabetes should still be regarded as candidates for therapeutic measures hitherto reserved for patients with established coronary heart disease – eg judicious use of aspirin, statins and antihypertensive drugs. A decision to intervene pharmacologically as primary prevention should be based on calculation of the absolute risk of cardiovascular events for the individual concerned.

> Patients with type 2 diabetes should be regarded as candidates for therapeutic measures used in patients with established coronary heart disease

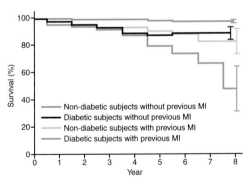

Figure 7.3
Kaplan–Meier estimates of the probability of death from coronary heart disease in subjects who had not had a previous myocardial infarction. 1059 type 2 diabetic vs 1378 non-diabetic subjects. Reproduced with permission from Haffner SM *et al. N Engl J Med* 1998; **339**: 229-34.

Acute myocardial infarction

The prognosis for patients with type 2 diabetes who survive a myocardial infarction is poor and the incidence of recurrent coronary events high. In the 4S study, approximately half of all placebo-treated patients with diabetes who had had a myocardial infarction had sustained a major coronary event at five years. Mortality (both immediate in-hospital, and late) is also high. Even with the use of thrombolysis, the mortality rate of patients with diabetes after a myocardial infarction is approximately twice as high as that of their non-diabetic counterparts. Left ventricular failure and cardiogenic shock are the principal causes of death, but while various plausible hypotheses have been proposed, the continuing dismal prognosis of patients with diabetes has not been satisfactorily explained. For example, there is no conclusive evidence that infarct size is larger or that the histology of coronary heart disease differs appreciably in diabetic patients. However, it is recognized that coronary artery disease may progress more rapidly in those with diabetes and the existence of a specific diabetic cardiomyopathy has been postulated which may contribute to the development of cardiac failure (page 94) in some people.

> Immediate and later mortality rates following myocardial infarction are high in patients with type 2 diabetes

The symptoms of myocardial infarction may also be modified by diabetes. So-called clinically 'silent' infarcts are more common – neuropathy in the autonomic fibres that transmit pain sensation from the myocardium is held to be responsible. Since angina pectoris may also be less prominent, acute coronary ischaemia may present atypically with symptoms such as dyspnoea, syncope and, in the elderly, confusion. Electrocardiograms suggestive of ischaemia are more common in asymptomatic diabetic than non-diabetic patients.

> Acute myocardial infarction may present with minimal or atypical symptoms in diabetic patients

> The small risk of retinopathic intraocular haemorrhage should not deter use of streptokinase and tPA in diabetic patients who have suffered a myocardial infarction

Management

There is no evidence for diminished therapeutic efficacy of accepted cardiovascular interventions in patients with diabetes. The acute effect of aspirin, for example, is similar in subjects with and without diabetes. Due to their higher absolute risk, however, diabetic patients may derive even greater benefit from interventions such as thrombolysis and β-blockers, and there is evidence that these drugs are underused in this high-risk group.

> The benefits of thrombolysis and β-blockers may be greater in diabetic patients, as a result of their higher absolute risk

Thus, in addition to measures such as analgesia, the management of acute myocardial infarction in diabetic patients should include, as appropriate:

- *Aspirin* – to be given at presentation and in the long term if no contraindications exist (75 mg/day, enteric-coated).
- *Thrombolysis* – as for non-diabetics. The small risk of vitreous haemorrhage from streptokinase or tissue plasminogen activator (tPA) in patients with advanced retinopathy should not deter use of these agents. The beneficial effects outweigh any potential detrimental retinal effects.
- *Angiotensin converting enzyme (ACE) inhibitors* – these are indicated primarily for cardiac failure or impaired left ventricular function revealed on echocardiogram. The results of the MICRO-HOPE study (page 102) extended the indications for these agents.
- *β-blockers* – subgroup analyses have suggested that these agents may be particularly beneficial in diabetic patients.

Meticulous control of the metabolic disturbances associated with acute myocardial infarction may also help to reduce mortality in diabetic patients. The associated hormonal stress response, for example, includes a massive release of catecholamines, and has several potentially adverse metabolic consequences:

- Acute exacerbation of insulin resistance.
- Acute hyperglycaemia.
- Increased lipolysis – fatty acids increase infarct size and may be pro-arrhythmic. Decreased insulin secretion and elevated fatty acid levels conspire to increase myocardial oxygen requirements, which may be detrimental in the acutely ischaemic myocardium.
- Suppression of insulin secretion – this exacerbates the direct adverse effects of catecholamines and other stress hormones on carbohydrate and lipid metabolism.

A proportion of non-diabetic patients with acute myocardial infarction will develop transient hyperglycaemia as a consequence of this hormonal stress response. Acute left ventricular failure is particularly likely to lead to hyperglycaemia. Glycated proteins may be of some use in this situation. However, they are relatively insensitive for diagnostic purposes, particularly of minor degrees of glucose intolerance (chapter 4), if there is any continuing doubt, a 75 g oral glucose tolerance test (pages 39 and 176) performed approximately six weeks after infarct recovery will provide a definitive answer.

Glucose–insulin infusion

Even in the absence of diabetes, intravenous infusions of glucose/insulin/potassium reduce myocardial infarct size in experimental animal models. Convincing evidence for benefit in hyperglycaemic patients was also provided by a multicentre, randomized study from Sweden, the Diabetes Mellitus Insulin Glucose Infusion in Acute Myocardial Infarction (DIGAMI) study (Tables 7.1 and 7.2, Figure 7.4).

As a secondary prevention measure, and in cost-effectiveness terms, the glucose–insulin protocol used in the DIGAMI study compares favourably with established interventions such as thrombolysis. For the cohort as a whole, 11 patients were treated to save one life at 3.5 years. A second DIGAMI study has been

Table 7.1
The Diabetes Mellitus Insulin Glucose Infusion in Acute Myocardial Infarction (DIGAMI) study.

Study design
620 subjects, more than 80% of whom were considered to have type 2 diabetes, were randomly assigned to (a) intensive treatment with an intravenous insulin–glucose infusion on the coronary care unit followed by multiple daily insulin injections (*n*=306), or (b) to a control group who received insulin only if clinically indicated (*n*=314). Approximately 13% were previously undiagnosed. Thrombolysis, aspirin, ACE inhibitor and β-blocker use was similar between the groups. At discharge, 87% of the intensive treatment group, compared with 43% of the control group, were taking insulin. Although 15% of the intensive treatment group experienced hypoglycaemia, this was not associated with any adverse events.

Study results
HbA$_{1c}$ decreased significantly in both groups during follow-up, the reduction was greatest in the intensively treated group at three and 12 months.
- A relative reduction in mortality of 30% was observed in the intensively treated group during the first year of follow-up.
- A significant (*p*<0.05) reduction in absolute mortality of 11% was still evident after nearly 3.5 years. This was most pronounced in a pre-defined subgroup of patients who had not previously received insulin treatment and who had a lower predicted cardiovascular risk because they were younger (<70 years) with no previous history of myocardial infarction or congestive cardiac failure.

Table 7.2
Protocol used on coronary care units during the DIGAMI study.

Infusion = 500 ml 5% glucose with 80 units of short-acting insulin, ie ~1 unit insulin per 6 ml infusate. Initial infusion rate 30 ml/hour. Blood glucose should be checked after 1 hour. Infusion rate adjusted, aiming for 7–10 mmol/l. Glucose checked every two hours, or every one hour after infusion rate altered. If initial decrease in glucose is >30% and blood glucose is >11 mmol/l, infusion rate should be left unchanged. It should be reduced by 6 ml/hour if blood glucose is 7–10.9 mmol/l. It should be reduced by 50% during the night, if blood glucose is stable at <11 mmol/l after 2200 hours, and intermittent monitoring continued.

Blood glucose (mmol/l)	Action
>15	Give 8 units insulin as iv bolus and increase infusion rate by 6 ml/hour.
11–14.9	Increase infusion rate by 3 ml/hour.
7–10.9	Leave infusion rate unchanged.
4–6.9	Decrease infusion rate by 6 ml/hour.
<4	Stop infusion for 15 minutes. Test blood glucose every 15 minutes until ≥7 mmol/l. If symptoms of hypoglycaemia are present, administer 20 ml of 30% glucose iv. Restart infusion with the rate decreased by 6 ml/hour when blood glucose is ≥7 mmol/l.

NB: careful monitoring by trained staff is required for safe protocol implementation.

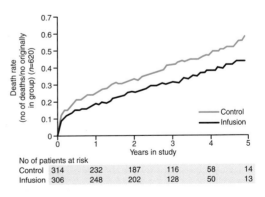

No of patients at risk

Control	314	232	187	116	58	14
Infusion	306	248	202	128	50	13

Figure 7.4
Actuarial mortality curves during long-term follow-up in patients receiving insulin–glucose infusion followed by subcutaneous insulin, and controls. Reproduced with permission from Malmberg K *et al*. *Br Med J* 1997; **314**: 1512-5.

designed to separate the effects of the early insulin–glucose infusion from subsequent subcutaneous insulin administration. The mechanism responsible for the improvement in survival remains unclear, but acute insulin-mediated suppression of plasma fatty acid levels (page 21) may be relevant. Another intriguing, but largely theoretical, possibility is that the reduced mortality in the intensively treated patients might at least partly have resulted from sulphonylurea withdrawal. The impressive results of the subgroup analysis may reflect the higher intrinsic cardiovascular risk of patients previously treated with oral antidiabetic agents. Concerns about the cardiovascular safety of sulphonylureas were initially raised by the findings of the University Group Diabetes Program in the US in the 1970s. Although this controversial study has since been strongly criticised, it reported an increased risk of cardiovascular mortality in patients randomized to tolbutamide. More recently, the United Kingdom Prospective Diabetes Study did not demonstrate any difference in risk of coronary heart disease between patients treated with sulphonylureas and those treated with insulin. While the cardiovascular safety of sulphonylureas has been requestioned from time to time, there is no clear evidence to deter sulphonylurea use in the pursuit of metabolic control in type 2 patients. Sulphonylureas are considered further in chapter 9.

> Intravenous infusion of insulin and glucose followed by subcutaneous insulin injection reduces mortality in diabetic patients who have had a myocardial infarction

> In the DIGAMI study, patients with type 2 diabetes considered to be at relatively low risk of cardiovascular death showed the greatest benefit from insulin therapy

The intravenous insulin–glucose infusion should be continued for 24 hours, at which stage the patient should be moved on to small doses of subcutaneous insulin. Whether twice-daily insulin is as effective as multiple daily injections is not yet known, but it is almost certainly more acceptable to most patients. Long-term therapy may not be feasible in some – recurrent hypoglycaemia with small daily doses may necessitate withdrawal, for example – but, otherwise, insulin should probably be continued as long as possible. Metformin should be withdrawn in patients with acute ischaemic heart disease because of the potential for lactic acidosis in the setting of tissue hypoxia (page 146).

Revascularization procedures

In general, revascularization procedures (angioplasty, coronary artery bypass grafting) seem to be less effective in patients with type 2 diabetes – both graft and patient survival rates are lower. Restenosis following angioplasty seems to be more common in diabetic patients. In a recent analysis of the Bypass Angiography Revascularization Investigation (BARI), survival was better in diabetic subjects after a myocardial infarction if they had previously undergone coronary artery bypass grafting rather than coronary angioplasty. Therapeutic developments, such as increasing use of intracoronary stents and new agents directed against platelet aggregation, are being evaluated.

Cardiac failure

Studies in diabetic animals and humans provide support for a specific defect in myocardial function independent of atheroma of the coronary vasculature. Subclinical echocardiographic abnormalities of left ventricular function have been reported in diabetic patients. Microangiopathy and fibrosis of the myocardium are histological features to which systemic hypertension may contribute. These abnormalities may help to explain the well documented excess incidence of cardiac failure in diabetic patients – up to five times higher than in non-diabetic individuals. The Hypertension in Diabetes Study (page 99) documented a significant reduction in the incidence of cardiac failure with tight blood pressure control. Insulin resistance is a feature of cardiac failure and its role is being examined with respect to possible novel therapeutic strategies.

> Type 2 diabetes is associated with an increased risk of cardiac failure

Peripheral arterial disease

Together with neuropathy and infection, peripheral arterial disease contributes to foot disease in diabetic patients (page 77). The incidence of peripheral arterial disease is about twice as high in diabetic patients. Abnormalities of circulating lipids, hypertension and smoking are all recognized risk factors for peripheral arterial disease.

> The prevalence of peripheral arterial disease is approximately doubled in diabetic patients

Clinical features

In people with type 2 diabetes, atherosclerosis has a predilection for the distal vessels, ie those below the popliteal fossa. The typical presentation is a palpable femoral pulse, but there may be no pulse below this level. The condition is asymptomatic until significant arterial stenoses develop. Symptoms, which depend on site and degree of stenosis, may then include:

- *Intermittent claudication* – classic calf claudication on walking, which is rapidly relieved by rest
- *Rest pain* – this denotes critical ischaemia, usually distal disease
- *Leriche's syndrome* – buttock and leg claudication, and erectile dysfunction due to major stenosis of the aortofemoral vessels
- *Ischaemic foot lesions* – in isolation, ischaemia accounts for <10% of diabetic foot ulcers, but it is a significant co-pathology in the neuroischaemic lesions that accompany about 50% of all ulcers

- *Impaired functional capacity* – this is less well defined but may also occur.

Co-existing vascular disease may impede the healing of ulcers that are predominantly neuropathic in origin, particularly when there is deeper infection in soft tissues or bone. This combination of pathologies is particularly common in elderly people with type 2 diabetes. Occasionally, atherosclerosis may also lead to functional renal artery stenosis, which is relevant to the pathogenesis and treatment of hypertension.

> Atherosclerosis has a predilection for vessels below the popliteal fossa in diabetes

Assessment of peripheral vasculature

Clinical evaluation

The history should enquire about: claudication, rest pain in limbs, features of Leriche's syndrome, past or present foot ulcers, smoking history, family history of premature atherosclerosis, and personal history of atherosclerosis including history of myocardial infarction, transient ischaemic attacks, stroke and lipid status, if known.

Physical examination

Physical examination should include manual palpation of peripheral pulses and auscultation for bruits. Trophic changes in the skin should be sought and limb temperature assessed. While a limb will be pale and cold in the presence of significant ischaemia, limbs may also appear red where blood flow is critically impaired ('sunset foot'). Buerger's sign may be positive: ie the limb blanches on being raised from the horizontal, but assumes a dusky red colour when dependent (over the edge of the bed). Evidence of additional risk factors for atherosclerosis, including corneal arcus, xanthelasma and hypertension, should be sought, as should aggravating disorders such as anaemia.

Doppler studies

Doppler studies are readily performed at the bedside with a hand-held probe, but interpretation will require experience; there is potential for misinterpretation in patients with diabetes. The ratio of the Doppler-measured ankle pressure to the Doppler-measured brachial artery pressure is normally 1.0, values less than 0.5 indicate severe disease. It should be noted that the ratio may be falsely elevated by arterial calcification in subjects with chronic neuropathy, which renders the vessels resistant to compression by the ankle pressure cuff. The quality of the Doppler signal may be a helpful pointer: normally three components are discerned and the signal is said to be triphasic, but arterial calcification may lead to a bi- or monophasic signal instead. Further assessment is then indicated.

Duplex scanning

Duplex scanning is a non-invasive technique that combines ultrasound imaging with Doppler assessment to provide information about the haemodynamic significance of a lesion. Once again, calcification may limit the quality of the information obtained. Duplex scanning is usually a prelude to angiography when contemplating surgery.

Oxygen tension

Oxygen tension can be measured transcutaneously on the dorsum of the foot using a laser Doppler probe to confirm critical ischaemia. The technique is not widely available.

Angiography

Angiography is used to delineate the site and extent of the lesions which often affect the distal arterial tree. Digital subtraction of bone improves the quality of the imaging of below-knee vessels. There is also the major advantage of being able to perform angioplasty or give thrombolytic agents simultaneously. Care should be taken to ensure adequate hydration of patients with renal impairment. Metformin should be omitted on the day of angiography (assuming normal renal function). Since iodinated radiographic contrast can sometimes cause acute renal impairment, it should only be reinstated when normal renal function has been confirmed.

Management

The management options for peripheral vascular disease include aspirin, foot care, vasodilating agents, surgical sympathectomy, reconstructive surgery or angioplasty, amputation and rehabilitation. It should be remembered that patients with peripheral arterial disease are at high risk of cardiovascular events; this reflects generalized atheroma.

- *Aspirin* – reduces mortality from cardiovascular disease and should be given where there are no contraindications. Always control blood pressure first in patients with severe hypertension.
- *Foot care* – is of great importance and patients should receive appropriate instruction. Regular inspection by a trained professional and timely podiatry may avert the development of more serious lesions.
- *Vasodilators* – Oral agents are usually ineffective but iv praxilene and low molecular-weight dextran may sometimes be helpful in selected inpatients with severe ischaemia.
- *Surgical sympathectomy* – in the lumbar region is ineffective for intermittent claudication. Patients with severe co-existing neuropathy will often already have clinical features suggestive of sympathetic denervation.
- *Reconstructive surgery or angioplasty* – may preserve limbs and avoid major amputation. Where there is proximal disease – patients with weak femoral pulses, and absent pulses more distally – angioplasty (localized short stenoses are most suitable) or arterial bypass grafting (aortofemoral and femoropopliteal) may help. Distal disease – normal femoral and popliteal pulses with absent foot pulses – is,

however, more commonly encountered in diabetes and much more difficult to treat by either route, particularly when there is diffuse disease below the level of the popliteal fossa.

- *Amputation* – may need to be radical, ie below knee, if it is required for major arterial occlusion. Above-knee is avoided where possible because rehabilitation is more difficult.
- *Rehabilitation* – prospects after major amputation are often overestimated and old age and serious co-morbidity are major limiting factors. The aim must be to preserve a functionally useful limb wherever possible.

Patients with peripheral arterial disease are also at high risk of coronary events. Thus, measures aimed at reducing cardiovascular risk, including statins, antihypertensive therapy and aspirin, should be considered.

> Patients with peripheral vascular disease are at high risk of coronary heart disease

Cerebrovascular disease

Stroke is the second most common cause of death among people with type 2 diabetes. The incidence of cerebrovascular disease is roughly doubled in diabetic patients. A role for the central nervous system in the regulation of glucose metabolism has long been recognized: Claude Bernard described *piqûre* diabetes – glycosuria following transfixion of the medulla oblongata – in rabbits as long ago as the 19th century. Transient hyperglycaemia may be observed after an acute stroke in much the same way that it is observed after acute myocardial infarction, but limited observational studies suggest that hyperglycaemia at presentation with acute stroke is an independent marker of adverse clinical outcome, principally mortality, within the first month.

> Cerebrovascular disease is the second most common cause of death in subjects with type 2 diabetes

Transient defects associated with acute metabolic derangements

Hemiplegia

In addition to atheromatous cerebrovascular disease, transient hemiplegia has a recognized but rare association with hypoglycaemia in insulin-treated diabetic patients.

Other focal neurological deficits

Reversible focal neurological lesions are also recognized in patients presenting with non-ketotic, hyperosmolar pre-coma or coma.

Convulsions

Epilepsy may occasionally be triggered in susceptible patients by hyperglycaemia, especially if there is hyperosmolarity.

Cognitive dysfunction

Atherosclerotic dementia may contribute to impaired psychomotor performance, learning and memory in older diabetic individuals. Correlations between psychological dysfunction and hyperglycaemia have been reported in elderly subjects – hypertension and other factors are also implicated. There is some evidence suggesting that better glycaemic control may improve cognition, but further studies are required.

Atrial fibrillation

Diabetes is regarded as an additional risk factor for stroke (along with hypertension and advancing age) in individuals with atrial fibrillation. In the United Kingdom Prospective Diabetes Study, atrial fibrillation was identified as a major risk factor for stroke in subjects with type 2 diabetes.

Dyslipidaemia

Some statins, eg pravastatin and simvastatin, are licensed for the prevention of stroke in subjects who have already sustained a myocardial infarction, but there are no data specifically relating to diabetes.

> Atrial fibrillation is a major risk factor for stroke in patients with type 2 diabetes

Hypertension

Hypertension is a common, important and modifiable risk factor for both the micro- and macrovascular complications of diabetes. Although prevalence rates are highly dependent on specific definitions, numerous studies have shown that hypertension is more common in diabetic than in non-diabetic individuals; it is present in 50–80% of patients with type 2 diabetes, according to modern definitions (ie ≥140/90 mmHg). It is well recognized that obesity increases blood pressure; the effect attributable to gender is less clear – some studies suggest that women are at higher risk. While hypertension is more common in patients with type 2 diabetes, the prevalence essentially reflects the general background of the population concerned; black patients, for example, are at particular risk. Hypertension is closely associated with insulin resistance (page 21) in type 2 diabetes patients, but the strength and nature of the association is still unclear.

Hypertension is an important modifiable risk factor for several micro- and macrovascular complications of type 2 diabetes

There is considerable evidence that hypertension is both underdiagnosed and inadequately treated in patients with diabetes. Regular and accurate monitoring of blood pressure is an important and undervalued aspect of diabetes care.

Haemodynamic abnormalities in diabetes

Abnormal haemodynamics in patients with type 2 diabetes may increase the risk of tissue damage attributable to hypertension. The implication is that, for any level of systemic blood pressure, patients with diabetes are more susceptible to tissue damage. Postulated mechanisms include:

- *Autoregulation* – when this is interrupted (through hyperglycaemia) in vulnerable

vascular beds such as those of the retina and renal glomeruli, systemic blood pressure is transmitted directly to the microvasculature.

- *Decreased vascular compliance* – of major vessels such as the aorta, perhaps resulting from non-enzymatic glycation (page 65), may lead to the transmission of higher pressures to distal vascular beds. This abnormality may also contribute to isolated systolic hypertension in patients with type 2 diabetes.

- *Increased blood pressure variability* – has been reported during 24-hour ambulatory recordings.

- *Reduced decline in nocturnal blood pressure* – failure of the nocturnal decline in blood pressure (during sleep) is a reported early feature associated with microalbuminuria. 24-hour blood pressure exposure of vulnerable tissues is increased as a result.

Assessment of the diabetic patient with hypertension

Secondary hypertension should be excluded, target organ damage identified and other cardiovascular risk factors otherwise assessed in all diabetic patients with hypertension. A history and physical examination will usually reveal any endocrine or other cause of hypertension (Table 7.3). Most endocrine causes, with the exception of thyrotoxicosis, are uncommon. Signs of target organ damage include left ventricular hypertrophy, arterial bruits, absent pedal pulses (increased risk of renal artery stenosis) and hypertensive retinal changes.

Investigations

For most patients these should include:

- *Urinalysis* – to identify microalbuminuria or clinical grade proteinuria.

- *Renal function and electrolytes* – for renal impairment, hypokalaemia (usually due to diuretic use), Conn's syndrome (due to aldosterone excess) and hyperkalaemia (renal impairment and type III renal tubular acidosis).

Table 7.3
Endocrine causes of hypertension.

- Thyrotoxicosis – common and usually clinically evident.
- Acromegaly – uncommon, with characteristic appearance.
- Cushing's syndrome – uncommon, with typical clinical features.
- Conn's syndrome – may be asymptomatic hypokalaemia, often unrecognized.
- Phaeochromocytoma – uncommon, with typical clinical features.
- Primary hyperparathyroidism – common, associated with insulin resistance and hypertension.

Note that these disorders may be accompanied by glucose intolerance or type 2 diabetes.

- *Electrocardiogram* – for evidence of left ventricular hypertrophy (which indicates an adverse prognosis; echocardiography is more sensitive), ischaemia (may be subclinical), and atrial fibrillation (relatively common; suggests increased risk of stroke).
- *Plasma lipids*.
- *Ambulatory blood pressure monitoring* – the role of home measurements has not been delineated clearly, but ambulatory measurements may be useful if there is unusual variability in clinic pressures, hypertension apparently resistant to three or more drugs, symptoms suggestive of hypotension, or a suspicion of 'white coat hypertension'. The 1999 British Hypertension Society guidelines suggest an optimal mean daytime ambulatory pressure or home measurement of <130/75 in diabetic subjects.

Other investigations such as exercise testing and isotope studies (eg captopril renogram) to exclude renal artery stenosis may be indicated in some.

> Hypertension in type 2 diabetes is regarded as a component of the insulin resistance syndrome

Hypertension in Diabetes Study

In 1987, a randomized study of blood pressure control, the Hypertension in Diabetes Study, was embedded within the main United Kingdom Prospective Diabetes Study using a factorial design (UKPDS 38 and 39). The study provided important confirmation of the adverse effect of hypertension in patients with type 2 diabetes and Table 7.4 summarizes its key points. Whether any particular class of antihypertensive drug is associated with advantages or disadvantages for diabetic patients remains unclear, but considerable evidence suggests that the most important consideration is the level of blood pressure attained, rather than the agent used. Atenolol and captopril were shown to have similar efficacy in the Hypertension in Diabetes Study. The study did not have sufficient statistical power to identify real differences between these two classes.

> In type 2 diabetes, the blood pressure level attained appears to be more important than the type of antihypertensive drug used to attain it

Metabolic effects of antihypertensive drugs

Much debate has surrounded the influence of antihypertensive agents on the risk factors for cardiovascular disease. While the clinical significance of such effects remains unclear, it is obvious that antihypertensive treatment with β-blockers and thiazides has not led to the reductions in mortality from coronary heart disease that were expected. It has been suggested that adverse metabolic effects might have offset the beneficial effects of these two classes of drug in the trials concerned.

Insulin action

β-blockers (particularly non-selective agents) and high-dose thiazide diuretics aggravate insulin resistance (in contrast, ACE inhibitors and α-blockers may improve insulin action). Interestingly, during the first few years of the Hypertension in Diabetes Study, HbA$_{1c}$ levels

Table 7.4
The Hypertension in Diabetes Study (UKPDS 38 and 39).

Methodology
This prospective, randomized, multicentre, double-blinded study of type 2 diabetic patients compared (a) tight control of blood pressure (target <150/85, n=758) either with the ACE inhibitor captopril (25–50 mg bid, n=400) or atenolol (50–100 mg/day, n=358) plus additional agents as necessary (suggested sequence: frusemide, slow-release nifedipine, methyldopa and prazocin) with (b) less tight (<180/105, n=390) control.

Results (UKPDS 38)
- Mean blood pressure was reduced to 144/82 vs 154/87 mmHg (a difference of 10/5 mmHg) for the tight and less tight control groups, respectively ($p<0.0001$).
- Multiple drug therapy (three or more agents) was required more often in the tight control group (29% vs 11%, respectively). However, at nine years only 56% of patients in the tight control group had attained the target blood pressure of <150/85.
- Tight control reduced diabetes-related endpoints (fatal or non-fatal) by 24% ($p=0.0046$; Figure 7.5), diabetes-related deaths by 32% ($p=0.019$), stroke by 44% ($p=0.013$) and microvascular disease by 37% ($p=0.0092$).
- The reduction in microvascular complications was predominantly attributable to a reduced risk of photocoagulation for retinopathy; there were associated reductions in the progression of retinopathy (34%, $p=0.0004$). In addition, a measure of visual loss (equivalent of a reduction from 6/6 to 6/12 or 6/9 to 6/18 on the Snellen chart) was reduced, suggesting prevention of maculopathy, the main cause of visual impairment in type 2 diabetes (47%, $p=0.004$).
- A transient reduction in microalbuminuria ($p=0.009$) at six years in the tight control group was not sustained at nine years; there was no difference in clinical grade proteinuria or serum creatinine between the groups by the end of the study.
- All-cause mortality was not significantly reduced (18%, $p=0.17$) by tight blood pressure control. However, there was a 34% reduction in combined macrovascular endpoints (ie myocardial infarction, sudden death, stroke and peripheral vascular disease, $p=0.019$).
- Although the reduction in myocardial infarction (21%) was not statistically significant ECG Q-wave abnormalities were reduced by 48% ($p=0.007$). In addition, the risk of cardiac failure was reduced by 56% ($p=0.0043$).

Results (UKPDS 39: Atenolol vs captopril for hypertension)
- Captopril and atenolol were equally effective in reducing the incidence of diabetic complications (although study not adequately powered to detect small differences).
- The mean weight gain was higher in the atenolol group (3.4 vs 1.6 kg) while glycated HbA_{1c} concentrations were slightly higher over the first four years. No difference in the rate of severe hypoglycaemia was observed between the drugs.
- Captopril was better tolerated than atenolol with 78% vs 65% of patients still taking their allocated drug at their last clinic visit ($p<0.0001$).

were significantly higher in the atenolol-treated group than in the captopril-treated group – accordingly, more antihyperglycaemic therapy was required in the atenolol-treated patients. In longitudinal studies, both β-blockers and thiazides, particularly in combination, have been implicated in the pathogenesis of type 2 diabetes in patients with essential hypertension, but the nature of the association remains uncertain.

Dihydropyridine calcium antagonists with a short duration of action, such as nifedipine,

may impair insulin action, while longer-acting drugs (eg amlodipine) and modified-release preparations, together with non-dihydropyridine drugs (eg diltiazem and verapamil) appear to have neutral effects. In contrast, several classes of more recently introduced antihypertensive agent may have beneficial effects of insulin sensitivity:

- *ACE inhibitors* – are either neutral or may improve insulin sensitivity in non-diabetic and diabetic patients. ACE gene polymorphisms may have implications for

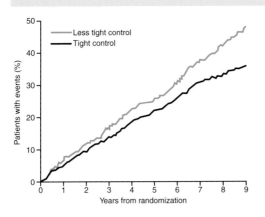

Figure 7.5
The Hypertension in Diabetes Study: effect of tight control of blood pressure on diabetes-related endpoints (fatal and non-fatal). Reproduced with permission from *Br Med J* 1998; **317**: 703-17.

insulin action (chapter 2) as well as the blood pressure response to ACE inhibitors.

- *Angiotensin II₁ receptor antagonists* – improved insulin action has been reported with use of these agents.
- *α₁-receptor blockers* – doxazosin can improve insulin sensitivity and plasma lipid profiles, but was withdrawn from the multicentre comparative Antihypertensive and Lipid Lowering treatment to prevent Heart Attack Trial (ALLHAT) because it was less effective in preventing cardiac failure than diuretic-based therapy.
- *Selective imidazoline-receptor agonists* – moxonidine improves insulin action in animal models and in obese hypertensive patients. Rilmenidine has also been reported to improve glucose metabolism in animals and humans and to have minor effects on lipid metabolism.

Lipids

The adverse effects of β-blockers and thiazide diuretics on plasma lipid levels (increased very low-density lipoproteins and hypercholesterolaemia, respectively) have also received attention.

Associated haemostatic abnormalities such as increased fibrinogen, factor VII levels and plasminogen activator inhibitor-1 activity may contribute to atherogenesis.

Hypokalaemia

There have been reports of an increased risk of sudden death in diabetic and non-diabetic patients with electrocardiographic abnormalities who have been treated with thiazide diuretics. The metabolic effects of thiazides can be minimized by the use of lower doses (eg bendrofluazide ≤2.5 mg/day). Higher doses have limited additional antihypertensive effects and carry greatly increased risks of adverse effects.

Other considerations

Several other large, randomized studies (Table 7.5) have demonstrated substantial benefits from treating hypertension in type 2 diabetes. These trials have used regimens based on thiazide diuretics and long-acting calcium antagonists and suggested that therapeutic benefit was greater in diabetic than non-diabetic subgroups, reflecting the higher absolute risk associated with diabetes. Reductions in both systolic and diastolic blood pressure are important. The difference between systolic and diastolic pressures (ie the pulse) is a superior indicator of vascular events than either systolic or diastolic pressure alone.

There have been reports of higher cardiovascular event rates in patients treated with calcium antagonists than other agents, but a lack of placebo comparisons and use of secondary endpoints complicate the interpretation of such findings. The Nordic Diltiazem (NORDIL) study and the International Nifedipine Study: Intervention as a Goal in Hypertension Treatment (INSIGHT) confirmed that the efficacy of these two agents was similar to that of diuretic- or β-blocker-based therapy.

Concerns about another long-running controversy, the 'J-shaped curve' (ie the

Table 7.5

Other randomized clinical trials of antihypertensive therapy in patients with type 2 diabetes.

1. SHEP (Systolic Hypertension in the Elderly Program)
JAMA 1996; **276**: 1886-92.
Total *n*=4736; diabetic *n*=583. Duration: 5 years.
Chlorthalidone ± atenolol or reserpine vs placebo.
Findings:
34% reduction in major cardiovascular events (cerebral and cardiac) with active treatment vs placebo. Greater benefit in diabetic subgroup reflecting higher absolute risk of these patients.

2. HOT (Hypertension Optimal Treatment)
Lancet 1998; **351**: 1755-62.
Total *n*=18790; diabetic *n*=1501. Duration: 3.8 years.
Felodipine + other agents (vs placebo) as required to attain diastolic blood pressure targets.
Findings:
Reduction (by 50%) in major cardiovascular events with target diastolic of 80 mmHg vs 90 mmHg in diabetic patients. Additional benefit of aspirin.

3. SYST-EUR (Systolic Hypertension in Europe)
Lancet 1997; **350**: 757-64 and *N Engl J Med* 1999; **340**: 677-84.
Total *n*=4695; diabetic *n*=492. Duration: 2 years (median).
Nitrendipine + enalapril or thiazide vs placebo.
Findings:
Excess risk of diabetes almost completely eliminated by antihypertensive therapy with major reductions (approx 70%) in cardiovascular mortality and all cardiovascular endpoints. Similar results to the Chinese study SYS-CHINA.

4. HOPE (Heart Outcomes Prevention Evaluation)
N Engl J Med 2000; **342**: 145-53.
Total with pre-existing coronary heart disease, stroke or peripheral vascular disease *n*=9297; 38% had diabetes. Duration: 4.5 years.
Ramipril (as well as other agents) vs placebo.
Findings:
Overall, 25% reduction in risk of cardiovascular death, 20% for myocardial infarction and 32% for stroke with ramipril vs placebo. For diabetic subgroup, 17% risk reduction in diabetic complications. New cases of diabetes reduced by 32%. This was not a treat-to-target (blood pressure) study; other agents were permitted as required.

5. MICRO-HOPE (Microalbuminuria, Cardiovascular, and Renal Outcomes) Lancet 2000; **355**: 253-59.
n= 3577 patients with diabetes (subgroup of HOPE) aged >55 years, with a previous cardiovascular event or one other cardiovascular risk factor (hypertension, raised cholesterol, low HDL-cholesterol, smoking or microalbuminuria. Duration: 4.5 years.
Ramipril (in addition to other agents) vs placebo.
Findings:
Ramipril reduced the primary combined outcome (myocardial infarction, stroke, cardiovascular death) by 25%, myocardial infarction by 22%, stroke by 33%, cardiovascular death by 37% and overt nephropathy by 24%. Risk reduction was in excess of that anticipated for reduction in blood pressure (2.4/1.0 mmHg).

suggestion that very low blood pressure is associated with adverse effects), have also been largely allayed. We may now conclude that the lower the blood pressure attained, the greater the clinical benefit (UKPDS 36). Studies in non-diabetic individuals have not suggested any significant differences between the major classes of antihypertensive agent to date and the 1999 World Health Organization International Society for Hypertension guidelines stated that any of the main classes of antihypertensive drug are suitable as first-line therapy. However, the MICRO-HOPE study (Table 7.5) showed benefits for ramipril on microvascular and macrovascular events in (type 2) diabetic patients. In this – and the main HOPE study – the benefits were disproportionate to the observed reductions in blood pressure, and raised the possibility of an endothelial protective effect for this drug (ramipril). The incidence of self-reported new cases of diabetes was reduced in the main HOPE cohort, as it was in the Captopril Prevention Project (CAPPP) and INSIGHT study.

> The lower the blood pressure, the greater the benefit in patients with type 2 diabetes

Cautions and contraindications

Diabetic patients are at risk of developing long-term tissue complications which may render certain antihypertensive drugs unsuitable (Table 7.6). Initially, the most appropriate drug should be selected (Table 7.7).

Risk of hypoglycaemia

Problems of impaired recognition of warning symptoms of and recovery from hypoglycaemia with β-blockers are uncommon with the cardioselective drugs such as atenolol. Insulin treatment should not generally be regarded as a contraindication to the use of cardioselective β-blockers, which are of proven benefit in diabetic patients. Reports of an increased risk of

Table 7.6
Cautions and contraindications to antihypertensive therapy in diabetic patients.

Caution or contraindication	Drugs to avoid
Dyslipidaemia	β-blockers, thiazide diuretics (high doses)
Erectile dysfunction	β-blockers, thiazide diuretics
Gout	Thiazide diuretics
Peripheral vascular disease	β-blockers
Renal artery stenosis	ACE inhibitors, AII_1 receptor antagonists

Table 7.7
Indications for particular antihypertensive drugs in type 2 diabetic patients.

Indication	Drugs of choice
Nephropathy	ACE inhibitors (+ loop diuretics), non-dihydropyridine calcium antagonists
Ischaemic heart disease	β-blockers, long-acting calcium antagonists
Cardiac failure	ACE inhibitors, AII_1 receptor antagonists, loop diuretics, β-blockers (certain agents in selected patients)

hypoglycaemia with ACE inhibitors in insulin-treated patients remain unsubstantiated: the United Kingdom Prospective Diabetes Study showed no difference in risk of severe hypoglycaemia between atenolol- and captopril-treated groups.

Renal artery stenosis

A minority of patients with type 2 diabetes, mainly those with evidence of peripheral vascular disease, have clinically significant renal artery stenosis. Certain drugs, such as the ACE inhibitors and angiotensin II receptor antagonists should be used with caution in such patients because of the risk of precipitating an acute deterioration in renal function. This occurs as a consequence of the effects of these drugs on intraglomerular haemodynamics. Where there are significant functional stenoses of both renal arteries, glomerular filtration is maintained by the vasoconstrictor effect of angiotensin II on efferent glomerular arterioles. Removal of this effect may lead to major reductions in the capacity for glomerular filtration. Under certain circumstances (patients with congestive cardiac failure with generalized atherosclerosis) unilateral renal artery stenosis may also lead to deterioration in renal function. The risk may be somewhat overstated, but it is prudent to remeasure plasma creatinine and electrolytes within a week of starting ACE inhibitor or angiotensin II_1 receptor antagonist therapy.

Effect of ethnicity on response to treatment

Hypertensive patients of African ethnicity, who tend to have low plasma renin levels, respond better to β-blockers and calcium antagonists than to ACE inhibitors. Similarly, it makes sense to select metabolically neutral drugs (page 99) as first-line agents in South Asian patients with multiple components of the insulin resistance syndrome. However, no clear evidence of the superiority of these drugs has yet been demonstrated within these ethnic groups.

Strategies for the management of hypertension in diabetes

Non-pharmacological strategies include attainment of ideal body weight, reduced dietary salt intake, and appropriate duration and severity of aerobic physical exercise (chapter 8). When blood pressure targets are not being achieved, start with the most appropriate drug for the particular patient. Add or substitute drugs in logical combinations (for example, ACE inhibitor plus diuretic, or long-acting calcium channel antagonist plus β-blocker) and use low doses of each agent to minimize the unwanted effects. Avoid potentially hazardous combinations such as ACE inhibitor and spironolactone (risk of hyperkalaemia), or diltiazem with a β-blocker. Diuretics are often useful, since hypertension in diabetic patients is associated with an expanded plasma volume. Loop diuretics are often necessary for patients with renal impairment (in whom hypertension may be particularly difficult to control).

Patients with diabetes will often require a multiplicity of drugs – for example, oral antidiabetic agents, lipid-lowering agents and aspirin – and since hypertension is largely asymptomatic, once-daily dosing and use of well-tolerated drugs are likely to improve compliance (which is recognized to be fairly poor). The angiotensin II_1 receptor antagonists appear to be particularly well tolerated; they do not lead to the cough that is induced in a proportion of patients treated with ACE inhibitors. Omapatrilat, a combined inhibitor of

ACE and neutral endopeptidase, may be more effective than many conventional classes of antihypertensive agent but, in pre-registration trials, it has been associated with serious angio-oedema in a few (<1%) patients.

Dyslipidaemia

Quantitative and qualitative alterations in plasma lipid levels alter the risk of atheromatous complications in patients with type 2 diabetes. The impact of dyslipidaemia is also magnified by the presence of diabetes and the development of microvascular complications. Thus, diabetic nephropathy is associated with additional disturbances of plasma lipids that exacerbate any existing risk. Common genetic dyslipidaemias, such as familial combined hyperlipidaemia, are just as common among diabetic as non-diabetic individuals. The rare syndromes of lipodystrophic diabetes are associated with marked hyperlipidaemia, but the most common plasma lipid abnormalities encountered in type 2 diabetes patients are hypertriglyceridaemia and a reduced HDL-cholesterol level. Hypertriglyceridaemia is associated with tissue insulin resistance (page 21). Elevations in total and LDL-cholesterol levels are not as prevalent, with total cholesterol, in general, being similar to that in the non-diabetic population.

Antidiabetic agents may improve lipid metabolism through several mechanisms, all of which reflect improved insulin action in target tissues involved in the regulation of lipid metabolism:

- the stimulatory effect of insulin on the endothelial lipoprotein lipase hydrolyses circulating triglycerides in very low-density lipoproteins (VLDL) and chylomicrons, leading to a secondary reduction in LDL-cholesterol levels
- the suppression of adipocyte lipolysis (via hormone-sensitive lipase) reduces the release of non-esterified fatty acids for metabolism by the liver and muscle
- the direct suppression of hepatic VLDL-lipoprotein production.

In type 2 diabetes, reduced breakdown of VLDL (consequent to insulin deficiency or insulin resistance) increases the circulating concentration of atherogenic triglyceride-rich particles. Low HDL-cholesterol levels are closely associated with hypertriglyceridaemia because of increased transfer of cholesteryl ester from HDL to VLDL and chylomicrons by cholesteryl ester transfer protein. LDL-cholesterol particle size is reduced by increased activity of hepatic lipase, which produces smaller, more dense, apoprotein-rich LDL particles (the so-called pattern B on electrophoresis) regarded as having enhanced atherogenicity. These abnormalities seem to be about twice as prevalent in subjects with type 2 diabetes.

However, any specified level of cholesterol has a greater impact on coronary risk in the presence of diabetes, and epidemiological data indicate that the risk of a coronary event is particularly high when all of the following are present: low HDL-cholesterol, a high ratio (>5.0) of total cholesterol to HDL cholesterol, and hypertriglyceridaemia. While this profile is also associated with a disproportionately increased risk of cardiovascular disease in non-diabetic individuals, it is suggested that the atherogenicity of disordered lipid metabolism in diabetes may be further increased by:

- *Glycation of lipoproteins* – apoprotein B, the major protein component of LDL, is susceptible to non-enzymatic glycation, which reduces the affinity of LDL for its tissue receptors, thereby reducing LDL clearance from plasma.
- *Oxidative modification* – the uptake of LDL by scavenger pathways which lead to atherosclerosis may be increased by oxidation, which may, in turn, be increased by glycation.

> Any level of cholesterol has a greater impact on coronary risk in the presence of diabetes

As already mentioned, nephropathy has a major impact on lipids. The development of diabetic nephropathy leads to an aggravated dyslipidaemia with elevated levels of total cholesterol, LDL-cholesterol and triglycerides combined with a reduced level of cardioprotective HDL-cholesterol. In addition, the plasma concentration of lipoprotein(a), an independent risk factor for coronary heart disease, will increase as a result of impaired renal catabolism.

Management

The greatly increased risk of atherosclerotic disease in patients with type 2 diabetes has led to an increased awareness of the importance of detecting and treating dyslipidaemia. This should be done in the context of total risk factor management, and based on a calculation of absolute cardiovascular risk. Although fasting plasma lipids are usually measured (in order to include triglycerides and HDL-cholesterol) there are practical difficulties involved in patients on insulin and increasing research attention is being focused on post-prandial lipid status. In patients with type 2 diabetes, post-prandial clearance of lipoproteins from the circulation is impaired and it is hypothesized that this post-prandial hyperlipidaemia contributes to atheroma development. Although many subtle alterations in plasma lipid levels have been described, therapeutic decisions rest on measurement of some or all of the following: total cholesterol concentration, triglycerides (fasting), LDL-cholesterol (calculated with reasonable accuracy using the Friedewald formula when triglycerides are <4.5 mmol/l), and HDL-cholesterol (which also allows calculation of the ratio of total cholesterol:HDL cholesterol).

Therapeutic targets in diabetic dyslipidaemia

Although observational studies suggest that low HDL-cholesterol and hypertriglyceridaemia may be more predictive than elevated LDL-cholesterol levels, the results of interventional clinical trials using statins strongly favour LDL-cholesterol lowering as the primary therapeutic aim (Table 7.8). Other markers, such as

Table 7.8
Trials demonstrating benefits of lowering LDL-cholesterol concentrations in patients with diabetes.
Sourced from *Diabetes Care* 1997; **20**: 614-20 and *Circulation* 1998; **98**: 2513-9.

The Scandinavian Simvastatin Survival Study (4S)
Significant (55%) reduction in the incidence of major coronary events in diabetic men with high LDL-cholesterol levels (5.5–8.0 mmol/l) and previous coronary heart disease. Mean follow-up duration: 4.5 years. *Diabetes Care* 1997; **20**: 614-20.

The Cholesterol and Recurrent Events (CARE) study
Pravastatin significantly reduced the incidence of coronary heart disease events in diabetic patients with average LDL-cholesterol levels and previous coronary disease over 5 years. *Circulation* 1998; **98**: 2513-9.

Note: results are derived from analyses of diabetic subgroups in each trial. The AFCAPS/TEXCAPS and LIPID studies also included diabetic subgroups.

Table 7.9
Comparison of suggested targets for plasma lipids and other coronary risk factors in diabetic patients.
Sourced from *Heart* 1998; **80**(2): S1-29 and *Diabetes Care* 2000; **23**(1): S57-60.

1. Joint British Societies recommendations on prevention of coronary heart disease in clinical practice
Targets for (a) patients (diabetic or non-diabetic) with coronary heart or other major atherosclerotic disease or (b) high-risk groups (coronary risk >15% over next 10 years) such as diabetic patients with no clinical evidence of atherosclerosis (particularly when risk factors are present in combination).

Risk factor	Target
Total cholesterol	<5.0 mmol/l
LDL-cholesterol	<3.0 mmol/l
Blood pressure	<130/80 mmHg

Also recommended: good glycaemic control (with use of insulin during and immediately after myocardial infarction), aspirin and other cardioprotective drugs as indicated (eg β-blockers, ACE inhibitors).
Heart 1998; **80**(2): S1-29.

2. American Diabetes Association, 2000
LDL-cholesterol thresholds for initiation and targets of drug therapy in diabetes:

	No evidence	Evidence (of macrovascular disease)
Initiation level	<3.4	<2.6
LDL-cholesterol goal	<2.6	<2.6

(All levels in mmol/l. To convert to mg/dl multiply by 39.)

Macrovascular disease includes clinically evident coronary heart, cerebrovascular or peripheral vascular disease. Note: Initiation levels may be lower for patients with no evidence of macrovascular disease but with evidence of multiple risk factors (low HDL-cholesterol, hypertension, family history of cardiovascular disease, microalbuminuria or clinical grade proteinuria). Diabetic men and women are considered to be at equal risk.
Diabetes Care 2000; **23**(1): S57-60.

apoprotein B and lipoprotein(a), are not routinely available in most institutions.

> Reduction of LDL-cholesterol concentrations is currently regarded as the primary therapeutic aim of lipid-lowering therapy

To date, no studies have been published which are confined to diabetic patients – both the 4S and CARE studies (Table 7.8) contained relatively small diabetic subgroups – and clinical guidelines produced by expert committees are being updated regularly as trial evidence accumulates. Current guidelines for secondary prevention with lipid-modifying drugs should be followed in diabetic patients with established cardiovascular disease, but primary prevention is less clearcut and differences in recommendations between expert groups have generated confusion. Examples of two recent guidelines, those of the Joint British Societies (1998) and those of the American Diabetes Association (2000) are presented in Table 7.9.

The magnitude of benefit derived from well-tolerated drugs such as the hydroxymethyl glutaryl coenzyme A (HMG-CoA) reductase

inhibitors (statins) depends on the absolute cardiovascular risk. The available data suggest that diabetic patients should be considered at high risk. In the CARE study, for example, in high-risk patients with diabetes and established coronary heart disease, 22 new coronary events were prevented in every 100 patients treated with simvastatin for five years. In contrast, only about one event per 100 patients was prevented over five years during a primary prevention trial in non-diabetic men in the West of Scotland with no risk factors other than LDL-cholesterol levels of 4.5–6.0 mmol/l who received similar treatment with pravastatin. Calculation of absolute cardiovascular risk should be approached logically, the aim being to target drug therapy to those at highest risk of events. It has been suggested that some of the available risk factor assessment tables can underestimate risk in diabetic patients and that risk cut-off levels are ultimately arbitrary. Once again, there are inconsistencies between the published guidelines. The 1998 Joint British Guidelines (Table 7.9) attempt to identify those at highest coronary risk (>30% risk over next 10 years) as a priority, but also set targets for lipids and blood pressure (including drug use where necessary) in patients whose risk is >15% over 10 years. The UK Government's endorsement of an intervention for primary prevention level of 3% per year has attracted fierce criticism as being little more than an exercise in rationing statin use. Some authorities argue that statins are no less cost-effective than other antidiabetic therapies but, in any case, patent expiry should result in cheaper generic alternatives becoming available in the near future.

Non-pharmacological approaches to treatment

Dietary measures

Dietary measures include attainment of ideal body weight and reduction in total fat consumption to around 30% of total calorie intake, and in saturated fat to <10% of total calorie intake. Excessive alcohol must also be curbed – alcohol can exacerbate hypertriglyceridaemia. The United Kingdom Prospective Diabetes Study (UKPDS 45) showed that three months' dietary therapy (hypocaloric for overweight patients, total maximum fat intake <35% with substitution of polyunsaturated for saturated fats) in newly diagnosed patients reduced mean plasma triglyceride levels (17% in men, 10% in women)

and led to marginal improvements in total cholesterol and cholesterol subfractions. Body weight was reduced by a mean of 5% and fasting plasma glucose by 3 mmol/l over the three-month period. A Mediterranean diet has been shown to be beneficial after myocardial infarction.

Aerobic physical exercise

Aerobic physical exercise can be useful in reducing hypertriglyceridaemia and LDL-cholesterol and raising HDL-cholesterol levels.

Optimization of metabolic control

Hepatic LDL receptors, the major regulators of plasma LDL level, are dependent on insulin, and total and LDL-cholesterol levels may therefore decline with improved glycaemia. Elevated triglyceride levels may respond even more to the use of insulin to attain good glycaemic control.

Avoidance of drugs that exacerbate dyslipidaemia

β-blockers as well as higher doses of thiazide diuretics exacerbate dyslipidaemia, but clinical indications such as angina pectoris and post-myocardial infarction should take precedence. Moreover, the Hypertension in Diabetes Study found no consistent trends in lipid levels between the atenolol- and captopril-based treatments. Post-menopausally, low-dose oestrogen replacement therapy tends to improve the plasma lipid profile. However, the mode of delivery (oral vs transdermal) and the co-administration of progesterone are important modulators of response – hypertriglyceridaemia may be exacerbated by oral preparations and synthetic progestogens may have deleterious effects that detract from the beneficial effects of oestrogen. Pre-treatment lipid levels also seem to influence the response. Oestrogen and norethisterone acetate (a progestogen) may improve aspects of carbohydrate metabolism and insulin action, but at present, the risks and benefits of oestrogen and progestogen replacement therapy remain largely unclear, particularly in post-menopausal women with established coronary heart disease.

Exclusion of other factors

Hepatic dysfunction, renal impairment and hypothyroidism may all cause or exacerbate dyslipidaemias and should be excluded.

> The effects of post-menopausal oestrogen and progestogen replacement therapy on the lipid profile are variable

Pharmacological approaches to treatment

If the above measures prove inadequate, specific lipid-lowering drugs will be indicated for many patients.

Statins

The HMG-CoA reductase inhibitors (statins) reduce intracellular cholesterol synthesis, thereby upregulating the expression of hepatic LDL receptors and leading to increased clearance of LDL-cholesterol from the circulation. LDL-cholesterol and apoprotein B concentration then decline by about 25–30%. The statins are generally very well-tolerated drugs with an excellent safety record and large clinical trials have clearly demonstrated their beneficial effect on LDL-cholesterol levels. Reductions of approximately 25% have generally been observed in coronary events. Higher-dose statins, in particular, may also reduce elevated plasma triglyceride levels, and other effects, such as improved endothelial function and stabilization of atheromatous plaques may also be important. Improvements (ie increases) in low HDL-cholesterol concentrations are less marked, but current clinical trial evidence favours statins as first-line drugs for patients with established coronary heart disease and a total cholesterol concentration >5.0 mmol/l (195 mg/dl). The most recent data indicate that the effects of these drugs are additive to those of oestrogen and progesterone in post-menopausal women. Although their effects on insulin resistance remain unclear, there is some evidence suggesting improvements in carbohydrate metabolism and other, more potent, statins are in development. Recent data from the West of

Scotland study showing that pravastatin reduced the risk of new cases of type 2 diabetes by 30% has broader public health implications.

> Statins are currently regarded as first-line drugs for diabetic patients with established coronary heart disease or raised LDL-cholesterol concentrations

Fibric acid derivatives

The fibrates represent a logical alternative, particularly for mixed dyslipidaemia treatment, although the current evidence from clinical trials is less convincing than that for the statins. These drugs reduce triglyceride levels and increase HDL-cholesterol levels, but to a lesser extent. Glycaemic control may be slightly improved by lowering plasma fatty acid levels and reducing the activity of the glucose–fatty acid (Randle) cycle, but this is rarely clinically apparent. However, some fibrates also seem to decrease plasma fibrinogen levels, an independent risk factor for atherosclerosis, and several trials have reported variable rates of reduction in coronary events in non-diabetic and diabetic patients (Table 7.10). It is worth noting that LDL-cholesterol concentrations were not altered by gemfibrozil in the Veterans Administration HDL Intervention Trial (VA-HIT), suggesting there may be another mechanism of action for these drugs. The Diabetes Atherosclerosis Intervention Study (DAIS) was performed exclusively in men and women with type 2 diabetes who had the typical lipid phenotype discussed above. This angiographic study showed a significant reduction in the progression of focal coronary lesions with fenofibrate, but was not powered to demonstrate a reduction in clinical events.

The choice between statins and fibrates in diabetic patients is the topic of several large comparative clinical trials currently in progress. Further information on efficacy and safety will emerge in the next few years. Combination therapy using statins and fibrates together is presently not generally recommended since the risk of myositis may be increased (although clinically evident myositis is uncommon).

Table 7.10

Placebo-controlled trials of effects of fibrates on coronary events. Sourced from *N Engl J Med* 1987; **317**: 1237-45, *Diabetes Care* 1992; **15**: 820-5, *N Engl J Med* 1999; **341**: 410-8 and data presented at the European Society of Cardiology meeting, 1998 and the XIIth International Symposium on Atherosclerosis, 2000.

1. Helsinki Heart Study
n=4081 men; n=135 diabetic men.
Non-significant reduction in coronary heart disease in diabetics with gemfibrozil *vs* placebo. *N Engl J Med* 1987; **317**: 1237-45; *Diabetes Care* 1992; **15**: 820-5.

2. Veterans Administration HDL Intervention Trial (VA-HIT)
n=2531 men with coronary heart disease; 25% diabetic. Mean HDL-cholesterol at entry 0.8 mmol/l. Reduction in combined non-fatal and fatal coronary events (22%, p=0.006) and stroke (27%, p=0.05) with gemfibrozil *vs* placebo. Median follow-up 5.1 years. *N Eng J Med* 1999; **341**: 410-8.

3. Bezafibrate Infarction Prevention Study (BIP)
n=2855 men, n=367 women (mean age 60 years). Patients with diabetes largely excluded, duration 5+ years. Benefits for subgroup with hypertriglyceridaemia, ie 40% reduction in combined coronary endpoints (p=0.03) with bezafibrate *vs* placebo. No significant reduction in events for the total cohort. Data presented at European Society of Cardiology meeting, 1998.

4. Diabetes Atherosclerosis Intervention Study (DAIS)
n=418 men and women with type 2 diabetes and dyslipidaemia. Fenofibrate 200 mg/day *vs* placebo. Mean duration of follow-up 38 months. Angiographic measurement of progression of coronary atherosclerosis. Significant 40% reduction in progression of focal lesions. Non-significant 23% reduction in clinical events. Data presented at the XIIth International Symposium on Atherosclerosis Stockholm, June 2000.

Other pharmacological options include:

- *Resins* – such as cholestyramine are unpalatable and may increase triglyceride levels. Their use has declined in line with the introduction of statins, but a new tablet form has recently been introduced in the US.
- *Niacin* – has modest effects on LDL-cholesterol levels, but concomitant tolerability problems, because of flushing,

for example. There is an FDA-approved preparation in the US.

- *Nicotinic acid* – reduces triglyceride levels but is contraindicated in diabetes because hyperglycaemia may be exacerbated after an initial transient reduction in glucose concentrations.
- *Acipimox* – is a nicotinic acid analogue that reduces triglyceride levels. There is some evidence that it also improves insulin sensitivity, but no evidence that it reduces clinical events.
- *Fish-oil supplements* – reduce triglyceride levels and mortality in survivors of myocardial infarction, but deterioration in glycaemic control has also been reported.
- *Plant sterols* – these can lower plasma cholesterol levels. There are no drug preparations, but some food products contain them. Their effects are minor compared with those of potent agents such as the statins.
- *Antioxidants* – while there is considerable evidence that oxidized LDL particles have enhanced atherogenicity *in vitro*, the effects of antioxidants (such as high-dose vitamin E) have been generally disappointing in clinical intervention studies to date. There is a lack of data concerning the impact of antioxidant supplementation in type 2 patients.

Specialist advice should be sought in the management of major or resistant dyslipidaemias. Combinations of drugs, eg statin plus resin, are logical and may have synergistic effects.

Further reading

Adler AI, Stratton IM, Neil HAW *et al*. Association of systolic blood pressure with macrovascular and microvascular complications of type 2 diabetes (UKPDS 36): prospective observational study. *Br Med J* 2000; **321**: 412-19.

American Diabetes Association. Management of dyslipidaemia in adult with diabetes. *Diabetes Care* 2000; **23**(1): S57-60.

Capes SE, Hunt D, Malmberg K, Gerstein HC. Stress hyperglycaemia and increased risk of death after myocardial infarction in patients with and without diabetes: a systematic overview. *Lancet* 2000; **355**: 773-8.

Curb JD, Pressel SL, Cutler JA *et al* for the systolic hypertension in the elderly program cooperative research group. Effect of diuretic-based antihypertensive treatment on cardiovascular disease risk in older patients with systolic hypertension. *JAMA* 1996; **276**: 1886-92.

Detre KM, Lombardero PHMS, Brooks MM *et al*. The effect of previous coronary artery bypass surgery on the prognosis of patients with diabetes who have acute myocardial infarction. *N Engl J Med* 2000; **342**: 989-97.

Edmunds E, Lip GYH. Cardiovascular risk in women: the cardiologists' perspective. *Q J Med* 2000; **93**: 135-45.

Frick MH, Elo O, Haapa K *et al*. Helsinki heart study: primary prevention trial with gemfibrozil in middle-aged men with dyslipidemia. *N Engl J Med* 1987; **317**: 1237-45.

Gaede P, Vedel P, Parving H-H, Pedersen O. Intensified multifactorial intervention in patients with type 2 diabetes mellitus and microalbuminuria: the Steno type 2 randomized study. *Lancet* 1999; **353**: 617-22.

Gerstein HC, Yusuf S. Dysglycaemia and risk of cardiovascular disease. *Lancet* 1996; **347**: 949-50.

Goldberg RB, Mellies MJ, Sacks FM *et al*. Cardiovascular events and their reduction with pravastatin in diabetic and glucose intolerant myocardial infarction survivors with average cholesterol levels: subgroup analyses in the cholesterol and recurrent events (CARE) trial. *Circulation* 1998; 2513-9.

Gress TW, Nieto FJ, Shaha E *et al*. Hypertension and antihypertensive therapy as risk factors for type 2 diabetes mellitus. *N Engl J Med* 2000; **342**: 905-12.

Groeneveld Y, Petri H, Hermans J, Springer MP. Relationship between blood glucose level and mortality in type 2 diabetes mellitus: a systematic review. *Diabetic Med* 1999; **16**: 2-13.

Guidelines subcommittee. 1999 World Health Organization - International Society for Hypertension guidelines for the management of hypertension. *J Hypertens* 1999; **17**: 151-83.

Haffner SM, Lehto S, Ronnemaa T, Pyörälä K, Laasko M. Mortality from coronary heart disease in subjects with type 2 diabetes and in non-diabetic subjects with and without prior myocardial infarction. *N Engl J Med* 1998; **339**: 229-34.

Hansson L, Zanchetti A, Carruthers SG *et al* for the HOT study group. Effects of intensive blood-pressure lowering and low-dose aspirin in patients with hypertension: principal results of the hypertension optimal treatment (HOT) randomized trial. *Lancet* 1998; **351**: 1755-62.

Joint British recommendations on prevention of coronary heart disease in clinical practice. *Heart* 1998; **80**(2): S1-29.

Kannel WB, McGee DL. Diabetes and glucose tolerance as risk factors for cardiovascular disease: the Framingham study. *Diabetes Care* 1979; **2**: 120-6.

Koskinen P, Manttari M, Manninen V *et al*. Coronary heart disease incidence in NIDDM patients in the Helsinki heart study. *Diabetes Care* 1992; **15**: 820-5.

Laakso M. Glycemic control and the risk for coronary heart disease in patients with non-insulin-dependent diabetes mellitus. The Finnish studies. *Ann Intern Med* 1996; **124**: 127-30.

Lithell HO. Effect of antihypertensive drugs on insulin, glucose, and lipid metabolism. *Diabetes Care* 1991; **14**: 203-9.

Malmberg K for the DIGAMI (Diabetes Mellitus, Insulin Glucose Infusion in Acute Myocardial Infarction) Study Group. Prospective randomized study of intensive insulin treatment on long term survival in patients with diabetes mellitus. *Br Med J* 1997; **314**: 1512-5.

Mason RP, Mason PE. Calcium antagonists and cardiovascular risk in diabetes. *Diabetes Care* 1999; **22**: 1206-8.

Ramsay LE, Williams B, Johnston DG *et al*. Guidelines for management of hypertension: report of the third working party of the British Hypertension Society. *J Hum Hypertens* 1999; **13**: 569-92.

Rubins HB, Robins SJ, Collins D *et al*. Gemfibrozil for the secondary prevention of coronary heart disease in men with low levels of high-density lipoprotein cholesterol. *N Eng J Med* 1999; **341**: 410-8.

Staessen JA, Fagard R, Lutgarde T *et al* for the systolic hypertension in Europe (Sys-Eur) trial investigators. Randomized double-blind comparison of placebo and active treatment for older patients with isolated systolic hypertension. *Lancet* 1997; **350**: 757-64.

Tuomilheto J, Rastenyte D, Birkenhäger WH *et al* for the systolic hypertension in europe trial investigators. Effects of calcium-channel blockade in older patients with diabetes and systolic hypertension. *N Engl J Med* 1999; **340**: 677-84.

Turner RC, Millins H, Neil HAW *et al*. Risk factors for coronary artery disease in non-insulin dependent diabetes mellitus: United Kingdom prospective diabetes study (UKPDS: 23). *Br Med J* 1998; **316**: 823-8.

UK Prospective Diabetes Study Group. Tight blood pressure control and risk of macrovascular and microvascular complications in type 2 diabetes (UKPDS 38). *Br Med J* 1998; **317**: 703-13.

UK Prospective Diabetes Study Group. Efficacy of atenolol and captopril in reducing risk of macrovascular and microvascular complications in type 2 diabetes (UKPDS 39). *Br Med J* 1998; **317**: 713-20.

UK Prospective Diabetes Study (UKPDS) Group. Effects of three months' diet after diagnosis of type 2 diabetes on plasma lipids and lipoproteins (UKPDS 45). *Diabetic Med* 2000; **17**: 518-23.

Yudkin JS. Which diabetic patients should be taking aspirin? *Br Med J* 1995; **311**: 641-2.

Yudkin JS. Managing the diabetic patient with acute myocardial infarction. *Diabetic Med* 1998; **15**: 276-81.

8. Non-pharmacological treatment

Treatment targets
Treatment algorithm
Diet
Exercise
Body weight control

Treatment targets

The importance of controlling metabolic and other risk factors is central to the reduction of diabetic complications. Treating with the aim of achieving the best possible targets (ie with the lowest risk of complications) is now emerging as an important part of most diabetes care plans.

Glycaemic control

Any decrease in hyperglycaemia will decrease the risk and severity of diabetic complications (chapters 6 and 7). Benefits will continue to accrue until blood glucose concentrations are returned to within normal limits. The United Kingdom Prospective Diabetes Study has demonstrated that each 1% decrease in HbA_{1c} over 10 years reduces the risk of a myocardial infarction by about 14% and the risk of a microvascular complication by about 25%.

> Decreasing hyperglycaemia prevents or delays the onset and reduces the severity of diabetic complications

The European Diabetes Policy Group has recommended a graded system of glycaemic targets based on vascular risk (Table 8.1a), while the American Diabetes Association has essentially defined its goal as a return to a value within the normal glucose range (Table 8.1b). Their messages are more consistent than

they sound: glycaemic control should attempt to achieve glucose values as near normal as possible, given the circumstances of the individual patient. A fasting plasma glucose (FPG) level <7.0 mmol/l (126 mg/dl) and an HbA_{1c} level <7.5% would be acceptable, but, ideally, where appropriate, attempts should be made to achieve an FPG <6.0 mmol/l (110 mg/dl) and an HbA_{1c} <6.5%.

Over-rigorous efforts to achieve ideal targets may lead to hypoglycaemic episodes in some patients, despite careful attention to the treatment regimen and all reasonable precautions. In these patients less-than-ideal may have to suffice.

Blood lipid profile

The blood lipid profile provides a well-recognized link with cardiovascular disease. Raised circulating concentrations of total cholesterol, low-density lipoprotein (LDL)-cholesterol and triglyceride are all associated with increased cardiovascular risk, as is a lowered circulating concentration of high-density lipoprotein (HDL)-cholesterol. In line with its approach to targets for glycaemic control, the European Diabetes Policy Group has recommended a graded system of lipid targets based on the extent of vascular risk (Table 8.2a). A similar approach has been taken by the American Diabetes Association (Table 8.2b). Several authorities have, however, produced more complicated guidelines based on the ratios of total cholesterol to HDL-cholesterol, or LDL-cholesterol to HDL-cholesterol. A recommendation produced by the Joint British Societies provides a graduated assessment for risk of coronary heart disease, taking into account gender, age, smoking, total cholesterol to HDL-cholesterol ratio, and systolic blood pressure (Figure 8.1).

> Treatment should be intensified to achieve targets for glucose, lipids and blood pressure that confer low risk for the development of diabetic complications

Table 8.1

Targets for glycaemic control suggested by (a) the European Diabetes Policy Group and (b) the American Diabetes Association.

(a) European targets (*Diabetic Med* 1999; **16**: 716-30)

	Low risk	Arterial risk	Microvascular risk
HbA_{1c} %	≤6.5	>6.5	>7.5
Venous plasma glucose			
Fasting/pre-prandial			
mmol/l	≤6.0	>6.0	≥7.0
mg/dl	<110	≥110	≥126
Self-monitored blood glucose*			
Fasting/pre-prandial			
mmol/l	≤5.5	>5.5	>6.0
mg/dl	<100	≥100	≥110
Post-prandial or peak			
mmol/l	<7.5	≥7.5	>9.0
mg/dl	<135	≥135	>160

*Fasting capillary blood glucose is about 1.0 mmol/l (18 mg/dl) lower than venous plasma blood glucose. Post-prandial capillary blood glucose is about the same as venous plasma blood glucose.

(b) American targets (*Diabetes Care* 2000; **23**: S32-42)

	Non-diabetic	Goal	Additional action suggested
Pre-prandial plasma glucose (mg/dl)	<110	90–130	<90/>150
Bedtime glucose (mg/dl)	<120	110–150	<110/>180
HbA_{1c} (%)	<6	<7	>8

These values are guidelines for non-pregnant individuals and may need modification in the light of factors such as age, co-morbidity, etc. Subsequent action will depend on individual patient circumstances. HbA_{1c} is referenced to a non-diabetic range of 4.0–6.0% (mean 5.0%, SD 0.5%). To convert mg/dl to mmol/l, divide by 18.

Decisions on whether to treat dyslipidaemia in diabetic patients should take account of the number and extent of concomitant vascular risk factors, and the Joint British Societies assessment offers a valuable guide. Note that such tables are not appropriate for people with familial dyslipidaemia. As a very general indicator, an ideal lipid profile will have a fasting total serum cholesterol level <5 mmol/l (193 mg/dl), a total:HDL-cholesterol ratio <4, and a fasting serum triglyceride level <1.7 mmol/l (150 mg/dl).

> Cardiovascular risk is increased by raised LDL-cholesterol, raised triglyceride, or reduced HDL-cholesterol, and particularly by all three in combination

Blood pressure

The United Kingdom Prospective Diabetes Study demonstrated the substantial benefits of blood pressure control in type 2 diabetic patients, and recognized that these benefits increased in line with blood pressure reduction until a normal blood pressure had been achieved. The benefits were reflected in both macrovascular and microvascular complications, and diabetes-related deaths were reduced by about 30% for every 10 mmHg decrease in systolic blood pressure over a nine-year period.

The European Diabetes Policy Group has recommended an ideal blood pressure target of <140/85 mmHg for type 2 diabetic patients. The American Diabetes Association equivalent is <130/85 mmHg. Some authorities, however,

Table 8.2
Targets for blood lipids control suggested by (a) the European Diabetes Policy Group, and (b) the American Diabetes Association.

(a) European target: risk of macrovascular disease

	Low risk	At risk	High risk
Serum total cholesterol			
mmol/l	<4.8	4.8–6.0	>6.0
mg/dl	<185	184–230	>230
Serum LDL-cholesterol			
mmol/l	<3.0	3.0–4.0	>4.0
mg/dl	<115	115–155	>155
Serum HDL-cholesterol			
mmol/l	>1.2	1.0–1.2	<1.0
mg/dl	>46	39–46	<39
Serum triglycerides			
mmol/l	<1.7	1.7–2.2	>2.2
mg/dl	<150	150–200	>200

(b) American target: blood lipid risk categories for coronary heart disease

	Acceptable	Borderline	High
Plasma LDL-cholesterol (mg/dl)	<100	100–129	≥130
Plasma HDL-cholesterol (mg/dl)	>45	35–45	<35
Plasma triglycerides (mg/dl)	<200	200–399	≥400

have questioned whether such targets reflect the available evidence accurately.

Reducing hypertension reduces morbidity and mortality in type 2 diabetes

---

Body weight

It is well-recognized that excess adiposity is a risk factor for type 2 diabetes and other components of the insulin resistance or metabolic syndrome. There is also a wealth of evidence to suggest that reducing adiposity in overweight and frankly obese patients will improve both metabolic control and life expectancy. Any reduction in adiposity down towards the normal weight range is strongly recommended.

Excess visceral adiposity is an important cardiovascular risk factor

---

Obesity is usually defined as a body mass index (BMI) >30. (BMI is calculated by dividing weight in kg by height in m^2, ie kg/m^2.) Overweight has been defined by the World Health Organization (WHO) as a BMI between 25 and 30 kg/m^2, and 'normal' as a BMI within the range 18.5–25 kg/m^2. However, BMI provides an estimate of whole-body size and does not take account of fat distribution. Since visceral (abdominal) obesity rather than generalized or lower body subcutaneous obesity has been recognized as an important cardiovascular risk factor, it has been suggested that girth measurements at the waist and hip (enabling calculation of the waist:hip ratio) may be more useful. Waist-to-hip ratio should be:

- <0.95 for men
- <0.80 for women.

Other targets

Ideal goals for glycaemic control, lipid profile, blood pressure and body weight offer helpful benchmarks, even if they are neither

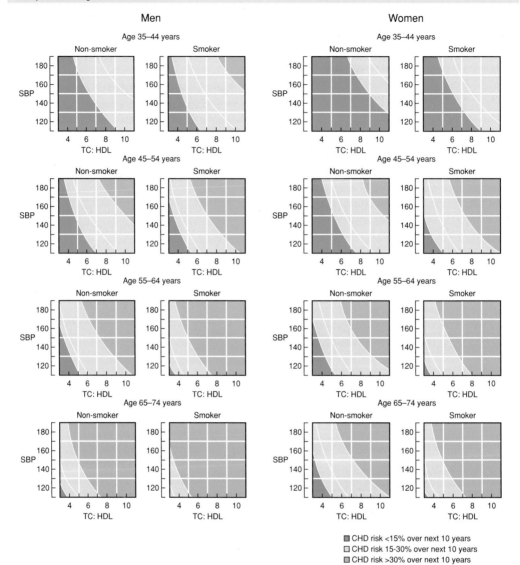

Figure 8.1
Joint British Societies' (British Cardiac Society, British Hypertension Society, British Hyperlipidaemia Association, British Diabetic Association) estimated risks of coronary heart disease (CHD) over next 10 years, based on systolic blood pressures (SBP), TC:HDL ratios, age, and smoking habit.

TC = total cholesterol; HDL = high-density lipoprotein cholesterol. Reproduced with permission from the Joint British Societies and *Heart* 1998; **80**(2): S1-29.

realistically attainable nor sustainable in many patients. In such cases it may be appropriate to lay greater emphasis on the means employed to work towards these goals – reducing snacking, walking a defined distance each day, or even re-doubling efforts to take all medication and

attend all clinic appointments – than the goals themselves. It cannot be overstated that progression towards these targets, however modest, will reap rewards in terms of offsetting both the onset and severity of long-term vascular and neuropathic complications.

Treatment algorithm

The standard procedure for treatment of type 2 diabetes follows a stepwise progression starting with non-pharmacological measures, ie diet, exercise, weight control and health education. If these do not achieve or sustain targets for metabolic control, an oral antidiabetic agent is then introduced. If targets are still not achieved a second (and possibly a third) differently acting oral agent is introduced. Patients who still fail to achieve and maintain targets should be switched to insulin – an oral agent may be added back if appropriate. Alternatively, the most suitable oral agent may be continued and insulin added-in, initially as a single injection before bed. This algorithm is summarized in Figure 8.2.

> Rapid progression through a treatment algorithm may be necessary to achieve optimal glycaemic control

This treatment algorithm can be adapted readily to suit particular groups of patients (eg the obese or elderly) through the choice of therapeutic agent(s). The targets can also be adjusted to accommodate individual circumstances. The presence of diabetic complications and the concurrent use of other medications will inevitably restrict the choice of antidiabetic agent, potentially reducing the scope for achieving targets.

Type 2 diabetes is highly variable in its presentation and usually progressive, presenting different problems at different stages of its natural history. The fundamental features of insulin resistance and defective insulin secretion, and the metabolic disturbances created in muscle, liver and adipose tissue will gradually change. Accordingly, type 2 diabetes constitutes a moving target that requires a selection of different agents to treat different aspects at different stages of the disease process.

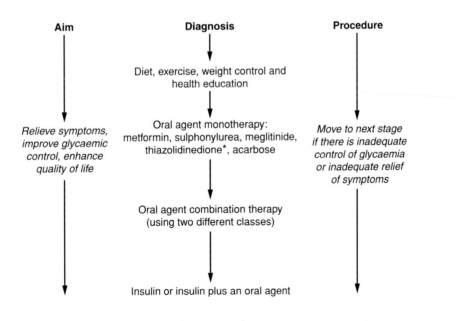

| Aim | Diagnosis | Procedure |

Diagnosis → Diet, exercise, weight control and health education → Oral agent monotherapy: metformin, sulphonylurea, meglitinide, thiazolidinedione*, acarbose → Oral agent combination therapy (using two different classes) → Insulin or insulin plus an oral agent

Aim: Relieve symptoms, improve glycaemic control, enhance quality of life

Procedure: Move to next stage if there is inadequate control of glycaemia or inadequate relief of symptoms

Figure 8.2
An algorithm for the treatment of type 2 diabetes mellitus. The progressive hyperglycaemia of type 2 diabetes requires a stepped care approach with treatment being modified and added to over time. Late introduction of combinations of oral agents is often a prelude to insulin treatment.
*Note that in Europe thiazolidinediones are presently available only for use in combination with other types of oral antidiabetic agents.

Type 2 diabetes presents a therapeutic 'moving target' due to the progressive course of its natural history

Given the proven advantages of effective metabolic control, it is important not to delay movement through the treatment algorithm if control at any particular step is clearly unsatisfactory. Non-pharmacological measures should be reinforced at every opportunity – they are seldom fully exploited. For patients who present with severe hyperglycaemia and/or severe symptoms it may be necessary to proceed very rapidly through the algorithm – even beginning with oral combination or insulin therapy in some cases. Some patients require insulin initially but may subsequently be satisfactorily controlled using oral agents.

Controlling body weight, blood pressure, lipids and glycaemia retards the onset and severity of diabetic complications

Diet

Diet is the cornerstone of treatment for type 2 diabetes. Every patient should receive detailed advice from a dietician, explaining the types and amounts of food that will enable dietary compliance. Dietary recommendations should be reinforced by all members of the care team whenever the opportunity arises. In fact, the 'diabetic' diet is nothing more than a normal balanced diet should be – ie rich in complex high-fibre carbohydrates and low in saturated fats and cholesterol. Meals should be taken regularly, and the total energy content adjusted in an effort to maintain body weight within the normal range. Ideally >55% of the total energy content will come from complex carbohydrate, while <30% will come from fat (Table 8.3).

Diet is the cornerstone of treatment for type 2 diabetes

Table 8.3
Recommended dietary composition for patients with diabetes. Major nutrients are given in terms of their percentage contribution to the total energy content of the diet.*

	European Diabetes Policy Group[+]	American Diabetes Association
Carbohydrate[a]	>55%	55–60%
– added sugar	<25 g/day	–
– total sugar	<50 g/day	–
Fat	<30%	<30%
– saturated	<10%	<10%
– mono-unsaturated	10–15%	<12%
– polyunsaturated	<10%	6–8%
Protein	10–15%	0.8 g/kg body weight
Fibre	>30 g/day	40 g/day[e]
Salt	<6 g/day[b]	<3 g/day
Cholesterol[c]	<300 mg/day	<300 mg/day
Alcohol[d]	<30 g/day	<4 equivalents/week

*A typical daily diet might comprise about 2000 kcal (8400 kJ) – more for active individuals, slightly less for highly sedentary individuals, and <1500 kcal (6300 kJ) for those on an energy-restricted diet.
[+]Where explicit values are not stated in the recommendations, appropriate values from Diabetes UK have been inserted.
[a]Carbohydrates should be mainly fibre-rich and complex, with little (<50 g/day) as simple sugars.
[b]Salt intake should be <3 g/day if patient is hypertensive.
[c]Cholesterol should be substantially less than 250 mg/day if patient is dyslipidaemic.
[d]Alcohol intake should be <20 g/day in women and only taken with meals. Equivalents are 1 fl oz spirit, 4 fl oz wine, and 12 fl oz beer.
[e]Fibre intake should be about 25 g/day on a low-energy diet.

It seems that visualizing meal structures in terms of a 'healthy eating pyramid' (Figure 8.3) can help some patients translate these dietary recommendations into eating habits. The pyramid emphasizes that fatty foods and sugars should be reduced or eliminated from the diet wherever possible, and that snacking between main meals is discouraged unless required to alleviate symptoms or prevent an anticipated episode of hypoglycaemia. Lean meats and fish are encouraged in moderation so that total daily protein intake (about 0.8 g/kg body weight; typically about 50–70 g) is responsible for about 10–15% of the total energy content of the diet. The mainstay of every meal is food rich in complex carbohydrate.

An example of the implementation of the healthy eating pyramid is given in Figure 8.4 and further represented as a daily meal plan in Table 8.4. It often proves necessary to illustrate physically to patients the amount that constitutes a serving, and to introduce some patients to a greater variety of vegetables, fruits, beans, etc, which they might otherwise ignore. Equally, it can be helpful to point out the increasing range of 'low-fat' products available and to practise devising balanced but varied and appetizing menus that comply with the general dietary recommendations.

If food intake is spread out into three or four discrete meals a day, it can often be combined more effectively with drug treatment regimens and help to facilitate control of day-time hyperglycaemia. Further, introducing this kind of routine will assist compliance and highlight any variance from the expected norm. Most people seem to consume most of their energy in their evening meal at the end of the day, but the use of some drug treatments is facilitated if energy intake is more evenly distributed among the three or four main meals.

Reducing fat

Avoiding fatty foods, confectionery and snacking are key messages to include from the outset in any programme of dietary advice.

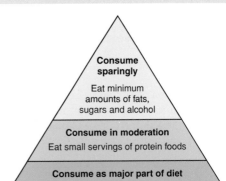

Butter, margarine, cooking fat, oil, cream, high-fat cheeses
Cakes, sweet biscuits, pastries
Processed or fatty meat (eg bacon, sausage, salami, pâté)
Fried foods
Snack foods (eg crisps, dips, nuts)
Chocolate
Ice cream
Mayonnaise, salad dressings
Confectionery
Soft drinks (except 'diet' drinks)
Alcohol
Sugar
Honey
Jam
Diabetes 'speciality' foods

Fish, seafood
Lean meat
Eggs
Tofu
Low-fat cheeses
Yoghurt
Milk (preferably skimmed)

Legumes and pulses (eg lentils, kidney beans, haricot beans)
Bread, especially containing a large amount of grains
Breakfast cereals, preferably whole grain (rolled oats and bran)
Spaghetti and pasta
Fresh friut
Barley and rice
Vegetables, mushrooms
Salad (undressed)

Figure 8.3
Healthy eating pyramid for a diabetic diet.
Foods rich in fat and sugar should be consumed very sparingly. Lean meat, fish and other foods rich in protein, as well as low-fat dairy produce, should be eaten in moderation. Foods with a high complex carbohydrate content such as bread, rice, pasta, potatoes and other garden vegetables can be eaten liberally, along with ample amounts of fresh fruit.

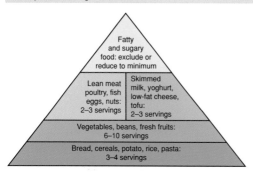

Figure 8.4
An example of a healthy eating pyramid, reflected in numbers of servings daily.

An approximate guide to servings sizes is: meat, poultry, fish about 2 oz (50 g) after cooking; 1 egg; nuts about 1.5 oz (40 g); milk, yoghurt, tofu about 200 ml or 200 g; cheese 1–2 oz (25–50 g); fresh vegetables, fruit and beans about 2–4 oz (50–100 g); bread 1–2 slices; cereals about 1–2 oz (25–50 g); potatoes, rice, pasta about 3–5 oz (80–130 g).

Recognizing fatty foods and finding alternatives are useful skills in the conversion to a starch-based diet. The importance of reducing fat (including cholesterol) intake is usually expressed in terms of reducing the overall risk of macrovascular complications, but significant improvements in insulin sensitivity can also result. Since fat is more than twice as energy-dense as carbohydrate or protein (Table 8.5), reducing fat intake is an effective approach to weight-control. It is always worth clarifying the energy content of different food types: an individual striving to achieve a total daily intake of 2,000 calories (kcal) (8,400 kJ) might try to consume about 280–320 g carbohydrate, 50–65 g fat, and 50–70 g protein (Table 8.5).

Table 8.4
An example of a daily meal plan, based on healthy eating pyramid use.

Meal	Food	Amount/Type
Breakfast	Egg	1
	Bread	2 slices
	Milk	200 ml
	Fruit	Peach
Lunch	Lean meat	2 oz
	Rice	4 oz
	Vegetables	3 oz
	Beans	3 oz
	Yoghurt	150 ml
Snack	Fruit	Apple
Dinner	Salad	Green
	Fish	2 oz
	Potato	4 oz
	Vegetables	2 x 3 oz
	Fruit	Pear
Supper	Cereal	2 oz

Please cross-refer to Figures 8.2 and 8.3. 1 oz = 28.3 g. NB some ethnic groups will require modified advice, but the relevant teaching materials should be available in the appropriate languages.

Saturated fatty acids

Saturated fatty acids, eg palmitic acid, contain no double-bonds and are the predominant components of animal fat. Their intake should be minimized, certainly to <10% of the total daily energy intake. This reduction will also facilitate a reduction in serum cholesterol, especially in patients with raised cholesterol levels.

Table 8.5
The energy content of foods – illustrating that fats are more than twice as energy-dense as carbohydrates and proteins – and recommended daily intake of each for an average diabetic patient

	Energy content		Recommended daily intake*			
	kcal/g	kJ/g	g	kcal	kJ	% total energy
Carbohydrate	4	17	285	1140	4790	57
Fat	9	38	65	580	2440	29
Protein	4	17	70	280	1170	14

*total energy content 2000 kcal (8,400 kJ).

Polyunsaturated fatty acids

Polyunsaturated fatty acids, eg linoleic acid, contain two or more double-bonds, and are mainly derived from plant sources (especially vegetable oil). Their intake should be restricted, although small quantities of some polyunsaturates are essential (they cannot be synthesized by the human body). γ-linolenic acid, derived from evening primrose oil, is said to be helpful in the treatment of neuropathy. Small amounts of polyunsaturated fish oils can reduce triglyceride concentrations and decrease platelet aggregability, but large quantities may impair glycaemic control.

Monounsaturated fatty acids

Monounsaturated fatty acids, eg oleic acid, contain one double-bond and are also derived from vegetable sources (eg olive oil). These fats can assist in the reduction of saturated fats and there is tentative evidence that modest amounts of monounsaturated fatty acids can reduce the risk of macrovascular disease (whether or not this is largely due to their replacement of dietary saturated fats is not yet clear).

Complex carbohydrate and fibre intake

The rationale for consuming complex carbohydrate is mainly the time taken to digest this food type into absorbable sugar. It slows digestion which, in turn, slows the rate at which sugars, principally glucose, enter the circulation. Although glucose uptake by the liver and peripheral tissues is always outpaced by glucose absorption after a meal, the slower the latter, the greater the reduction in post-prandial hyperglycaemia. The different types of carbohydrate and the presence of other nutrients and fibre within the food ingested will each impact on overall rate of digestion and subsequent hyperglycaemic effect. The hyperglycaemic potential of different foods is sometimes expressed as the 'glycaemic index', a measure of the area under the blood glucose curve for up to three hours after ingestion of 50 g of the foodstuff compared with 50 g of glucose (some calculations are alternatively based on 50 g of white bread):

$$\text{Glycaemic index (\%)} = \frac{\text{Area under glycaemic curve of foodstuff}}{\text{Area under glycaemic curve of glucose}}$$

Use of the glycaemic index has been limited by variations in composition of different varieties and different sources of the same foodstuff, but the similarly low glycaemic indices of cereals, rice, pasta and potatoes, provide the basis for recommending a large amount of complex carbohydrate in the diet.

> Soluble fibres are particularly effective in reducing post-prandial hyperglycaemia

Dietary fibre further slows the digestion of carbohydrate and absorption of sugars. Fibre traps carbohydrates within its matrix and forms a diffusional barrier which impedes access by digestive enzymes and slows the release of sugars. Most dietary fibres are non-digestible plant polysaccharides. Some of these are soluble and form viscous gels, others are insoluble. Soluble fibres such as gums, pectins, hemicellulose and mucilages are generally more effective in reducing post-prandial hyperglycaemia than insoluble fibres such as celluloses and wheat bran.

The fibre content of a diabetic diet (>30 g/day, Table 8.3) is usually achieved by the patient eating a good selection of vegetables and pulses, in addition to the main sources of complex carbohydrate. Fibre supplements such as guar gum (a galactomannan from the Indian cluster bean *Cyamopsis tetragonoloba*) have a modest additional antihyperglycaemic effect in some patients and can improve the lipid profile, but they can also cause abdominal discomfort and flatulence, and interfere with the absorption of other micronutrients and drugs. A diet naturally rich in fibre from vegetables, fruit and cereals is most appropriate.

Artificial sweeteners

Non-nutritive sweeteners are already widely used in food and drink. To avoid consuming extra sugars, non-nutritive sweeteners such as aspartame, saccharin and acesulphame K provide a valuable alternative in beverages, particularly in 'diet' soft drinks for thirst-quenching. Previous concerns in the US about the putative carcinogenicity of saccharin seem to have been misplaced, and this sweetener is no longer scorned.

Diabetic speciality foods

'Diabetic foods' typically contain fructose or sorbitol for sweetening and bulking. They are generally *not* recommended, because large quantities can have unwanted effects. For example, excess fructose can cause hypertriglyceridaemia and diarrhoea.

Salt

Sodium consumption should be restricted to reduce the risk of hypertension. A daily salt consumption of <3 g is strongly recommended in hypertensive patients. Potassium chloride may be an appropriate substitute, but care must be taken in patients using potassium-sparing antihypertensive agents and in those with renal impairment.

Alcohol

Diabetic patients are advised to consume alcohol strictly in moderation and preferably with food. This is especially pertinent for those on antidiabetic drug treatment, because alcohol can cause hypoglycaemia. Alcohol is also a significant energy (calorie) source. Alcohol abuse is unacceptable and dangerous, because hypoglycaemia can pass undiagnosed in inebriated patients. In Europe, <30 g/day in men and <20 g/day in women are the recommended maxima; the US recommendation is less than four 'equivalents'/week (one 'equivalent' is approximately 1 fl oz spirit, 4 fl oz wine, or 12 fl oz beer). There is evidence that *low* but regular alcohol intake (eg one glass of wine a day) may reduce cardiovascular risk in diabetic and non-diabetic individuals.

Vitamins and minerals

Vitamin deficiencies are not a recognized problem in diabetes, but this condition may be associated with reduced concentrations of water-soluble vitamins. It has been tentatively claimed that supplements of the antioxidant vitamins (C, E and β-carotene) might combat insulin resistance, reduce glycation and atherogenesis, but more thorough studies are required.

Deficiencies of some of the minerals required for glucose metabolism have been noted in type 2 diabetic patients and appropriate supplementation is usually beneficial. Hypomagnesaemia (plasma levels more than 2 SD below normal), usually due to increased magnesium excretion, is found in about 25% of diabetic patients, and magnesium supplementation ($\geq$350 mg/day) in this subgroup can help to improve insulin sensitivity and glycaemic control and thus, possibly, cardiovascular prognosis.

Chromium levels are often reduced in diabetic patients, especially the elderly, probably as a result of poor diet. Supplements of trivalent chromium ($\geq$200 μg/day) in such patients have been shown to improve glycaemic control and reduce total cholesterol concentration.

Reduced zinc levels are not uncommon in diabetic patients. Absolute zinc deficiency is rare, but supplementation has proven helpful in some patients with liver disease.

Vanadium is not known to be deficient in type 2 diabetic patients, but preliminary trials have shown that vanadium supplements improve glycaemic control without stimulating insulin secretion. The potential toxicity of vanadium salts has stimulated research into more potent vanadium compounds which can be used at much lower dosages and carry less risk. Several other trace elements (eg molybdenum and selenium) produce insulin-like effects or enhance insulin action, and general mineral supplements which contain the recommended daily allowances of these substances may be helpful in those with poor nutrition.

Exercise

Physical exercise, particularly aerobic exertion, improves insulin sensitivity and glycaemic control in type 2 diabetes. Regular exercise also helps to maintain muscle mass, reduce adiposity and improve the blood lipid profile. Clearly, exercise can be a valuable therapeutic approach, provided that the patient is willing and able to participate (Table 8.6). Recommendations must, however, be based on a thorough clinical assessment to evaluate potential contraindications. Activities can then be selected that are appropriate for the individual's medical circumstances, age, ability and interest. Even very modest amounts of exercise can benefit a previously sedentary individual, and even apparently trivial activities may be usefully introduced in some cases.

> Aerobic exercise improves insulin sensitivity and glycaemic control

Since subclinical cardiovascular disease is not uncommon in patients with type 2 diabetes, a cautious approach to starting an exercise programme is warranted. High-risk patients might be considered for exercise treadmill testing. Once on a programme, patients should build up the intensity and duration of their exercise gradually. Examples of commonly enjoyed exercise types are brisk walking once or twice daily for more than 15 minutes, swimming, cycling, and gentle jogging. If there is any prospect of inducing hypoglycaemia, however, exercise should be carefully integrated with both dietary intake and drug therapies. It may also be advisable, particularly during the escalation of exercise, to check blood glucose levels both before and after the workout. The patient should always carry glucose and fluid replacement with them, drink regularly, wear suitable clothing, especially comfortable footwear, and warm-up and warm-down slowly. Normal warnings for insulin-treated patients should always be reinforced – notably that exercise can increase the absorption of insulin injected close to muscle, so it is better not to take strenuous exercise soon after an insulin injection or at the time of peak absorption. Likewise, advice on the timing of exercise in relation to dietary intake and on the need to carry identification and glucose and to be aware of hypoglycaemic symptoms should be given.

Isometric exercises that increase intrathoracic pressure should be avoided, especially where there is hypertension or retinopathy. Pulse rate can be checked by the patient and exercise intensity then adjusted so that heart rate is ideally raised to between 50 and 70% of the range between basal and maximum (maximum estimated as 220 minus age). Appropriate precautions must be taken for patients with

---

Table 8.6
Establishment of an exercise programme for a type 2 diabetic patient.

- Assess contraindications and gauge suitability.
- Design a realistic programme with the patient – jointly select type, duration and intensity of exercise. Aerobic exercise, for example, might involve walking briskly for >15 minutes once or twice a day (which should raise heart rate to more than halfway between basal and maximum levels).
- Provide general advice – that intensity and duration should be built up gradually, that it is important to warm-up and warm-down, and that exercise should be timed to fit in with drug treatment and eating patterns.
- Identify risks and explain precautions – hypoglycaemia and the need for good foot care, the dangers of isometric exercise, the special considerations that apply to cardiovascular diseases, and the need to avoid strenuous exercise during times of peak insulin absorption.
- Remind the patient that they should always carry glucose and identification with them, quench thirst appropriately, and avoid overexertion.

hypertension, any evidence of heart disease and a potentially high susceptibility to stroke. The risk of foot damage, delayed hypoglycaemia and dehydration must also be appreciated, in order to ensure that exercise does not do more harm than good in high-risk patients.

Maximum heart rate for aerobic exercise	= 220 – age

Body weight control

When body weight either falls rapidly without active intervention or declines to the lower end of the normal range, it is often a sign of uncontrolled hyperglycaemia, and may warrant insulin therapy. Body weight usually increases when insulin therapy is introduced, and total energy intake should then be adjusted to achieve and consolidate body weight within the normal range. A low body weight may indicate over-obsessive dietary management, sometimes poor diet (particularly in the elderly), an undiagnosed concurrent illness (such as tuberculosis), or a malabsorption syndrome.

Excess adiposity, especially visceral adiposity, is commonplace among type 2 diabetic patients – more than 70% are obese on diagnosis in the US. Combining a low-energy diet and exercise can be very effective in obese patients and patients with lesser degrees of overweight (ie BMI 25–30 kg/m^2) or a high waist:hip ratio (>0.95 in men and >0.80 in women).

Low-energy diets

Energy-restricted diets can usually be designed by cutting out snacks, reducing the sizes of servings and altering the selection of foods within the normal balanced diet. A moderate energy deficit about 500–1,000 kcal (2,100–4,200 kJ) less than the estimated energy requirement for the individual concerned is usually sufficient to improve glycaemic control rapidly and weight loss more gradually. However, it must be appreciated that weight loss will usually be accompanied by increased metabolic efficiency, so that body weight will tend to level out, despite adherence to a low-

energy diet. (The compensation is due to reduced resting energy expenditure, typically consequent to loss of lean tissue.) Energy-restricted diets should reduce fat content whenever possible and ensure adequate consumption of vitamins, minerals, fibre and protein.

Very low calorie diets ('VLCDs'), typically providing about 400–800 kcal/day (1,680–3,360 kJ/day), are available as formula-based preparations including vitamin and mineral supplementation. While a very low energy intake is generally correlated with faster and greater weight loss, it must be ensured that lean body mass (including cardiac muscle) is not decreased. Patients with heart disease must approach these diets with extra caution, and thyroid hormones should not be used as a means of weight loss for the same reason. Non-nutritive 'bulking' agents are occasionally helpful in energy-reduced diets.

Reducing the energy content of a normal diet by 500–1,000 kcal (2,100–4,200 kJ) will usually cause weight loss of about 2 kg (4.5 pounds) in the first week, diminishing thereafter to level out at one to three months when 5–15 kg (about 11–33 pounds) have been lost (corresponding to 5–10% of initial body weight). Sustained weight loss of this magnitude is likely to reduce HbA$_{1c}$ by about 0.5%, and lower serum triglyceride and total cholesterol levels by 10%. Greater weight loss is usually associated with greater improvement in metabolic control. In fact, each kg of sustained weight loss increases average life expectancy by three to four months. Weight loss through diet and exercise provides a fundamental treatment strategy for every overweight or obese type 2 diabetic patient.

Reinforce dietary and exercise advice to optimize weight loss before considering antiobesity drugs

Antiobesity drugs

One of the most widely used antidiabetic drugs, metformin, does not cause weight gain, and may assist with modest weight loss. α-glucosidase inhibitor drugs used in the treatment of post-prandial hyperglycaemia are also unlikely to cause weight gain. However, this is not the case with other antidiabetic agents, further complicating treatment for the obese type 2 diabetic patient. Antiobesity drugs have not generally been included in most algorithms for diabetes treatment, due mainly to safety concerns. However, safer agents are emerging, and these may have a place in the treatment of some overweight patients, most likely those who have already responded to an energy-reduced diet but require further weight control (and who are not contraindicated). Current antiobesity agents include orlistat and sibutramine, but the latter is not presently available in most European countries. Given the benefits that can be realized with sustained weight reduction in obese and overweight type 2 diabetic patients, it is appropriate to consider these agents.

> The antidiabetic drugs metformin and the α-glucosidase inhibitors do *not* promote weight gain

Orlistat

Orlistat is a gastrointestinal lipase inhibitor which slows the rate of triglyceride digestion by binding to the active site of intestinal lipases. This can reduce the amount of fat absorbed from the intestine by up to 30% and increase weight loss by about 2–4 kg more than is achieved by energy restriction alone. Trials with orlistat in obese type 2 diabetic patients found that more patients achieved a significant reduction in body weight than without this agent, and that those who maintained a weight loss of >6 kg also showed a decrease in HbA$_{1c}$ of >0.5%. Orlistat may inadvertently provide a means of assisting dietary compliance due to the inevitable problem of excess fat passing through to the faeces. More frequent defaecation, loose oily stools, diarrhoea and

even faecal incontinence may become a problem, especially if the fat content of the diet is not maintained at a low level. The possibility of impaired absorption of fat-soluble vitamins and concomitant medications should be borne in mind.

Sibutramine

Sibutramine enhances the satiety response by acting centrally as a serotonin and noradrenaline (norepinephrine) reuptake inhibitor. It may also increase energy expenditure by increasing sympathetic stimulation of thermogenesis. In obese type 2 diabetic patients, sibutramine, like orlistat, enhances weight reduction with a low-energy diet by an extra 2–4 kg. A corresponding improvement in HbA$_{1c}$ is also observed. In a recent multicentre trial, sibutramine, used as an adjunct to weight maintenance after weight loss, increased HDL-cholesterol levels and reduced triglycerides in non-diabetic subjects. Sibutramine may cause a small rise in pulse rate and blood pressure in some individuals, but this effect is usually more than countered by the decreased adiposity. However, sibutramine is not recommended for hypertensive patients. Unlike some previous satiety inducers, sibutramine is not a serotonin releaser, is not addictive and has no known effects on heart valves or pulmonary vascular function.

Further reading

American Diabetes Association. Position statement. Standards of medical care for patients with diabetes mellitus. *Diabetes Care* 2000; **23**: S32-42.

European Diabetes Policy Group 1998-1999. Guidelines for diabetes care. A desktop guide to type 2 diabetes mellitus. *Diabetic Med* 1999; **16**: 716-30.

James WP, Astrup A, Finer N *et al*. Effect of sibutramine on weight maintenance after weight loss: a randomized trial. *Lancet* 2000; **356**: 2119-25.

Scheen AJ, Lefèvre PJ. Management of the obese diabetic patient. *Diabetes Rev* 1999; **7**: 77-93.

UK Prospective Diabetes Study Group. Intensive blood-glucose control with sulphonylureas or insulin compared with conventional treatment and risk of complications in patients with type 2 diabetes (UKPDS 33). *Lancet* 1998; **352**: 837-53.

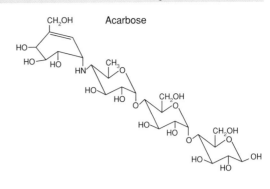

9. Pharmacological treatment I:

α-glucosidase inhibitors
Sulphonylureas
Meglitinide analogues
Future therapies to improve insulin
    secretion

When non-pharmacological treatments are unable to achieve or maintain adequate glycaemic control, oral antidiabetic drugs are indicated. Several differently acting classes are currently available, and this chapter considers the α-glucosidase inhibitors, the sulphonylureas and the meglitinides.

α-glucosidase inhibitors

Slowing the rate at which glucose enters the circulation after a meal reduces the extent of the post-prandial rise in glycaemia in type 2 diabetes. Inhibitors of intestinal α-glucosidase enzymes slow the rate of carbohydrate digestion and provide one means of reducing post-prandial hyperglycaemia.

> α-glucosidase inhibitors slow the rate of intestinal carbohydrate digestion

Brief history

The first α-glucosidase inhibitor, acarbose, was introduced in the early 1990s (Figure 9.1). Recently two further α-glucosidase inhibitors, miglitol and voglibose have been introduced in some countries, but not the UK. To date, this class of drugs has been used extensively in Germany, but not much elsewhere.

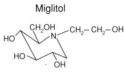
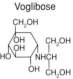

Figure 9.1
Chemical structures of the α-glucosidase inhibitors acarbose, miglitol and voglibose.

Pharmacokinetics

Acarbose and voglibose are absorbed in trivial amounts (acarbose <2% and voglibose <5%). Acarbose is degraded by amylases in the small intestine and by intestinal bacteria, and some of the degradation products are absorbed. Most of the acarbose and degradation products that are absorbed are eliminated over 24 hours in the urine. Miglitol is almost completely absorbed and eliminated unchanged in the urine (Table 9.1).

Mode of action

α-glucosidase inhibitors slow the process of carbohydrate digestion by competitively inhibiting the activity of α-glucosidase enzymes located in the brush border of the enterocytes lining the intestinal villi (Figure 9.2). Acarbose also causes a small reduction in the activity of α-amylase. The main α-glucosidases are glucoamylase, sucrase, maltase and dextrinase, and the inhibitors bind to these enzymes with high affinity, thus preventing the enzymes from cleaving their

Table 9.1
Dosage and pharmacokinetic features of the α-glucosidase inhibitors.

	Dosage	Amount absorbed	Plasma protein-bound	Elimination of absorbed drug and metabolites
Acarbose	Up to 3 x 100 mg/day	<2%	–	Urine
Miglitol	Up to 3 x 100 mg/day	>95%*	negligible	Urine
Voglibose	Up to 3 x 5 mg/day	<5%	–	Urine

* Where doses are submaximal, <70% of a maximum dose is absorbed.

normal disaccharide and oligosaccharide substrates into absorbable monosaccharides. The varying affinities with which the inhibitors bind to the enzymes give the inhibitors slightly different activity profiles. Acarbose shows greatest affinity for glycoamylase, then sucrase, then maltase, and then the dextrinases, while miglitol is an especially potent inhibitor of sucrase, and voglibose is generally more potent than acarbose on other α-glucosidases.

The consequence of inhibiting α-glucosidase activity is to defer the completion of carbohydrate digestion until the substrate is further along the intestinal tract. This, in turn, delays and spreads glucose absorption over a longer period, which reduces the height of the post-prandial hyperglycaemic peak, but prolongs its duration. Thus, α-glucosidase inhibitors must be taken with meals containing digestible carbohydrate (not monosaccharides). These inhibitors do not significantly affect the absorption of glucose itself, but miglitol does interfere slightly with sodium-dependent glucose transport across the brush border.

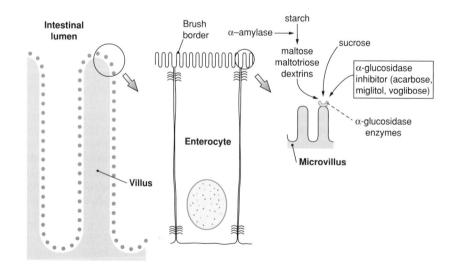

Figure 9.2
α-glucosidase inhibitors (acarbose, miglitol and voglibose) competitively inhibit the activity of α-glucosidase enzymes in the brush border of intestinal enterocytes.

Because the α-glucosidase inhibitors move glucose absorption more distally along the intestinal tract, they alter the release of intestinal hormones that are dependent on glucose absorption. Thus secretion of gastric inhibitory polypeptide (GIP), mainly from the jejunal mucosa, may be reduced by α-glucosidase inhibitors. In contrast, secretion of glucagon-like peptide-1 (7-36 amide) (GLP-1), mainly from the ileal mucosa, is increased by α-glucosidase inhibitors. Both GIP and GLP-1 enhance nutrient-induced insulin secretion, and these alterations probably balance each other out. Overall, the α-glucosidase inhibitors usually reduce post-prandial insulin concentrations because of the smaller rise in post-prandial glycaemia. Although lower concentrations of insulin and glucose during the post-prandial period imply a reduction in insulin resistance, euglycaemic hyperinsulinaemic clamp studies have demonstrated little improvement in insulin sensitivity.

Indications and contraindications

An α-glucosidase inhibitor can be used as adjunctive monotherapy for type 2 patients who are not adequately controlled by non-pharmacological measures. Because α-glucosidase inhibitors reduce post-prandial hyperglycaemia they can be a useful first-line monotherapy in patients who have only slightly raised basal glucose concentrations but more severe post-prandial hyperglycaemia. They can also be used as combination therapy in patients inadequately controlled with other classes of oral antidiabetic agent or insulin (Table 9.2).

When starting therapy with an α-glucosidase inhibitor, it is important to establish that the patient's meals are consistently rich in complex carbohydrate. The selected α-glucosidase inhibitor should always be taken with meals starting with a low dose and titrating up slowly. Monitoring of glycaemic control is recommended, although the post-prandially directed action of these agents is unlikely to induce hypoglycaemia. Thus, the α-glucosidase

Table 9.2
Clinical use of the α-glucosidase inhibitors.

Indications	Patients with type 2 diabetes inadequately controlled by non-pharmacological measures or other antidiabetic agents.
Type of therapy	Monotherapy, or in combination with any other antidiabetic agent.
Treatment schedule	Should be taken with meals rich in digestible complex carbohydrate. Dose should be titrated slowly to be compatible with meals.
Cautions and contraindications	Renal and hepatic disease; history of chronic intestinal disease.
Side-effects	Gastrointestinal disturbances (eg flatulence, abdominal discomfort and diarrhoea).
Adverse reactions	Gastrointestinal disturbances are occasionally severe. Very rarely associated with abnormal liver function.
Precautions	Serum creatinine and liver enzymes should be checked routinely if using high dosages.

inhibitors are antihyperglycaemic as opposed to hypoglycaemic agents. Limitations to their use are usually determined by tolerability to their gastrointestinal side-effects, which include flatulence. Patients who are already experiencing gastrointestinal problems – on metformin therapy, for example – are not good candidates for an additive α-glucosidase inhibitor, and treatment should not be given to patients with a history of chronic intestinal disease.

> Gastrointestinal side-effects are prominent with the α-glucosidase inhibitors

The hepatic effects of high doses of acarbose and its degradation products can occasionally increase liver enzyme concentrations, so it is recommended that alanine transaminase is checked regularly in patients receiving a maximum dose. If liver enzymes are raised, acarbose dosages should be reduced to a level at which normal enzyme concentrations are re-established. Since absorbed α-glucosidase inhibitors and their degradation products are largely eliminated in the urine, individuals with severe renal impairment are contraindicated.

Pregnancy and breast feeding are regarded as contraindications for *all* oral antidiabetic drugs, mainly due to caution and a lack of data, rather than evidence of any detrimental effect (page 46).

Efficacy

The main effect of the α-glucosidase inhibitors is to reduce post-prandial excursions of glycaemia. This, in turn, tends to smooth out the daily blood glucose profile, lowering post-prandial peaks and reducing interprandial troughs. Given as monotherapy to patients who comply appropriately with dietary advice, an α-glucosidase inhibitor will typically reduce peak post-prandial glucose concentrations by 1–3 mmol/l and occasionally by up to 4 mmol/l. The incremental area under the post-prandial plasma glucose curve can be halved in some individuals. Further, there is often a carry-over benefit of a small reduction in basal glycaemia of up to about 1 mmol/l. The accompanying decrease in HbA_{1c} is usually about 0.5%, but may be >1%, if a high dose of the drug is tolerated and dietary compliance maintained.

An α-glucosidase inhibitor can be used for additive efficacy in combination with any other class of antidiabetic agent, although there may then be a trivial reduction in the absorption of the initial drug. α-glucosidase inhibitors do not cause weight gain, can reduce post-prandial hyperinsulinaemia, and have been associated with a small lowering of triglyceride concentrations in some studies. Their ability to reduce interprandial hypoglycaemia and their generally good safety record are further advantages, but poor gastrointestinal tolerability has limited their use.

> The α-glucosidase inhibitors do not cause weight gain

Adverse effects

The most common problems experienced with the α-glucosidase inhibitors are gastrointestinal side-effects. If the dose is too high (relative to the amount of complex carbohydrate in the meal), then undigested oligosaccharides will pass into the large intestine, where they will be fermented by the resident bacteria, producing flatulence, meteorism, borborygmi, abdominal discomfort and, sometimes, diarrhoea. This is most likely to occur during the initial titration of the drug and can be minimized by slowing titration and ensuring that the patient complies with the dietary requirement of meals rich in complex carbohydrate. In some patients gastrointestinal symptoms gradually subside with time, which suggests that the gastrointestinal tract adapts.

Cases of raised liver enzyme concentrations with acarbose and voglibose do not seem to cause permanent abnormalities, and hypoglycaemic episodes are only likely to occur when an α-glucosidase inhibitor is used in combination with a sulphonylurea or insulin. No significant drug interactions are apparent.

> The α-glucosidase inhibitors are unlikely to cause hypoglycaemia as monotherapy

Sulphonylureas

Sulphonylureas have been the mainstay of oral treatment for type 2 diabetes for the past 40 years. This class of drug stimulates insulin secretion to lower blood glucose concentration (page 12).

> Sulphonylureas act principally by stimulating insulin secretion

Brief history

Sulphonamide antibacterial drugs were noted to cause hypoglycaemia in the early 1940s. Subsequent investigations into the chemical basis for this effect gave rise to the first sulphonylureas (carbutamide and tolbutamide) in the mid-1950s. By the 1960s, several so-called first-generation sulphonylureas as they were now known (eg acetohexamide, tolazamide and chlorpropamide) had become available, offering a range of different pharmacokinetic options. In the 1970s, however, a large multicentre trial in the US, the University Group Diabetes Program (UGDP), raised controversial questions about the possible detrimental cardiovascular effects of sulphonylureas. These findings have not been confirmed by long-term clinical experience, however, and a succession

of more potent 'second-generation' sulphonylureas (eg glibenclamide – also called glyburide – gliclazide and glipizide) emerged in the 1970s and 1980s. The latest, glimepiride, was introduced in the mid-1990s. Sulphonylureas currently used in the UK are illustrated in Figure 9.3.

Pharmacokinetics

The main differences between the individual sulphonylureas relate to their pharmacokinetics (Table 9.3). The duration of action varies from <12 hours (tolbutamide) to >24 hours (chlorpropamide), mainly due to differences in their rates of metabolism, metabolite activity and rates of elimination. All are well absorbed and most reach their peak plasma concentration within two to four hours. They are all

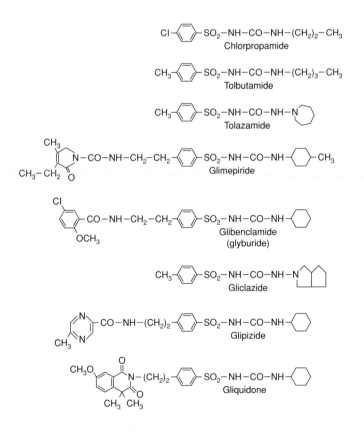

Figure 9.3
Chemical structures of the sulphonylureas chlorpropamide, tolbutamide, tolazamide, glimepiride, glibenclamide (glyburide), gliclazide, glipizide and gliquidone.

Table 9.3
Pharmacokinetic features of the sulphonylureas.

	Daily dosage (mg)[†]	Duration of action*	Activity of metabolites	Main elimination route
Chlorpropamide[1]	100–500	Long	Active	Urine >90%
Glibenclamide[§2]	2.5–15	Intermediate–long	Active	Bile >50%
Gliclazide[2a]	40–320	Intermediate	Inactive	Urine ~65%
Glimepiride[2]	1–6	Intermediate	Active	Urine ~60%
Glipizide[2b]	2.5–20	Short–intermediate	Inactive	Urine ~70%
Gliquidone[2]	15–180	Short–intermediate	Inactive	Bile ~95%
Tolazamide[1]	100–1000	Short–intermediate	Weakly active	Urine ~85%
Tolbutamide[†1]	500–2000	Short	Inactive	Urine ~100%

* Long = >24 hours; intermediate = 12–24 hours; short = <12 hours.
† Large dosages should be divided and related to meal pattern.
‡ Should be taken immediately before meals.
§ Glibenclamide is also known as glyburide (micronized formulation available in US).
[1] = first-generation sulphonylurea; [2] = second-generation sulphonylurea; [a] = modified-release formulation sulphonylurea (Diamicron MR, daily dose 30–120 mg); [b] = extended-release formulation (intermediate duration) sulphonylurea (Glucotrol XL).

metabolized by the liver, but their metabolites and routes of elimination vary considerably. Since all are highly protein-bound they can interact with other highly protein-bound drugs (eg the salicylates, sulphonamides, and warfarin), and there is then some potential for hypoglycaemia.

> Sulphonylureas are highly protein-bound in the circulation and there is increased potential for hypoglycaemia when they are administered with other protein-bound drugs

Mode of action

The sulphonylureas stimulate insulin secretion through a direct effect on the pancreatic β-cells. They bind to the sulphonylurea receptor (SUR) on these cells, which is a component of the transmembrane complex that houses the ATP-sensitive Kir 6.2 potassium channels (K-ATP channels). Binding of the sulphonylurea closes K-ATP channels, reducing potassium efflux and favouring membrane depolarization. In turn, depolarization opens voltage-dependent calcium channels, increasing calcium influx, raising intracellular calcium concentrations and activating calcium-dependent proteins that

control the release of insulin granules (Figure 9.4). In this way, the sulphonylureas lead to a prompt release of pre-formed insulin granules adjacent to the plasma membrane (first-phase insulin release). They subsequently increase the extended (second) phase of insulin release which begins about 10 minutes later as insulin granules are translocated to the membrane from deeper within the β-cell and new granules are formed. The increased release of insulin continues as long as drug stimulation continues, provided the β-cells are functionally capable. The sulphonylureas may also potentiate insulin release through SURs on insulin granules and through activation of protein kinase C. They can cause hypoglycaemia because they initiate insulin release when glucose concentrations are below the normal threshold for glucose-stimulated insulin release (about 5 mmol/l).

This class of drug also seems to exert some weak extra-pancreatic effects which suppress hepatic gluconeogenesis and potentiate insulin-mediated glucose uptake into muscle and adipose tissue. These actions generally require supra-therapeutic concentrations and are probably not clinically relevant. The sulphonylureas have been shown to transiently stimulate and then suppress glucagon secretion by isolated islets, but this effect is not considered to impact significantly on their clinical action. The hepatic extraction of insulin has been reduced by sulphonylureas in some studies, which could help to increase the systemic availability of insulin.

Indications and contraindications

Sulphonylureas have remained a popular first-line oral antidiabetic drug choice for type 2 patients who have not achieved or maintained adequate glycaemic control with non-pharmacological measures (Table 9.4). They are usually preferred for patients who are not overweight since they can cause weight gain,

but the availability of sulphonylureas with different pharmacokinetic properties has provided a choice of agent to accommodate the needs of patients with other medical conditions and contraindications or intolerance to other therapies. The sulphonylureas can be used in combination with any differently acting oral antidiabetic agent and have been used in combination with bedtime insulin in some, although this is not a widely accepted practice in the UK.

Starting sulphonylurea therapy, or indeed any other antidiabetic drug therapy, must be considered carefully within the context of the

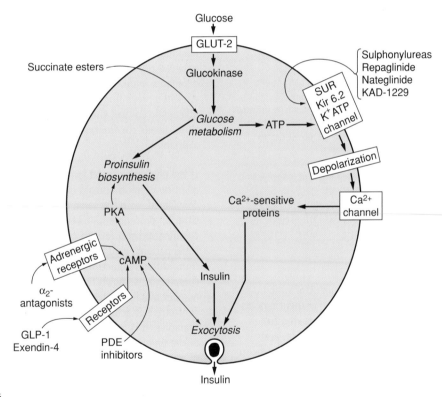

Figure 9.4

The insulin-releasing effect of sulphonylureas and other agents on the pancreatic β-cell. Sulphonylurea binds to the sulphonylurea receptor (SUR) within the plasma membrane of the pancreatic β-cell. This binding closes the Kir 6.2 potassium channels, reducing potassium efflux, depolarizing the cell, and opening voltage-dependent calcium influx channels. Subsequently, raised levels of intracellular calcium bring about insulin release. Sulphonylureas may also enhance nutrient-stimulated insulin secretion through other actions on the β-cell. GLUT-2 = glucose transporter isoform-2; GLP-1 = glucagon-like peptide 1 (7–36 amide); PDE = phosphodiesterase; cAMP = cyclic adenosine monophosphate; PKA = protein kinase A; Kir 6.2 K+ ATP channel = adenosine triphosphate-sensitive potassium inwardly-rectifying channel.

Table 9.4
Clinical use of the sulphonylureas.

Indications	Patients with type 2 diabetes inadequately controlled by non-pharmacological measures or other types of oral antidiabetic agents.
Type of therapy	Monotherapy, or in combination with other antidiabetic agents (except other insulin-releasing agents).
Treatment schedule	A low dose to begin with, escalated slowly. Schedule should be adjusted if necessary to minimize the risk of hypoglycaemia. Maximum effect may be achieved before the maximum permitted dose is reached.
Cautions and contraindications	Should be used cautiously in patients with hepatic or renal disease (see pharmacokinetics) or porphyria.
Side-effects	Occasional, usually transient, sensitivity reactions. Chlorpropamide can lead to facial flushing after alcohol has been consumed – rarely, it causes hyponatraemia.
Adverse reactions	Risk of hypoglycaemia, especially with high doses of longer-acting preparations.
Precautions	Interactions with other protein-bound drugs such as the salicylates and sulphonamides.

overall care plan. An assessment of which agent is most likely to achieve the therapeutic goals of the care plan must be made, taking full account of the accompanying medical and lifestyle circumstances and other commitments of the patient. Once an agent has been selected, contraindications should be checked again. The duration of action and route of elimination of the particular sulphonylurea may be important considerations if the prospect of interprandial hypoglycaemia is likely, or if renal or liver disease are a concern. Shorter-acting preparations and those without active metabolites are generally preferred for

individuals at risk of hypoglycaemia and the elderly. Transient sensitivity reactions can occur.

The starting dose should always be low and blood glucose monitored in an appropriate way (chapter 5) – for example, by a member of the care team every two weeks, preferably supplemented by home self-monitoring. Dosage may be increased at two- to four-week intervals as required, until the glycaemic target is achieved. If symptomatic hypoglycaemic episodes occur, an attempt should be made to confirm blood glucose level with home self-monitoring. In such cases, and where an increase in dosage produces no further improvement in glycaemic control, patients should be returned to their previous dose. It is not uncommon for the maximum blood glucose-lowering effect to be achieved far below the maximum permitted drug dosage – probably because the drug is already producing its maximum increase in insulin secretion for the patient's prevailing β-cell capability. Long-term glycaemic control should be checked using HbA_{1c} levels (or fructosamine if HbA_{1c} is not available).

If the glycaemic target is not achieved, the addition of another class of agent should be considered, with the same evaluation and titration procedure followed. If the new combination still fails to give adequate control, some patients may benefit from the addition of a third, differently acting, oral therapy, but compliance is known to deteriorate with the number of agents taken. If adequate glycaemic control is not achieved with a combination of oral therapies, it is quite likely that the natural history of the type 2 diabetes has progressed to a state of severe β-cell failure. It is then usually advised to switch to insulin therapy (page 161).

Always start with a low dose of sulphonylurea. Monitor blood glucose by an appropriate method and increase dosages at two- to four-week intervals as necessary until the glycaemic target is achieved

Efficacy

The blood glucose-lowering efficacy of sulphonylureas has been evaluated in many retrospective and prospective studies, and from over 40 years of clinical experience. Given as monotherapy in type 2 patients who are not adequately controlled by non-pharmacological measures, sulphonylureas usually reduce fasting plasma glucose (FPG) by 2–4 mmol/l, and this is usually associated with a decrease in HbA_{1c} levels of 1–2%. Since the hypoglycaemic effect of sulphonylureas is due mainly to increased insulin secretion, the effectiveness of sulphonylureas is dependent on adequate β-cell function, and is independent of age and body weight.

The progressive β-cell failure that occurs during the natural history of type 2 diabetes may require the sulphonylurea dosage to be increased when glycaemic control deteriorates. Rapid and uncontrollable deterioration of glycaemic control during sulphonylurea therapy, sometimes termed sulphonylurea failure, occurs in 5–10% of patients each year. The inability to maintain acceptable glycaemic control is generally similar for all sulphonylureas (and metformin), and reflects an advanced extent of β-cell failure. In other words, it is mainly disease progression, rather than drug failure and the term 'sulphonylurea failure' is something of a misnomer. However, some differences have been observed between individual sulphonylureas. In the UKPDS, the 'secondary failure' rate of chlorpropamide was higher than that of glibenclamide. Further, a five-year comparative study showed a lower secondary failure rate for gliclazide than either glibenclamide (glyburide) or glipizide. Individuals who have adequate β-cell function usually respond well to the sulphonylureas, and early use of sulphonylureas as first-line monotherapy in these patients is much more successful than late intervention in patients with little or no remaining β-cell reserve. Patients who respond well to the sulphonylureas tend to have less severe fasting hyperglycaemia on presentation.

Insulin concentrations during sulphonylurea therapy do not usually extend beyond the range observed in the non-diabetic population (including those with impaired glucose tolerance), and suggestions that sulphonylurea-induced hyperinsulinaemia might increase the risk of detrimental insulin-induced effects on the cardiovascular system remain unsubstantiated. Sulphonylurea therapy generally seems to have little effect on the blood lipid profile, although some studies have noted a small decrease in plasma triglyceride level and small improvements in other lipid parameters, possibly as a result of improved glycaemic control.

When a sulphonylurea is used in combination with another type of oral antidiabetic (that is not an insulin-releaser), the glucose-lowering efficacy of the sulphonylurea is approximately additive to the effect of the other agent (dependent, of course, on adequate β-cell function). Early use of combination therapy is indicated when optimal titration of a single agent does not achieve adequate glycaemic control. A combination of two different types of agent is more likely to achieve the glycaemic target and will also 'buy time' during which control is better maintained. If institution of combination therapy is only undertaken as a last resort after 'failure' of a single oral agent, it is likely that β-cell failure is already advanced and combination therapy will offer limited benefit.

Adverse effects

Hypoglycaemia is the most common and serious adverse event experienced with the sulphonylureas, and patients on sulphonylurea therapy should receive instruction as to how to recognize and prevent this side-effect, and how to react when the symptoms occur. Hypoglycaemia is more likely in patients on longer-acting preparations and with irregular eating habits. Hypoglycaemia is also more likely to occur in patients with good control. Estimates of the incidence of mild hypoglycaemia (ie hypoglycaemia not requiring assistance from another individual) are mostly based on patient-reported symptoms and are unconfirmed by blood glucose measurements. In the UKPDS, about 20% of patients treated with a sulphonylurea reported one or more episodes of hypoglycaemia a year and similar accounts have emerged from other studies. Glibenclamide (glyburide) causes mainly interprandial hypoglycaemia, while chlorpropamide reportedly causes hypoglycaemia mostly in the early mornings before breakfast. The typical symptoms of hypoglycaemia are listed in Table 9.5.

> Hypoglycaemia is the most common and severe adverse event associated with sulphonylurea therapy

The UKPDS reported that more severe hypoglycaemia (ie that requiring the assistance of another person or medical intervention) occurred in about 1% of sulphonylurea-treated patients a year. However, much lower rates – 0.2–2.5 episodes per 1,000 patient years – have emerged from adverse-event reports to the regulatory authorities and from physician questionnaires. The mortality risk associated with sulphonylurea-induced hypoglycaemia is about 0.014–0.033 per 1,000 patient years, with the longer-acting agents carrying the greatest risk. For comparison, the incidence of insulin-induced hypoglycaemia has been estimated as high as 100 per 1,000 patient years.

> Weight gain is a recognized feature of sulphonylurea therapy

Mild hypoglycaemic reactions require a reassessment not only of the choice of agent, but the treatment schedule, any intercurrent illness, any potential drug interactions (Table 9.6), and any modifiable features of the patient's lifestyle such as diet and meal patterns. Alcohol consumption can predispose to hypoglycaemia and should be reconsidered. The possibility of an acute cerebrovascular event should be excluded. Severe hypoglycaemic episodes causing neuroglycopenic coma should be treated in a similar manner to the insulin-induced severe hypoglycaemia (discussed in chapter 11 and opposite) but excluding the use of glucagon.

> Severe sulphonylurea-induced hypoglycaemia is a medical emergency

Table 9.5

Signs and symptoms of hypoglycaemia and actions to be taken by the patient.

Symptoms	Physiological mechanism	Onset occurs when blood glucose is: (mmol/l)*	Intervention required
Hunger, sweating, tremor, palpitations	Autonomic response to subnormal glycaemia	Below ~3.5	Take glucose-rich sweets, drink, or food
Cognitive dysfunction, incoordination, atypical behaviour, speech difficulty, drowsiness, dizziness	Neuroglycopenia (brain deprived of glucose)	Below ~2.8	Take glucose-rich sweets or drink, and seek assistance
Malaise, headache, nausea, reduced consciousness	Severe neuroglycopenia	Below ~2.0	Third party intervention required[+]
Convulsions, coma	Severe neuroglycopenia	Below ~1.5	Medical intervention essential[+]

*Approximate concentration of glucose in arterialized venous blood below which symptoms are induced by insulin infusion in non-diabetic individuals. Symptoms often seem to occur at higher glucose concentrations in diabetic patients.
[+]Glucagon is *not* suitable for treating hypoglycaemia in type 2 patients since it stimulates insulin secretion. Hospitalization is strongly recommended for patients with severe sulphonylurea-induced hypoglycaemia.

Table 9.6
Drugs able to potentiate the hypoglycaemic effect of sulphonylureas.

Displace them from plasma proteins:	Salicylates, sulphonamides, warfarin, phenylbutazone, fibrates
Decrease their hepatic metabolism:	Warfarin, monoamine oxidase inhibitors, chloramphenicol, phenylbutazone
Decrease their renal excretion:	Salicylates, probenecid, allopurinol
Intrinsic hypoglycaemic activity:	Salicylates, alcohol, monoamine oxidase inhibitors

Other adverse effects which can occur with sulphonylurea therapy are sensitivity reactions (usually rashes), but these are transient, reversible and rarely lead to erythema multiforme. Fever, jaundice and blood dyscrasias are very rare. Some sulphonylureas have been noted to precipitate acute porphyria. Chlorpropamide, in particular, can lead to facial flushing after alcohol consumption, and has been reported to cause photosensitivity. This drug may also increase renal sensitivity to antidiuretic hormone, which very occasionally leads to sufficient water retention to create hyponatraemia. Conversely, glibenclamide and tolazamide have a mild diuretic action. Weight gain is a recognized feature of sulphonylurea therapy – typically a gain of 1–4 kg which stabilizes after about six months. This is attributed to the increased insulin concentrations with their anabolic effects and reduced loss of glucose in the urine.

> Severe sulphonylurea-induced hypoglycaemia has a high case-fatality rate

Cardiac muscle and vascular smooth muscle express various isoforms of the SUR which bind sulphonylureas with much lesser affinity than the SUR expressed by the pancreatic β-cells. Thus, while very high concentrations of sulphonylureas can cause contraction of these muscles, this is not considered likely to be clinically significant at therapeutic concentrations.

> Longer-acting sulphonylureas, such as chlorpropamide and glibenclamide should be avoided in the elderly

Management of sulphonylurea-induced hypoglycaemia

Recurrent symptoms suggestive of hypoglycaemia should prompt a reduction in dose or withdrawal of sulphonylurea therapy. The importance of the effects of alcohol may be underestimated in elderly patients and the potential for drug interaction must always be borne in mind. Presentation with altered conscious level or focal neurological signs may lead to an erroneous diagnosis of acute cerebrovascular event, but the possibility of hypoglycaemia should always be excluded in patients with type 2 diabetes presenting with any of these features.

> All sulphonylureas have the potential to cause severe hypoglycaemia

Patients with severe sulphonylurea-induced hypoglycaemia should be admitted to hospital quickly; relapse following initial resuscitation with oral or iv glucose is well recognized and may necessitate prolonged iv infusion of dextrose. An iv bolus of glucose leads to further release of insulin, especially in subjects whose β-cell function is relatively well preserved. This predictable consequence of treatment, combined with the long duration of action of drugs such as chlorpropamide and glibenclamide, explains the tendency for hypoglycaemia to recur.

> Relapse after resuscitation is common in severe sulphonylurea-induced hypoglycaemia

The antihypertensive agent diazoxide and the somatostatin analogue octreotide offer a more direct approach by inhibiting stimulated endogenous insulin secretion; but although these drugs have been used successfully as adjuncts to iv dextrose, neither is licensed for this indication in the UK.

- *iv dextrose* – remains the mainstay of therapy; continuous infusion of 5–10% dextrose may be required for several days.
- *Diazoxide* – antagonizes the actions of sulphonylureas by opening ATP-sensitive potassium channels in the membranes of β-cells (pages 12 and 30). However, associated adverse cardiovascular effects, including tachycardia and orthostatic hypotension, may be hazardous in elderly patients who may have compromised vasculature or impaired baroreceptor reflexes.
- *Hydrocortisone* – has been advocated, but there is scant evidence of efficacy and high doses may lead to hypokalaemia.
- *Glucagon* – stimulates endogenous insulin release and therefore cannot be recommended.
- *Mannitol* – is advocated for cerebral oedema; dexamethasone is a widely used alternative.
- *Octreotide* – has been shown to be an effective and well-tolerated inhibitor of sulphonylurea-induced hypoglycaemia under controlled experimental conditions, but clinical experience in this indication is limited.

Serum potassium should be monitored and iv supplements administered if hypokalaemia develops – high plasma insulin levels will increase potassium transport into cells. Where chlorpropamide accumulation is suspected, renal elimination may be greatly enhanced by forced alkaline diuresis. General supportive measures and correction of any underlying or contributory factors, eg acute renal impairment, are also necessary.

Meglitinide analogues

The first phase of glucose-stimulated insulin secretion is diminished or lost early in the natural history of type 2 diabetes. Consequently, the plasma insulin rise during digestion of a meal is delayed. An initial surge of insulin release is particularly important for the suppression of hepatic glucose production, and failure to accomplish this in type 2 diabetes makes a substantial contribution to post-prandial hyperglycaemia. It is difficult to organize sulphonylurea regimens that give maximum insulin release during meal consumption and minimum insulin release at other times, but a new group of agents, the 'prandial' insulin releasers, has emerged to produce a rapid but short-lived stimulation of insulin secretion. These, also known as the meglitinides, can be taken immediately before a meal so that the prompt stimulation of extra insulin release reinstates an initial surge of insulin and limits the raised insulin concentrations to the period of meal digestion. Repaglinide is the first of these new agents to become available for clinical use.

> Repaglinide is the first of a new class of rapid-acting secretagogues, the meglitinides, to become available

Brief history

The non-sulphonylurea portion of glibenclamide – a benzamido compound termed meglitinide – was shown to stimulate insulin secretion in the early 1980s. Derivatives of meglitinide, such as repaglinide, and related compounds, such as nateglinide, have been developed as rapid insulin releasers. Repaglinide was introduced in 1998 and nateglinide is currently being reviewed by the regulatory authorities.

Pharmacokinetics

Benzamido prandial insulin releasers differ from sulphonylureas in their structure (Figure 9.5) and most importantly in their pharmacokinetics. Repaglinide is rapidly and almost completely

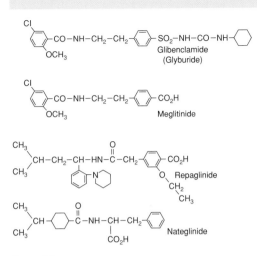

Figure 9.5
Chemical structures of meglitinide, repaglinide and nateglinide compared with glibenclamide (glyburide).

absorbed, with peak plasma concentrations achieved within an hour. It is then rapidly metabolized by the liver to inactive metabolites mainly excreted in the bile. When taken about 15 minutes before a meal, repaglinide produces a prompt insulin-releasing effect which is limited to a period of about three hours, thus coinciding with the duration of meal digestion.

Mode of action

The mechanism through which benzamido prandial insulin releasers stimulate insulin secretion is essentially the same as that of the sulphonylureas. These drugs also bind to the SUR on the plasma membrane of the β-cell – but at a different site. This binding closes the ATP-sensitive Kir 6.2 potassium channel, leading to depolarization, voltage-dependent calcium influx, and activation of calcium-dependent proteins that control insulin release (Figure 9.4).

> Repaglinide binds to a different site on the SUR to that of the sulphonylureas

Since the Kir 6.2 potassium channel is closed when either the benzamido binding site *or* the

sulphonylurea binding site on the SUR is bound with its respective agonist, there is no additive advantage in giving a prandial insulin releaser in addition to a sulphonylurea. (The pharmacokinetic differences would enable the 'prandial' benzamido compound to bind before the sulphonylurea but this has not been translated into a clinical advantage). Due to the short half-life of the prandial insulin releasers, the insulin-releasing effect of these agents predominantly enhances the first phase and early second phase of secretion, and is not sustained as long as that of the sulphonylureas. No other actions of the benzamido compounds on the β-cell, or extra-pancreatic effects, have yet been established.

Indications and contraindications

The indications for repaglinide as a monotherapy in type 2 patients inadequately controlled by non-pharmacological measures are essentially the same as those for a sulphonylurea. However a 'prandial' insulin releaser could be more appropriate for an individual with an irregular lifestyle in which meals are unpredictable and may be missed (Table 9.7). A prandial insulin releaser is also likely to benefit an individual who regularly experiences interprandial hypoglycaemia. Such cases require a reassessment of the choice of agent, taking full account of the pharmacokinetics, dosage and timing, and the potential for addition of an α-glucosidase inhibitor to help smooth out the daily glucose profile. Prandial insulin releasers can be used effectively in combination with any other differently acting oral antidiabetic (ie non insulin-releasing) agent, eg metformin or a thiazolidinedione. The protocol for starting repaglinide therapy is also similar to that for starting a sulphonylurea (page 131). Repaglinide should be taken 15–30 minutes before each main meal and begun at a low dose (eg 0.5 mg). The effect on glycaemic control should be monitored, and the dosage titrated up slowly to a maximum of 4 mg before each main meal if required. As with the sulphonylureas, if a titration step gives no further benefit or a

Table 9.7
Clinical use of repaglinide.

Indications	Patients with type 2 diabetes inadequately controlled by non-pharmacological measures or other types of oral agents that do not stimulate insulin secretion. Patients prone to interprandial hypoglycaemia on a sulphonylurea.
Type of therapy	Monotherapy, or in combination with other antidiabetic agents (except other insulin-releasing agents).
Treatment schedule	Repaglinide should be taken about 15 minutes before each main meal. The dose should be low (eg 0.5 mg) to begin with and escalated up slowly to 4 mg before each main meal.
Cautions and contraindications	Should be used with caution in patients with hepatic or severe renal disease.
Side-effects	Occasionally sensitivity reactions, usually transient.
Adverse reactions	Risk of hypoglycaemia.
Precautions	Possible interactions with erythromycin, rifampicin and some antifungal agents.

hypoglycaemic episode occurs, the patient should return to the previous dosage, and if glycaemic targets are not met, early introduction of combination therapy should be considered. The main contraindications to repaglinide are hepatic disease and severe renal impairment (see pharmacokinetics).

Efficacy

Clinical trials have noted that repaglinide (0.5–4 mg taken about 15–30 minutes before meals) increases insulin secretion and reduces post-prandial hypoglycaemia in a dose-related manner. A dose of 4 mg has been shown to reduce the incremental area under the post-prandial glucose curve by about one-third. With appropriate titration against the complex carbohydrate content of the diet, repaglinide's effect can be limited to the period of digestion. By timing the intake of repaglinide to about

15–30 minutes before the meal, the greatest stimulation of insulin secretion occurs during the early period (within about 30 minutes) of meal digestion, thus replacing the acute insulin response which is diminished or absent in type 2 diabetes and helping to suppress hepatic glucose production.

Chronic use of repaglinide has a carry-over effect to lower the basal glycaemia. Reductions in HbA_{1c} observed with repaglinide have been similar in magnitude to those observed with the sulphonylureas, ie 1–2%. Repaglinide usually shows a greater post-prandial glucose-lowering effect but a lesser reduction in fasting glycaemia, but has not been available long enough to enable comparisons with sulphonylureas over several years. Whether intermittent daily stimulation of β-cell function with such a prandial insulin releaser is different in the long term to more protracted daily stimulation of β-cell function remains to be seen.

Repaglinide has been used successfully in combination with metformin. Combination of prandial insulin releasers with metformin or a thiazolidinedione should help to reduce the risk of severe hypoglycaemia in patients with good glycaemic control. A small increase in body weight can be expected in patients starting antidiabetic therapy with repaglinide, but there is little change in weight among patients switched from sulphonylurea therapy. Plasma lipid profiles do not seem to be significantly affected by repaglinide.

Adverse effects

Despite the short duration of action of the prandial insulin releasers, hypoglycaemia remains the predominant adverse effect. However its incidence is much lower than with the sulphonylureas – the number of serious events, in particular, appears to be reduced. Reassessment of opportunities to minimize the risk of hypoglycaemia is recommended in any patient experiencing such episodes (page 134). Sensitivity reactions, usually transient, have been reported with repaglinide, and the manufacturers suggest caution over possible interactions with erythromycin, rifampicin and various antifungal agents. Since repaglinide has a lower binding affinity for isoforms of the SUR in cardiac and vascular smooth muscle, the possibility of clinically significant cardiovascular effects remains similarly putative for repaglinide as for the sulphonylureas.

> Repaglinide is associated with a lower incidence of serious hypoglycaemia than some of the longer-acting sulphonylureas

Nateglinide

Nateglinide is a benzamido prandial insulin releaser in clinical development due to become available in the US in 2001. Structurally, it is related to phenylalanine (Figure 9.5). Preclinical and initial clinical studies indicate that it has a slightly faster onset and shorter duration of action than repaglinide. A dose of 60 mg taken 20 minutes before an iv glucose tolerance test replaced the first phase of insulin release and lowered glucose concentrations.

Doses of 60 mg or 120 mg immediately before a meal have been shown to reduce post-prandial hyperglycaemia in type 2 diabetes. Nateglinide is likely to be used particularly effectively in combination with an agent that reduces insulin resistance.

Future therapies to improve insulin secretion

New sulphonylurea formulations

Changes in the formulation of some sulphonylureas have already been undertaken to modify their duration of action. For example, a micronized formulation of glibenclamide (glyburide) introduced in the US increases the rate of absorption and enables an earlier onset of action. A longer-acting ('extended release') formulation of glipizide (Glucotrol XL) has also been introduced.

A 'modified release' formulation of gliclazide (Diamicron MR) has been developed. While the duration of action of gliclazide is unchanged, this new formulation uses a hydrophilic matrix to match progressive delivery of gliclazide with the hyperglycaemic profile. Improved bioavailability enables once-daily dosing, while reducing the dosage from 80 mg per tablet to 30 mg per tablet. (If blood glucose remains inadequately controlled, the dose, which is given in the morning, can be increased as required.)

> Modified-release formulations of sulphonylureas with improved bioavailability allow dose reductions

New fixed-dose combinations of glibenclamide (glyburide) and metformin have now become available in the US. Fixed-dose combinations have long been available in a minority of countries. The new combinations, eg Glucovance, combine glibenclamide (G) and metformin (M) at dosages of G1.25:M250, G2.5:M500, and G5:M500 mg. It is envisaged that fixed-dose (single tablet) combinations might simplify combination therapy for many patients. Patients with particularly marked hyperglycaemia after non-pharmacological treatment would be candidates for initiation of drug therapy with a fixed combination sulphonylurea–metformin regimen. The precautions associated with both classes of agent would apply, and any dose escalation would follow the procedure described previously (page 132).

A slow-release formulation of metformin has recently become available in some countries to enable once-daily administration of this drug.

> Fixed-dose combination tablets containing glibenclamide (glyburide) and metformin are already available in some countries

Novel insulin releasers

A potential future approach to synchronizing insulin secretion with meal consumption involves the intestinal hormone glucagon-like peptide-1 (7-36 amide) (GLP-1). GLP-1 potentiates nutrient-stimulated insulin secretion via receptors in the pancreatic β-cell membrane which activate cyclic adenosine monophosphate (cAMP) and this increases the insulin response to a meal. It also enhances proinsulin biosynthesis and may additionally slow gastric emptying and induce satiety. Since GLP-1 is a rapidly degraded peptide, its therapeutic application requires injection or infusion. To obviate this problem, slow-release formulations, a sublingual preparation, and aerosol forms of GLP-1 are being evaluated. It may also be possible to prolong the plasma half-life of exogenous (and endogenous) GLP-1 by administration of agents that inhibit the dipeptidyl peptidase IV enzyme which degrades GLP-1. A more stable analogue of GLP-1, exendin-4, has been discovered in the saliva of an American lizard, which might provide another potential therapeutic option. Interestingly, GLP-1 and exendin-4 have recently been found to both stimulate division of β-cells and increase new β-cell formation from uncommitted progenitor cells in the exocrine pancreatic ducts.

A further novel approach to enhancing insulin secretion involves succinate esters which enhance the activity of the Krebs cycle in the β-cell. This stimulates proinsulin biosynthesis and insulin secretion. However, succinate esters can serve as a nutrient fuel in a range of tissues and provide a substrate for gluconeogenesis. Thus, this approach can only be exploited if the succinate esters are targeted predominantly at β-cells.

Imidazoline compounds can also stimulate insulin secretion, possibly both independently and through a mechanism involving closure of the Kir 6.2 potassium channels in the pancreatic β-cells. Imidazoline-binding sites have been identified in pancreatic β-cells, but are not yet fully characterized.

Pancreatic β-cells express several types of phosphodiesterase (PDE) and when some (eg type III) of these are inhibited, cAMP concentrations are increased and the initiation of insulin secretion (by other agents) is promoted. Again, specific targeting of the pancreatic β-cell would be required.

Further reading

Bailey CJ. Antidiabetic drugs. *Brit J Cardiol* 2000; **3**: 350–60.

Bailey CJ. New insulin secretagogues. *Diabetes Revs Int* 1998; **7**: 2-7.

Campbell IW. Antidiabetic drugs present and future. *Drugs* 2000; **60**: 1017-28.

Chiasson JL, Josse RG, Hunt JA *et al*. The efficacy of acarbose in the treatment of patients with non-insulin dependent diabetes mellitus: a multicenter controlled clinical trial. *Ann Intern Med* 1994; **121**: 928-35.

Groop LC. Sulphonylureas in NIDDM. *Diabetes Care* 1992; **15**: 737-54.

Harrower ADB. Comparative tolerability of sulphonylureas in diabetes mellitus. In: Krentz AJ, Ed. *Drug treatment of type 2 diabetes*. Auckland: Adis International, 2000; 77-84.

Krentz AJ, Ferner RE, Bailey CJ. Comparative tolerability profiles of oral antidiabetic agents. *Drug Safety* 1994; **11**: 223-41.

Landgraf R. Meglitinide analogues in the treatment of type 2 diabetes mellitus. *Drugs Ageing* 2000; **17**: 411-25.

Lebovitz HE. α-glucosidase inhibitors as agents in the treatment of diabetes. *Diabetes Rev* 1998; **6**: 132-45.

Lebovitz HE, Melander A. Sulphonylureas: basic aspects and clinical use. In: Alberti KGMM, Zimmet P, DeFronzo RA, Keen H (Eds). *International textbook of diabetes mellitus*, 2nd edn. Chichester: Wiley, 1997; 817-40.

Marbury T, Huang WC, Strange P, Lebovitz H. Repaglinide versus glyburide: a one-year comparison trial. *Diab Res Clin Pract* 1999; **43**: 155-66.

Nattrass M, Bailey CJ. New agents for type 2 diabetes. *Clin Endocrinol Metab* 1999; **13**: 309-29.

10. Pharmacological treatment II:

Metformin
Thiazolidinediones
Future therapies to improve insulin action

Insulin resistance is an important pathogenic feature of most presentations of type 2 diabetes, and a logical therapeutic target. The biguanide metformin and the thiazolidinediones (TZDs) rosiglitazone and pioglitazone are the main agents currently available to act directly against insulin resistance.

Metformin

Brief history

Galega officinalis (goat's rue or French lilac), historically used as a traditional treatment for diabetes in Europe, was found to be rich in guanidine. In 1918 guanidine was shown to have a blood glucose-lowering effect, and several derivatives (eg galegine and synthalin A) were introduced as antidiabetic drugs in the 1920s. These were discontinued and all but forgotten as insulin became widely available, and it was not until the late 1950s that three antidiabetic biguanides were reported: metformin and phenformin in 1957, and buformin in 1958 (Figure 10.1). Phenformin was withdrawn in many countries in the 1970s due to a high incidence of lactic acidosis, and buformin receives limited use in a few countries, leaving metformin as the main biguanide. Indeed metformin is currently the most extensively used oral agent for type 2 diabetes worldwide.

Pharmacokinetics

Metformin hydrochloride is a stable hydrophilic biguanide which is quickly absorbed and quickly eliminated unchanged in the urine (Table 10.1).

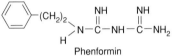

Guanidine

Galegine
(isoamylene guanidine)

Synthalin A
(decamethylene diguanidine)

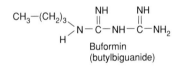

Phenformin
(phenethylbiguanide)

Buformin
(butylbiguanide)

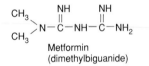

Metformin
(dimethylbiguanide)

Figure 10.1
Chemical structures of guanidine, galegine, synthalin A, phenformin, buformin and metformin.

Table 10.1
Pharmacokinetic features of the biguanide metformin.

Time to peak plasma concentration	1–2 hours
Plasma $t_{1/2}$	2–5 hours
Plasma protein-bound	Negligible
Metabolism	Not metabolized
Elimination	Urine (approximately 90% eliminated in urine in 12 hours)

Thus it is imperative that metformin is only prescribed to patients with sufficient renal function to avoid accumulation of the drug. Renal clearance of metformin is achieved more by tubular secretion than glomerular filtration, and the only significant interaction is competition with cimetidine which can increase plasma metformin concentration. There is little binding of metformin to plasma proteins, so metformin does not interfere with protein-bound drugs. Since it is not metabolized, it does not interfere with the metabolism of other drugs either. It is widely distributed, and high concentrations are retained in the walls of the gastrointestinal tract, providing a reservoir from which plasma concentrations are maintained. Nevertheless, peak plasma concentrations (about 2 µg/ml) are short-lived: in patients with normal renal function the plasma $t\frac{1}{2}$ for metformin is two to five hours, and almost 90% of the absorbed dose is eliminated within 12 hours.

Mode of action

Metformin has a variety of metabolic effects (Table 10.2). It acts partly by improving insulin action and partly by effects that are not directly insulin-dependent. Metformin lowers blood glucose concentrations without causing overt hypoglycaemia. Its clinical efficacy requires the presence of insulin, but the drug does not stimulate insulin release and typically causes a small decrease in basal insulin concentrations in hyperinsulinaemic patients. The most evident blood glucose-lowering mechanism metformin has is its reduction of excessive hepatic glucose production (Figure 10.2). It reduces hepatic gluconeogenesis mainly by increasing sensitivity to insulin. Additionally it reduces the hepatic extraction of certain gluconeogenic substrates (such as lactate) and opposes the effects of glucagon. It decreases the rate of hepatic glycogenolysis, and the activity of hepatic glucose-6-phosphatase.

> Metformin has multiple metabolic effects; reduction of excessive hepatic glucose production is thought to be the principal mode of action

Insulin-stimulated glucose uptake and glycogen formation in skeletal muscle are enhanced by metformin. These involve increased movement of insulin-sensitive glucose transporters into the cell membrane and increased activity of glycogen synthase. Metformin also acts in an insulin-independent manner to suppress fatty acid oxidation and reduce triglyceride levels in hypertriglyceridaemic patients – this reduces the energy supply for gluconeogenesis and improves the glucose–fatty acid (Randle) cycle. Finally, preclinical studies have shown that metformin increases glucose turnover in the splanchnic bed (independently of insulin), which is likely to contribute to its blood glucose-lowering effect; it also expends extra energy to help prevent weight gain.

Table 10.2
Metabolic and other effects of metformin.

Antihyperglycaemic	Suppresses hepatic glucose output. Increases insulin-mediated glucose use. Decreases fatty acid oxidation. Increases splanchnic glucose turnover.
Weight stabilization or reduction	–
Improved lipid profile	Reduces hypertriglyceridaemia. Lowers NEFAs, lowers LDL-C and raises HDL-C in some patients.
Decreased hyperinsulinaemia	–
Does not cause serious hypoglycaemia	–
Counters insulin resistance	Decreases the endogenous/exogenous insulin requirement.
Vascular effects	Increased fibrinolysis. Decreased PAI-1.

NEFAs = non-esterified fatty acids; LDL-C = low-density lipoprotein-cholesterol; HDL-C = high-density lipoprotein-cholesterol; PAI-1 = plasminogen activator inhibitor-1.

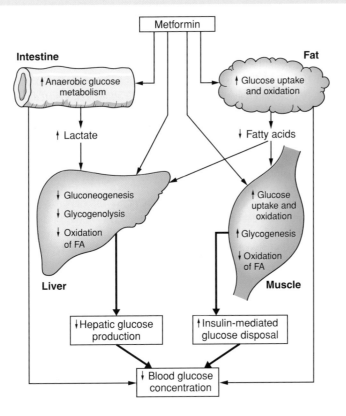

Figure 10.2
Mechanisms of action of metformin. FA = Fatty acids

At the cellular level, metformin can improve insulin sensitivity by increasing the insulin-stimulated tyrosine kinase signalling activity of the insulin receptor (page 18). Signalling is also increased through the enhanced activity of a range of post-receptor insulin-signalling pathways. Although metformin also increases insulin receptor binding when insulin receptor numbers are depleted, this is unlikely to have a significant impact on insulin action. The insulin-independent effects of metformin seem to result from changes in membrane fluidity in hyperglycaemic states and in the activities of certain metabolic enzymes. Collectively, the cellular effects of metformin counter insulin resistance and reduce glucotoxicity in type 2 diabetes.

> Metformin therapy also improves insulin action in skeletal muscle

Indications and contraindications

Metformin is customarily the therapy of choice for overweight and obese type 2 patients because it does not lead to weight gain. However, it is an equally effective antihyperglycaemic agent in normal-weight patients and is now used extensively as first-line monotherapy for type 2 diabetes inadequately controlled by diet, exercise, or lifestyle management. Metformin can be used in combination with any other class of oral antidiabetic agent or with insulin.

> Metformin does not lead to weight gain or serious hypoglycaemia

> Metformin is widely regarded as the drug of choice for overweight or obese patients with type 2 diabetes

Starting treatment with metformin should follow the same protocol as starting treatment with a sulphonylurea (page 131). The main contraindications are listed in Table 10.3. Patients are excluded if there is evidence of impaired renal function (eg serum creatinine >120–130 µmol/l or 1.4–1.5 mg/dl, dependent on lean body mass) to avoid the risk of drug accumulation. Cardiac or respiratory insufficiency, and any other condition predisposing to hypoxia or reduced perfusion (eg septicaemia) are further contraindications, as is liver disease, alcohol abuse, or a history of metabolic acidosis. Metformin can otherwise be used in the elderly, provided there is no renal insufficiency. It should be noted that the improved insulin sensitivity may cause ovulation to resume in cases of anovulatory polycystic ovary syndrome (PCOS).

Metformin should be taken with or immediately before meals to minimize the possibility of gastrointestinal side-effects. The starting dose should be 500–850 mg/day (or 500 mg twice a day; one tablet with each of the morning and evening meals). Blood glucose concentration should be monitored and the dosage increased slowly (one tablet at a time), at intervals of about two weeks, until the glycaemic target is attained. As with the other oral agents outlined (chapter 9), if the target is not attained and a higher dosage produces no greater effect, the dosage should be stepped down, and combination therapy considered (eg addition of a sulphonylurea, prandial insulin releaser or thiazolidinedione). The most effective dose is usually about 2000 mg/day in divided doses with meals, but the absolute maximum allowed is 2550–3000 mg, dependent on country. A slow-release formulation of metformin and a fixed-dose combination of metformin plus a sulphonylurea are now available in some countries (page 139).

Abdominal discomfort and other gastrointestinal side-effects are not uncommon during the introduction of metformin. Symptoms usually remit if the dose is reduced and re-titrated slowly, and only about 5–10% of patients cannot tolerate any dose at all. Unexplained diarrhoea in diabetic patients is sometimes linked to metformin. During long-term treatment, it is advisable to recheck yearly for contraindications, particularly a raised serum creatinine level. In patients with poor diet, metformin can reduce absorption of vitamin B_{12} and a haemoglobin measurement is also advised. Deficiency of vitamin B_{12} sufficient to cause megaloblastic anaemia is, however, very unusual. Treatment should be temporarily stopped during use of iv radiographic contrast media, surgery and any other situation in which the exclusion criteria could be invoked. Substitution with insulin may then be appropriate.

Table 10.3
Clinical use of metformin.

Indications	Patients with type 2 diabetes inadequately controlled by non-pharmacological measures or other oral antidiabetic agents.
Type of therapy	Monotherapy, or in combination with any other antidiabetic agent.
Treatment schedule	Metformin should be taken with meals and dose escalated slowly to a maximum of 2550 (or 3000*) mg/day.
Cautions and contraindications	Renal and hepatic disease; cardiac or respiratory disease or any other hypoxic condition; severe infection; alcohol abuse; history of acidosis; intravenous radiographic contrast media.
Side-effects	Gastrointestinal symptoms (eg diarrhoea); metallic taste; possibly reduced absorption of vitamin B_{12} and folic acid; ovulation in polycystic ovarian syndrome.
Adverse reactions	Risk of lactic acidosis if contraindications breached: risk of hypoglycaemia with combination therapy.
Precautions	Contraindications should be observed, especially renal function (eg creatinine level): interacts with cimetidine.

*Maximum dose varies between countries.

> About 5% of patients cannot tolerate any dose of metformin due to gastrointestinal side-effects

> The contraindications to metformin must be observed

Standard monitoring of glycaemic control by home blood glucose measurement, or measurement of fasting or random plasma glucose or HbA_{1c} at clinic visits is recommended with all diabetes treatment programmes. Since type 2 diabetes is a progressive disease, it may be necessary to increase the drug dosages or move to another stage in the treatment algorithm at any time. Metformin alone is unlikely to cause serious hypoglycaemia, but hypoglycaemia becomes an issue when metformin is used in combination with an insulin-releasing agent or insulin.

Efficacy

The long-term blood glucose-lowering efficacy of metformin is similar to that of the sulphonylureas, but the mechanism of action is different. Optimally titrated metformin monotherapy typically reduces fasting plasma glucose (FPG) by 2–4 mmol/l in type 2 patients inadequately controlled on non-pharmacological therapy, which corresponds to a decrease in HbA_{1c} of 1–2%. While metformin's effect is dependent on the presence of some endogenous β-cell function, it is independent of weight, age and duration of diabetes. (As the United Kingdom Prospective Diabetes Study illustrated, diabetes is characterized by a progressive increase in hyperglycaemia with time, principally due to deterioration of β-cell function, irrespective of the therapies used.)

Monotherapy with metformin offers several advantages. Its mechanism of action (it does not stimulate insulin secretion) means that it is unlikely to cause severe hypoglycaemia. Indeed, the reduction in insulin concentration, notably in hyperinsulinaemic patients, should actually improve insulin sensitivity by relieving the insulin-induced down-regulation of insulin receptors and suppression of post-receptor insulin pathways. Body weight tends to stabilize or decrease slightly during metformin therapy, and small improvements in the blood lipid profile may be observed in hyperlipidaemic patients. Thus, plasma concentrations of triglyceride, free fatty acids and low-density lipoprotein (LDL)-cholesterol tend to fall, while high-density lipoprotein (HDL)-cholesterol tends to rise. These effects appear to be independent of the antihyperglycaemic effect, although a lowering of triglyceride and free fatty acid levels is likely to improve insulin sensitivity and benefit the glucose–fatty acid cycle. In the United Kingdom Prospective Diabetes Study, patients who started oral antidiabetic therapy with metformin showed a reduced risk of myocardial infarction of 39% after 10 years. In addition to effects on body weight and lipid profile, several other potentially vasoprotective effects, including increased fibrinolysis and a reduced plasminogen activator inhibitor-1 (PAI-1) concentration, have been reported.

> Metformin significantly reduced the risk of myocardial infarction in the United Kingdom Prospective Diabetes Study

Combination of metformin with a sulphonylurea, repaglinide, acarbose or a thiazolidinedione produces an additive blood glucose-lowering effect, provided that the combination is instituted before severe β-cell failure. Although there is an increased risk of hypoglycaemia, the other effects of the two agents in combination are generally intermediate – the weight gain seen with a sulphonylurea is reduced in combination with metformin, for example, while the insulin reduction and improved lipid profile seen with metformin monotherapy are lessened in combination. Consistent with its ability to improve insulin sensitivity, when metformin is added to patients on insulin therapy, a reduction in insulin dosage is usually required. At the same time, most patients also show an improvement in glycaemic control. Metformin reduces the weight gain associated with insulin therapy, and decreasing the insulin dosage in itself decreases the risk of hypoglycaemic episodes. The regimen usually involves once-daily bedtime NPH or lente insulin or twice-daily NPH insulin with metformin at mealtimes.

> Metformin may be usefully combined with the sulphonylureas, repaglinide, the thiazolidinediones and insulin

Adverse effects

The most serious adverse event associated with metformin is lactic acidosis. The incidence is rare (about 0.03 cases per 1000 patient-years), but the associated mortality rate is about 50%. Since the background incidence of lactic acidosis among type 2 patients has not yet been established, it is likely that a proportion of cases are falsely attributed to the drug. Most cases in patients receiving metformin are due to malprescription. A commonly overlooked contraindication is renal insufficiency, which results in metformin accumulation. Excessive concentrations of metformin increase glycolysis to lactate, particularly in the splanchnic bed. The situation is aggravated by any co-existing hypoxic condition or impaired liver function. Although hyperlactataemia also occurs in cardiogenic shock and other illnesses that decrease tissue perfusion, metformin is usually an incidental factor in such cases. Metformin should be stopped in all cases of suspected or proven lactic acidosis, however, regardless of cause.

Severe lactic acidosis is typically characterized by a raised blood lactate concentration (eg >5 mmol/l), decreased pH (eg <7.25), and increased anion gap (eg $[Na^+] - [Cl^- + HCO_3^-]$ >15 mmol/l). Presenting symptoms are usually non-specific but often include hyperventilation, malaise and abdominal discomfort. Patients with suspected metformin-associated lactic acidosis should be admitted to hospital promptly and treatment with iv bicarbonate

commenced immediately, regardless of cause. If a raised plasma metformin concentration (eg >5 µg/ml) is found, circulating metformin can be removed by haemodialysis. Supportive measures to address any co-existing hypoxaemia or hypotension should also be initiated.

> Lactic acidosis is a rare but potentially lethal side-effect of biguanide treatment

Thiazolidinediones

The thiazolidinediones (TZDs) are agents which improve insulin sensitivity by stimulating a nuclear receptor known as the peroxisome proliferator-activated receptor-gamma (PPARγ). The TZDs are also referred to as PPARγ agonists, glitazones, insulin sensitizers and enhancers of insulin action.

> The thiazolidinediones are insulin-sensitizing drugs

Brief history

The antidiabetic activity of TZDs was described in the early 1980s and the first to become available for clinical use was troglitazone (Figure 10.3). Troglitazone was introduced in Japan and the US in 1997, but withdrawn in 2000 due to reports of fatal idiosyncratic hepatotoxicity. The drug was withdrawn by the UK distributor just weeks after its introduction in late 1997. Two other TZDs, rosiglitazone and pioglitazone, that have not been associated with this severe side-effect, were introduced in Japan and the US in 1999 and in Europe in 2000.

> Troglitazone, introduced in 1997, was withdrawn in 2000 following reports of fatal hepatotoxicity

Pharmacokinetics

Rosiglitazone and pioglitazone are quickly and almost completely absorbed (peak

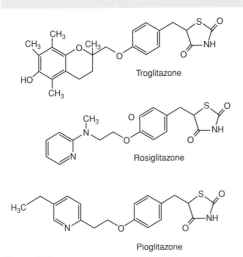

Troglitazone

Rosiglitazone

Pioglitazone

Figure 10.3
Chemical structures of the thiazolidinediones, troglitazone, rosiglitazone and pioglitazone.

concentration reached within one to two hours, slightly longer when taken with food) (Table 10.4). Both agents are extensively metabolized by the liver, rosiglitazone mainly to weakly active metabolites excreted more in urine than bile, pioglitazone to more active metabolites excreted mostly in bile. Rosiglitazone metabolism is undertaken mainly by CYP2C8, an isoform of cytochrome P450 which is not widely activated. Thus rosiglitazone does not interfere with the metabolism of other drugs. Pioglitazone is metabolized partly by CYP2C8, CYP3A4 and other isoforms of P450, and could potentially interfere with the metabolism of oral contraceptives and some other agents.

However, to date, no significant drug interactions have been reported, and the risk appears to be low. Although both TZDs are almost completely bound to plasma proteins, their concentrations are generally low and they have not been reported to interfere with other protein-bound drugs.

Mode of action

Stimulation of PPARγ appears to be the principal mechanism through which TZDs enhance insulin sensitivity. PPARγ is mostly (and strongly) expressed in adipose tissue where it operates in association with the retinoid X receptor to increase transcription of certain insulin-sensitive genes (Figure 10.4). These genes include lipoprotein lipase (LPL), the fatty acid transporter protein (FATP), the adipocyte fatty acid-binding protein (aP2), fatty acyl-CoA synthase and the insulin-sensitive glucose transporter, GLUT-4. Stimulation of PPARγ by a TZD will promote adipocyte differentiation and lipogenesis, and increase the local effects of insulin.

> Activation of PPARγ seems to be the principal mechanism through which the thiazolidinediones promote insulin action

PPARγ is weakly expressed in skeletal muscle and liver where it also appears to enhance certain insulin actions (Table 10.5). TZDs are reported to increase glucose uptake via GLUT-4 in muscle, and decrease gluconeogenesis in the

Table 10.4
Pharmacokinetic features of the thiazolidinediones rosiglitazone and pioglitazone.

	Rosiglitazone	Pioglitazone
Time to peak plasma concentration	Approximately 1 hour	<2 hours
Plasma $t_{1/2}$	Approximately 3.5 (100–150)* hours	3–7 (16–24)* hours
Plasma protein-bound	>99%	>99%
Hepatic metabolism	Mainly by CYP2C8 to several weakly active metabolites	Mainly by CYP2C8 and CYP3A4 to active metabolites
Elimination	Mainly urine (>60%)	Mainly bile (>60%)

* values in parentheses include metabolites.

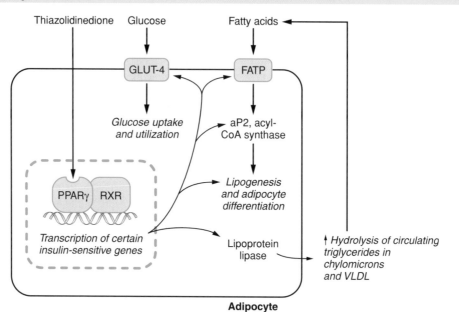

Adipocyte

Figure 10.4
Mechanism of action of a thiazolidinedione on an adipocyte PPARγ receptor (peroxisome proliferator-activated receptor gamma). RXR = retinoid X receptor; GLUT-4 = glucose transporter isoform 4; FATP = fatty acid transporter protein; aP2 = adipocyte fatty acid-binding protein; VLDL = very low density lipoproteins.

Table 10.5
Metabolic effects of the thiazolidinediones.

Adipose tissue	Muscle	Liver
↑ Glucose uptake	↑ Glucose uptake	↓ Gluconeogenesis
↑ Fatty acid uptake	↑ Glycolysis	↓ Glycogenolysis
↑ Lipogenesis	↑ Glucose oxidation	↑ Lipogenesis
↑ Differentiation	↑ Glycogenesis*	↑ Glucose uptake*

* = an inconsistent finding.

liver, possibly by reducing expression of phosphoenolpyruvate carboxykinase and increasing expression of glucokinase. Stimulation of lipogenesis via PPARγ reduces circulating non-esterified fatty acid (NEFA) concentrations which facilitates glucose use and reduces gluconeogenesis by correcting the glucose–fatty acid cycle. TZDs can also reduce the production and activity of cytokine tumour necrosis factor-α (TNFα) which has been implicated in the development of insulin resistance (page 21). The lowering of insulin

concentrations in hyperinsulinaemic patients, and the lowering of circulating triglyceride levels in some patients are further mechanisms which may help to improve insulin sensitivity.

TZDs, like metformin, are antihyperglycaemic, rather than hypoglycaemic, agents and require the presence of insulin to generate significant blood glucose-lowering effects. Their clinical efficacy is dependent on insulin levels sufficient to activate the genes listed above. They are not a substitute for the absence of insulin and they selectively enhance some effects of insulin on cellular metabolism and differentiation: they do not enhance all insulin effects. Thus TZDs act co-operatively with insulin to create an insulin-sparing and glucose-lowering effect linked to their lipogenic activity. Interestingly, the glucose-lowering activity of TZDs remains evident in animals devoid of adipose tissue, demonstrating the importance of the less prominent effects of the TZDs on other tissues.

Indications and contraindications

Rosiglitazone and pioglitazone are available for use as monotherapy in the US in non-obese and obese patients with type 2 diabetes inadequately controlled by non-pharmacological measures. They can also be used in combination with various other antidiabetic drugs in patients inadequately controlled by monotherapy. Rosiglitazone and pioglitazone are indicated for use in combination with metformin or a sulphonylurea in Europe, but not as monotherapy.

The general principles for initiating treatment with a TZD are essentially the same as those for initiating sulphonylurea or metformin treatment. The main cautions are listed in Table 10.6. Rosiglitazone and pioglitazone can lead to fluid retention with increased plasma volume, reduced haematocrit and a decrease in haemoglobin. The risk of oedema and anaemia should be appreciated, and patients with any evidence of congestive heart disease or heart failure are contraindicated (although precisely whom to exclude on the basis of cardiac status currently varies according to the different product labelling sheets in Europe and the US).

Haemoglobin should be checked before starting a TZD, bearing in mind that reductions of up to 1 g/dl may occur during therapy. No adverse effects on blood pressure have been noted, despite the increase in plasma volume. Liver function should also be checked – by measuring serum alanine transaminase (ALT) level – both before starting therapy and at intervals thereafter, especially during the first year of treatment. Pre-existing liver disease or the development of elevated ALT levels are contraindications, although hepatotoxicity has not been a major concern with either rosiglitazone or pioglitazone; two cases of non-fatal hepatocellular damage have been attributed to rosiglitazone during six months of use by more than 100,000 patients in the US. Precautionary monitoring of liver function remains a condition for TZD use because of the cases of fatal idiosyncratic hepatotoxicity seen with troglitazone.

Table 10.6
Clinical use of the thiazolidinediones.

Indications	Type 2 diabetic patients inadequately controlled by non-pharmacological measures or other oral antidiabetic agents.
Type of therapy	Monotherapy, or in combination with any other antidiabetic agents.*
Treatment schedule	Pioglitazone (15 or 30 mg/day); rosiglitazone (2 or 4 mg/day). Dose should be escalated gradually up to a typical maximum of 45 mg/day for pioglitazone† and 8 mg/day for rosiglitazone.
Cautions and contraindications	Congestive heart disease; heart failure‡; oedema; anaemia; impaired liver function.
Side-effects	Fluid retention; increased plasma volume; reduced haematocrit; decreased haemoglobin; ovulation in polycystic ovarian syndrome.
Adverse reactions	Risk of oedema and anaemia: risk of hypoglycaemia with combination therapy.
Precautions	Check for contraindications; monitor liver enzymes (eg alanine transaminase); potential effect on oral contraceptive activity (pioglitazone).

*Monotherapy and insulin combination not available in Europe.
†Maximum recommended daily dosage varies between countries.
‡Definition of heart failure in the product label varies between countries.

> Liver function tests must be undertaken both before and during treatment with the thiazolidinediones

The starting dose should always be low – 2 mg rosiglitazone once or twice a day or 15 mg pioglitazone once a day. Glucose monitoring and dosage titration are important, particularly bearing in mind that the TZDs exert a slowly generated antihyperglycaemic effect. In fact, full expression of the appropriate dosage may not occur until two to three months after first administration – rosiglitazone 4 mg twice-daily and pioglitazone 30 mg/day are commonly used dosages. If no effect is observed after three months, it is appropriate to consider the patient a non-responder.

Rosiglitazone and pioglitazone can be used in the elderly, provided there are no contraindications. In women with anovulatory polycystic ovary syndrome (PCOS) the improvement in insulin sensitivity may cause ovulation to resume.

Efficacy

The slowly generated blood glucose-lowering effect of TZDs in type 2 diabetes is explained by the substantial contribution of the nuclear effect, altering the expression of certain insulin-sensitive genes (Figure 10.4). Hence, maximal effect may take two to three months to occur, much longer than for other oral antidiabetic agents. Pre-registration trials with rosiglitazone and pioglitazone found that monotherapy with these agents reduced fasting plasma glucose (FPG) by about 3 mmol/l compared with baseline (Table 10.7). Some trial periods were too short to provide detailed information on HbA_{1c}, and overall, the suggestion was that the HbA_{1c} reduction was only about 0.6%. However, preliminary extension studies now suggest greater reductions with long-term use. It should be noted that not all patients respond to TZDs, and that the efficacy of this class of drug is highly dependent on adequate insulin concentrations being present.

> The thiazolidinediones require the presence of adequate quantities of insulin to exert their metabolic effects

Table 10.7
Blood glucose-lowering effects of rosiglitazone and pioglitazone in type 2 diabetic patients.
Data from published abstracts.

	Dose (mg/day)	Duration (weeks)	↓ FPG* (mmol/l)	↓ HbA_{1c}* (%)
Monotherapy				
Rosiglitazone	8	26	3.0	0.6
Pioglitazone	30	16	2.8	0.6
Combination with sulphonylurea[†]				
Rosiglitazone	4	26	2.1	0.9
Pioglitazone	30	16	2.9	1.2
Combination with metformin[†]				
Rosiglitazone	8	26	2.7	0.8
Pioglitazone	30	16	2.4	0.6
Combination with insulin				
Rosiglitazone	8	26	2.5	1.2[a]
Pioglitazone	30	16	2.7	1.2[b]

FPG = fasting plasma glucose; * = decrease from baseline; [†] = patients poorly controlled on existing treatment before rosiglitazone or pioglitazone added in; [a] = average decrease in insulin dose of 9 units/day; [b] = 16% of patients reduced their insulin dose by >25%.

Monotherapy with a TZD may produce a modest antihyperglycaemic effect, but the evidence suggests that efficacy is often enhanced when these drugs are combined with those from another class. Addition of rosiglitazone or pioglitazone to patients who are ill but stable on a sulphonylurea or metformin, for example, has consistently shown significant reductions in FPG and HbA$_{1c}$ (Table 10.7). Estimates of insulin sensitivity and endogenous β-cell function (based on analysis of basal glucose and insulin concentrations) have also indicated that TZD addition improves both these parameters.

In addition to improved glycaemic control, TZDs influence other aspects of metabolism. They invariably reduce circulating NEFA concentrations, one of the mechanisms, in fact, through which they can improve glycaemic control (page 148). Rosiglitazone seems to cause a small rise in total cholesterol levels, but this stabilizes within three to six months. This increase is accounted for by a rise in both the LDL-cholesterol and the HDL-cholesterol levels, which leaves the LDL:HDL and the total:HDL ratios little changed or slightly higher. HDL-cholesterol levels may continue to rise after six months. Pioglitazone appears to have little effect on total cholesterol, and has been shown to reduce triglyceride concentrations in some studies.

> Rosiglitazone and pioglitazone seem to have different effects on plasma lipids

Weight gain has been observed during TZD therapy, similar in magnitude to that seen during sulphonylurea therapy – typically 1–4 kg and stabilizing over six to 12 months. There is preliminary evidence that the distribution of body fat is also altered: visceral adipose depots may be reduced while subcutaneous adipose depots increase.

> Weight gain and oedema are prominent side-effects of the thiazolidinediones

Finally, there are provisional data to suggest that the TZDs exert a range of effects on vascular function which might reduce cardiovascular risk. They have been reported to down-regulate plasminogen activator inhibitor-1 (PAI-1) and to decrease urinary albumin excretion to a greater extent than would be expected by the improvement in glycaemic control. Preclinical studies have noted that chronic treatment of diabetic and glucose-intolerant animals with a TZD can preserve β-cell granulation and reduce β-cell failure.

Adverse effects

Rosiglitazone and pioglitazone have shown encouraging tolerability. The precautions related to heart disease, oedema, anaemia and liver function include intermittent monitoring in accordance with package labelling. Pioglitazone has rarely been associated with an elevation in creatine kinase concentration and myalgia. More than mild hypoglycaemia may occur when the TZDs are used in combination with other antidiabetic agents. If contraindications arise during treatment, monitoring should be intensified and then, if necessary, treatment discontinued.

Since PPARγ is expressed by many tissues, albeit at a low level, only time will tell if TZD stimulation has any unforeseen chronic effects. PPARγ activation in macrophages can reduce the production of some inflammatory cytokines and might increase transformation of monocytes to macrophages in the vascular wall. Stimulation of PPARγ in colon cells has been variously reported to increase and decrease cell division and differentiation in different animal and cell models.

> Pioglitazone and rosiglitazone have not been reported to cause severe hepatotoxicity compared with troglitazone

Future therapies to improve insulin action

Other PPARγ agonists

Several novel TZDs and other types of PPARγ agonists have been shown to improve insulin action in cultured cells and reduce insulin resistance in animal models of impaired glucose tolerance and type 2 diabetes. Some of these compounds have also been reported to improve glycaemic control during preliminary clinical trials in type 2 patients, and we expect these to be developed further. Several are agonists of both PPARγ and PPARα-mediated lipid oxidation. Stimulation of the latter nuclear receptor should confer a distinctive lipid-lowering effect.

Vanadium salts

Early clinical studies have confirmed that vanadium salts improve glycaemic control in type 2 patients. They act within two to three weeks to reduce fasting plasma glucose and improve glucose tolerance. They reduce hepatic glucose production and enhance insulin-mediated glucose use in muscle. These effects are brought about, at least in part, by an inhibitory effect on the phosphatases that dephosphorylate and deactivate the insulin receptor. Other cellular actions which could increase and mimic the effects of insulin have also been noted. Concern over the toxic effects of vanadium accumulation are a current challenge.

Insulin receptor-signalling enhancers

Other substances which enhance insulin receptor signalling by phosphatase inhibition or other mechanisms are currently being sought. The possibility of using insulin-like growth factor-1 (IGF-1) to stimulate insulin action via IGF-1 receptors is an option in rare cases of near-total disruption of insulin receptors, but its excess mitogenic and growth-promoting effects preclude more general use.

Several agents have been reported to stimulate post-receptor insulin-signalling intermediates and to increase translocation of insulin-sensitive GLUT-4 glucose transporters into the plasma membrane. Others have been shown to enhance the activity of enzymes of glycogenesis, glycolysis and glucose oxidation directly. Few of these options have proved suitable for further clinical evaluation, however. In contrast, lipoic acid, which has recently been tested for the

treatment of diabetic neuropathy, has been reported to improve both insulin sensitivity and glycaemic control in clinical trials.

Other agents

Deficiencies in certain minerals, notably chromium and magnesium, are associated with decreased insulin sensitivity, and patients with these deficiencies have shown improved glycaemic control after supplementation with magnesium salts or trivalent chromium. Extra intake of the antioxidant vitamins C and E has produced equivocal effects on glycaemic control in the limited trials to date. Agents designed to inhibit fatty acid oxidation, inhibit glucose-6-phosphatase, or suppress the secretion or action of counter-regulatory hormones such as glucagon have been described, but have not yet given rise to viable treatments. The amylin analogue pramlintide is an injectable peptide that has been shown to improve glycaemic control through several neurally mediated effects, including delayed gastric emptying, decreased glucagon secretion and a satiety action. Pramlintide reduces weight gain and is currently being considered as an adjunct to insulin therapy.

Further reading

Bailey CJ. New pharmacological approaches to glycaemic control. *Diabetes Rev* 1999; **7**: 94-113.

Bailey CJ. Potential new treatments for type 2 diabetes. *TIPS* 2000; **21**: 259-65.

Bailey CJ, Turner RC. Metformin. *N Engl J Med* 1996; **334**: 574-9.

Cusi K, DeFronzo RA. Metformin: a review of its metabolic effects. *Diabetes Rev* 1998; **6**: 89-131.

Day C. Thiazolidinediones: a new class of antidiabetic drug. *Diabetic Med* 1999; **16**: 1-14.

Evans AJ, Krentz AJ. Recent developments and emerging therapies for type 2 diabetes mellitus. In: Krentz AJ, Ed. *Drug treatment of type 2 diabetes*. Auckland: Adis International, 2000; 1-22.

Howlett HCS, Bailey CJ. A risk-benefit assessment of metformin in type 2 diabetes mellitus. In: Krentz AJ, Ed. *Drug treatment of type 2 diabetes*. Auckland: Adis International, 2000; 61-76.

Murphy E, Nolan JJ. Insulin sensitizer drugs. *Exp Opin Invest Drugs* 2000; **9**: 1347-61.

Schoonjans K, Auwerx J. Thiazolidinediones: an update. *Lancet* 2000; **355**: 1008-10.

Spiegelman BM. PPARγ: adipogenic regulator and thiazolidinedione receptor. *Diabetes* 1998; **47**: 507-14.

11. Pharmacological treatment III: insulin

Insulin preparations
Insulin species
Duration of insulin action
Starting insulin therapy
Insulin delivery systems
Unwanted effects of insulin therapy
Special situations
Patient acceptability
Combination therapy with oral agents
Discontinuation of insulin therapy

Insulin is life-sustaining in patients with type 1 diabetes because of the absence of endogenous insulin production due to near-complete β-cell destruction. Insulin is often used to improve metabolic control in patients with type 2

diabetes. The United Kingdom Prospective Diabetes Study (page 56) highlighted the progressive nature of type 2 diabetes, showing that a substantial proportion of patients will eventually require insulin to achieve and maintain their glycaemic target (Figure 11.1). Others will be treated with insulin rather than oral antidiabetic agents because complications such as advanced diabetic nephropathy make insulin the safest option (page 81). Clinical trial data have suggested that insulin is associated with decreased mortality after acute myocardial infarction (page 93) and insulin is often required temporarily in type 2 patients during other severe acute illnesses such as major sepsis, and surgery. Insulin is also regarded as the treatment of choice for gestational diabetes when dietary measures prove insufficient.

In the UK, about 20–25% of type 2 diabetic patients are estimated to require insulin within 10 years of diagnosis, although a greater proportion of patients, namely those who are inadequately controlled on other therapies, would probably benefit. In the US, 30–40% of type 2 patients are currently receiving insulin, partly because there was previously a smaller range of oral agents available in the US, but

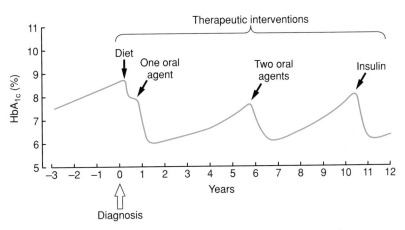

Figure 11.1
Typical changes in HbA$_{1c}$ values during treatment of a patient with type 2 diabetes requiring diet, then one oral antidiabetic agent, then two differently acting oral antidiabetic agents, and eventually insulin therapy, to control the progressive natural history of the disease.

also because the US has a greater proportion of severely obese type 2 patients (whose condition cannot be controlled with sulphonylureas).

In recent decades, developments in insulin manufacture have led to successive refinements, initially with improvements in purity, and then with the mass production of human sequence insulin. These advances have been coupled with advances in injection devices, making the practicalities much less daunting and more comfortable. Even after decades of experience, however, the optimal use of insulin and avoidance of its major unwanted side-effect – hypoglycaemia – remain elusive targets. The reality is that subcutaneous insulin injection can only ever approximate to the exquisitely sensitive response of a normal healthy individual's islet β-cells to glucose and other endogenous regulators (chapter 2). Further, there are fundamental problems with exogenous insulin use:

- Delivery into the systemic rather than portal circulation causes plasma insulin concentrations to be equally high in both circulation systems (in the physiological situation, portal levels are much higher), so that hyperinsulinaemia is a common occurrence.
- Systemic delivery delays the onset of action, and results in a relatively prolonged effect, compared with endogenously secreted insulin; there is a suboptimal matching of delivery peak and decline of insulin concentrations relative to meals. In particular, it is difficult to mimic the endogenous surge of insulin into the portal circulation at the beginning of a meal, which normally promptly suppresses hepatic glucose production.
- There is no scope for reducing plasma insulin levels in response to fasting or exercise once an injection has been given.
- It is difficult to control the fasting plasma glucose concentration (by suppressing hepatic glucose production) without inducing hypoglycaemia during the night.

- There is day-to-day variability in the absorption of intermediate-duration insulin in individual patients – more than is generally appreciated.
- There is an accompanying need for dietary restriction, including consuming an approximately similar quantity of carbohydrate at a set (meal) time each day and the need for between-meal snacks to prevent interprandial hypoglycaemia in some patients.

Certain clinical situations present further considerations:

- Obese patients with inadequately controlled type 2 diabetes (common) and those with additional causes for insulin resistance (page 21) have higher insulin requirements.
- Insulin clearance is impaired by complications such as renal impairment (relatively common) or the presence of hepatic cirrhosis.

A selection of short-, intermediate- and long-acting insulins, as well as mixtures of these three are available (Table 11.1). Recently, the range of mixed formulations has been increased by the introduction of the rapid-acting insulin analogues lispro (Humalog, Eli Lilly) and aspart (Rapitard, Novo Nordisk). In 2000, the first soluble long-acting analogue, glargine (Lantus, Aventis), was also approved for use in patients with type 1 and type 2 diabetes. Finer needles, new types of power injectors and mini-pumps now facilitate insulin administration.

Most patients will be started on insulin under the guidance of the local hospital diabetes resource centre or clinic. Some – the elderly, senile or infirm, for example – may be unable to self-administer insulin, in which case a responsible relative or district nurse is called in. Insulin therapy should always be accompanied by self-monitoring of capillary blood glucose by the patient where possible (page 60).

Table 11.1
Synopsis of insulin preparations*

Category	Rapid	Short	Short–intermediate	Intermediate	Long
Generic type		Regular ('soluble')†	Regular isophane (NPH) mixture	Isophane (NPH)	Crystalline zinc suspensions
Examples	Aspart Lispro	Actrapid Humulin S	Mixtard Humulin M1-5	Insulatard Humulin I	Ultratard Humulin Zn
Onset of action (minutes)	10–20	15–60	15–60	60–120	120–240
Duration of action (hours)	3–5	4–8	12–18	12–18	18–>24

*Times for onset and duration of action are approximate ranges that vary between individuals, with dose and site of subcutaneous injection and pathophysiological state.
†The term 'soluble' is no longer exclusively applicable to short-acting insulins. NPH = neutral protamine Hagedorn.

Insulin preparations

The variety of insulin preparations is daunting, but the types and methods of delivery can be summarized quite succinctly. Insulins are usually classified according to their onset and duration of action (Figure 11.2), but also vary in terms of:

- species and method of manufacture (animal-derived, semi-synthetic or synthetic)
- modifications which prolong duration of action
- designated mode of delivery (syringe, pen injector, or infusion device, for example)

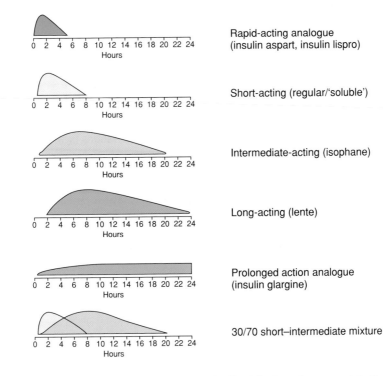

Rapid-acting analogue (insulin aspart, insulin lispro)

Short-acting (regular/'soluble')

Intermediate-acting (isophane)

Long-acting (lente)

Prolonged action analogue (insulin glargine)

30/70 short–intermediate mixture

Figure 11.2
Approximate times of onset and durations of action of various insulins following subcutaneous injection.

- strength – in the UK, all insulin preparations contain 100 units/ml (U100). Other strengths (U40, U80 and U500) are available in some other countries (or can be obtained by special request to the manufacturer).

Insulin species

Therapeutic insulin is derived from three sources:

Bovine

Bovine insulin is extracted from cattle pancreas. It is effectively obsolete but still available for patients who have been using it for many years. Long-term use is often associated with the presence of anti-insulin antibodies. Bovine insulin differs from human insulin (Figure 2.1) in three amino acids: A8 alanine, A10 valine and B30 alanine.

Porcine

Porcine insulin differs from human insulin in a single amino-acid (alanine replaces threonine at B30). It is reserved mainly for patients with type 1 diabetes who have experienced a decrease in the warning symptoms for hypoglycaemia with human insulin.

Human and genetically engineered

Human insulin is by far the most commonly used and now manufactured predominantly using recombinant DNA technology. Chemical (enzymatic) modification of porcine insulin (emp) is still employed by one major manufacturer (Novo Nordisk) in the production of so-called 'semi-synthetic' insulin. The method of manufacture is always stated on the bottle:

- prb – produced from the precursor molecule proinsulin and synthesized using recombinant DNA by bacteria containing the human proinsulin gene
- pyr – produced recombinantly from a precursor synthesized by yeast
- ge – genetically engineered – a more generic label.

Animal-derived insulins are unacceptable to devout followers of Islam and Judaism and to strict vegans.

The recently introduced insulin analogues (the rapid-acting lispro and aspart, and the prolonged duration insulin glargine) are genetically engineered:

Insulin lispro

Insulin lispro differs from human insulin by the transposition of two amino acids on the B chain of the molecule; from B28 proline and B29 lysine to B28 lysine and B29 proline (lys–pro becoming 'lispro').

Insulin aspart

In insulin aspart, aspartate replaces proline at position B28.

Insulin glargine

Two additional arginine molecules (B31 arginine and B32 arginine) are located at the C-terminus of the B-chain, conferring additional positive charges and thereby altering the isoelectric point. In addition, asparagine is replaced by arginine at A21, to confer stability.

Duration of insulin action

Short-acting insulins

Short-acting insulins (synonyms: soluble, regular, neutral, unmodified) differ slightly in their pharmacokinetics according to species. Onset of action following subcutaneous injection is fastest for human, followed by porcine, then bovine insulin.

> Human sequence short-acting insulins have a slightly faster onset and shorter duration of action than animal insulins

These differences, which may reflect lipophilic properties, are minor. For insulin to exert its effects in target tissues it must be absorbed from the subcutaneous injection site and diffuse from the interstitial space into the circulation. The rate at which this occurs is the principal determinant of the speed of onset of action, but other factors that influence pharmacokinetics include:

- site of injection – absorption from abdominal wall is faster than from thigh
- volume injected – smaller volumes are more quickly absorbed
- local mechanical factors – massage of injection site or exercise of local muscles will increase absorption rate.

Insulin can become denatured and lose efficacy if exposed to extremes of high or low temperature; storage at 4°C in a domestic refrigerator is usually recommended, freezing is not. Following subcutaneous injection of a human short-acting insulin preparation, the action profile is likely to be:

- onset around 30 minutes
- peak at one to three hours
- duration of four to eight hours.

When injected intravenously, the plasma half-life of a short-acting insulin is less than five minutes; continuous infusion is therefore required to maintain plasma levels. The only notable exceptions are when an iv bolus is required in a diagnostic endocrine test (eg the insulin tolerance test), when possible severe insulin resistance is being assessed, or for research purposes. Short-acting insulins are, in fact, the only preparations suitable for iv administration – modified insulins must be injected subcutaneously.

> Only unmodified, short-acting insulins are suitable for iv use

Pharmacokinetic properties dictate the timing of injections of short-acting insulin. Ideally, injections should take place 30–45 minutes before meals, in order to match peak action to glucose absorption from the gastrointestinal tract – but this is not always practical. A delayed meal carries the risk of hypoglycaemia. For an elderly patient, possibly senile, or reliant on a third party for insulin administration, it may be safer to ensure that the meal has been eaten first (tight glycaemic control is not usually an objective of treatment for such patients, and pharmacokinetic considerations are less of a concern). In contrast, patients using pen injection devices may prefer to take their insulin as the meal is served – although this applies more to rapid-acting insulins.

Rapid-acting insulins

The amino acid substitutions within these insulin molecules (opposite) reduce the tendency of the molecules to self-associate (as dimers and hexamers). This results in more rapid absorption into the bloodstream after subcutaneous injection (Figure 11.3). Compared with human short-acting insulin, rapid-acting insulins are characterized by an earlier peak and reduced duration of action:

- onset at 10–20 minutes
- peak at 40–60 minutes
- duration of three to five hours.

The rapid-acting analogues are an alternative to short-acting insulin, designed for use immediately before (or even just after) meals (Figure 11.4). Compared with human short-acting insulin, they produce an additional reduction in post-prandial peak glucose concentration of about 1–2 mmol/l. In patients with type 2 diabetes, they are most conveniently administered as pre-mixed preparations suitable for twice-daily use.

Twice-daily mixtures

Short-acting insulins may be mixed in the syringe with longer-acting preparations (isophane or, less commonly, lente). If insulins are mixed at home or in the surgery, the short-acting preparation *must* be drawn into the syringe before the longer-acting preparation to avoid contaminating the short-acting vial with protamine or zinc. Fixed, premixed combinations are also available: 10/90 (eg Humulin M1, Human Mixtard 10) through to 50:50 ratios of short to isophane (eg Humulin M5, Human Mixtard 50). This book uses the

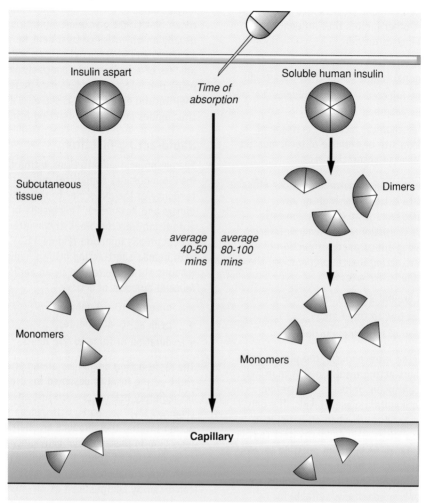

Figure 11.3
Rapid-acting insulin aspart dissociates into monomers more quickly than regular short-acting ('soluble') insulin.
Reproduced with permission from Heller S. *Prescriber* 2000; **11**: 47-53.

European nomenclature, which states the percentage of the shorter-acting insulin before the percentage of the longer-acting component. A 30/70 mixture twice daily is often favoured in the UK (Figure 11.5). If the glucose profile suggests it might be advantageous, it is acceptable to use a different preparation for the morning and evening injection. A pre-mixed preparation (Humalog Mix 25) comprising the analogue lispro and neutral protamine lispro (25% and 75%, respectively) has been designed for administration immediately before (or in some circumstances just after) meals.

> The nomenclature for premixed insulins varies from country to country.
>
> In Europe the percentage of the shorter-acting insulin ingredient is stated first; in the US the percentage of the longer-acting ingredient is stated first

Multiple daily injections

Another approach is to administer a short-acting insulin injection approximately 30 minutes before breakfast, lunch and dinner, and

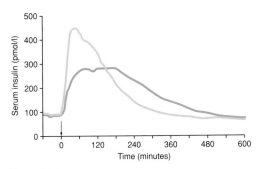

Figure 11.4
Serum insulin levels rise and fall rapidly with insulin aspart. Reproduced with permission from Heller S. *Prescriber* 2000; **11**: 47-53. ⎯⎯ = insulin aspart; ⎯⎯ = short-acting insulin.

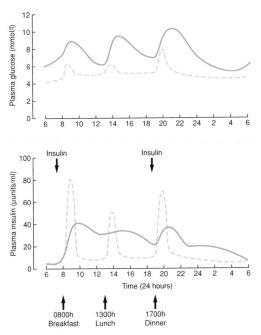

Figure 11.5
Daily plasma glucose and insulin profiles of a non-diabetic individual (- - - -) and a patient with type 2 diabetes (⎯⎯⎯). The type 2 diabetic patient was treated twice daily with a mixture of short- and intermediate-acting insulin. A slightly larger dose of both was given in the morning before breakfast than in the evening before dinner.

to then administer a longer-acting insulin at bedtime (around 2200 hours) to provide control until the following morning. Coupled with frequent blood glucose testing, this regimen forms the basis for so-called intensified insulin therapy in pursuit of a near-normal daily glucose profile, and is encouraged, where appropriate, in type 1 patients. It may also be useful in some type 2 patients, particularly those who require insulin during pregnancy (once-daily injection of a medium- or long-acting insulin is rarely sufficient). Multiple injections may be unsuitable for elderly or infirm patients, in whom excellent glycaemic control is not the primary objective. Increasing insulin dose to reduce fasting hyperglycaemia increases the risk of hypoglycaemia during interprandial periods, especially at night. A general guide is that if the patient requires a total daily dose of ≥30–40 units, this is split into two or more injections. The exception is when insulin is administered solely at bedtime to type 2 patients whose principal aim is to control a severely raised fasting plasma glucose concentration. Insulin glargine may prove to be more useful to such patients, with its potential to stabilize insulin throughout a 24-hour period and lessen the risk of hypoglycaemia (page 160).

Intermediate-duration insulins; isophane

Insulin is complexed with the fish sperm protein protamine to produce an isophane preparation. Isophane preparations have a slower onset and longer duration of action than unmodified short-acting insulins and are known generically as isophane or neutral protamine Hagedorn (NPH). They are well-established and widely used and have the following action profile:

- onset at about one to two hours
- peak at four to eight hours
- duration of 12–18 hours.

Once-daily NPH or lente insulin regimens seldom provide adequate glycaemic control: twice-daily regimens are more effective

Such preparations (eg Humulin I, Human Insulatard) may be used twice daily as monotherapy. In type 2 patients who have been inadequately controlled with oral agents, a single morning dose is seldom enough. More commonly, morning and evening administration is required. The morning dose is often given in conjunction with a short-acting insulin and pre-mixed preparations, often termed 'biphasic' or 'short–intermediate', are usually preferred in this respect. An alternative approach is to give an intermediate-acting insulin as monotherapy at bedtime, and to supplement it with an oral agent during the day. The principal aim of this type of regimen is to control pre-breakfast hyperglycaemia by suppressing overnight hepatic glucose production. The insulin-mediated suppression of fatty acid release from adipocytes may help to reduce glucose output from the liver by reducing the energy source for gluconeogenesis. However, waning of insulin action in the pre-breakfast period, possibly coupled with an intrinsic tendency for fasting plasma glucose concentrations to creep up at this time (the so-called 'dawn phenomenon') are factors that may detract from successful control. Because increasing the insulin dose carries a risk of night-time hypoglycaemia, a second injection pre-breakfast is often required. Increasingly, a single bedtime dose of isophane (NPH) is used in combination with daytime oral agents (page 172).

Long-acting insulins; PZI and lente preparations

Protamine zinc insulin (Hypurin bovine PZI, CP Pharmaceuticals) is not used much nowadays, although some patients have been successfully maintained on it for many years. It is a long-acting (>24 hours) insulin, but presents problems if mixed with short-acting analogues (excess protamine will tend to convert some of the short-acting into longer-acting insulin). Patients need not be transferred if this does not present a problem, but increasing the zinc content of the insulin preparation will result in amorphous (micro-crystalline) and crystalline insulins with prolonged action:

- onset at two to four hours
- peak at six to 18 hours
- duration of 18–>24 hours (amorphous, 18 hours; semilente, ie 30% amorphous, 70% crystalline, 18–24 hours; crystalline, >24 hours.

Examples of lente insulins include Human Monotard (Novo Nordisk) and Humulin Lente (Lilly); these are best used twice daily. Lente insulins contain an excess of zinc which can modify the action of a short-acting insulin if mixed in the same syringe. Although this should, in theory, delay the rise in plasma insulin concentration, in practice it seems to be of minor clinical significance as long as the mixture is prepared and injected without delay. Combinations of lente and short-acting insulins are not suitable for pre-mixed biphasic (short–intermediate mixed) preparations. Lente insulins have become less popular with the emergence of the biphasics.

Prolonged-action soluble insulins

The first example of a prolonged-action soluble insulin analogue, insulin glargine (Lantus, Aventis) became available in 2000. This analogue was designed to avoid the peak insulin concentration typically observed with conventional longer-acting insulins such as lente. Insulin glargine shows the following action profile (Figure 11.6):

- onset at about 90 minutes
- prolonged plateau, rather than peak
- duration of about 24 hours or longer.

While insulin glargine is soluble at acid pH in the vial, when injected subcutaneously it forms a microprecipitate at the injection site (because the latter is at a slightly alkaline, physiological pH). The stability of this microprecipitate slows absorption of insulin into the circulation, which means that a single daily injection can provide a fairly stable level of insulin for most of a 24-hour period, more closely mimicking the basal component of insulin secretion in healthy subjects. 'Basal' insulin secretion accounts for about half of all

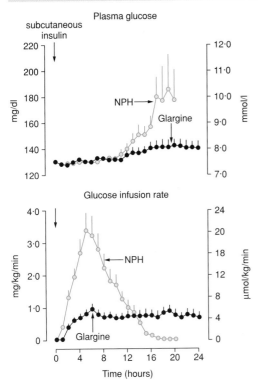

Figure 11.6
Plasma glucose and rates of glucose infusion required to maintain plasma glucose concentration at the target of 7.2 mmol/l in 20 patients with type 1 diabetes following injection of either 0.3 units/kg insulin glargine or NPH
Reproduced with permission from Bolli GB, Owens DR. *Lancet* 2000; **356**: 443-4.

daily insulin secretion, the rest being secreted in response to meals. Further studies are required in type 2 patients, but the peakless action of insulin glargine offers potential for reducing the incidence of hypoglycaemia (especially nocturnal episodes).

> Insulin glargine is a clear solution – the era when all clear preparations were short-acting insulins has passed

Another preparation with prolonged action, NN 304 (Insulin detemir, Novo Nordisk) represents a different approach; a fatty acyl group is

attached to the B chain (B29 lysine) of the insulin molecule which binds to albumin in the circulation. Clinical trials are in progress.

Starting insulin therapy

Indications

Insulin treatment should be considered in patients in whom glycaemic control has remained unsatisfactory with non-pharmacological measures and a combination of differently acting, optimally titrated, oral agents. It should also be considered for symptomatic patients with serious co-morbidity and for patients contraindicated for, or intolerant of, other oral therapies.

Procedure

The insulin starting dose is dependent on the extent of existing hyperglycaemia, whether or not the patient is obese, concomitant therapies and co-morbidity. If the HbA$_{1c}$ is >8% on current therapy:

- consider starting at 10 units/day
- monitor fasting plasma glucose (eg by self-monitoring)
- titrate up by two units/day to achieve target control
- if patient is obese, consider adding one unit/day to starting dose for each BMI unit >30
- if there is renal or hepatic impairment consider starting at a lower insulin dose.

If the HbA$_{1c}$ is <8% on current therapy, consider starting at six units/day and then monitor, titrate and adjust as above.

Selection of regimen

The insulin regimen should be tailored to the individual patient's circumstances. Twice-daily isophane (NPH) is a popular choice. The total daily dose is divided: about two-thirds is given before breakfast and one-third before dinner/at bedtime. Alternatively, a mixture of short-acting and intermediate-acting insulins, eg pre-mixed 30/70, might be appropriate.

More complicated regimens should only be used if necessary. These might include:

- bedtime intermediate-acting or long-acting insulin with pre-meal supplements of rapid-acting or short-acting insulin
- bedtime intermediate-acting or long-acting insulin with day-time oral agents
- pre-meal supplements of rapid-acting or short-acting insulin plus an oral insulin action enhancer such as metformin or a thiazolidinedione at bedtime and in the morning if required.

Note that a combination of insulin with a thiazolidinedione is not presently permitted in Europe. Other regimens are discussed elsewhere in this chapter.

Insulin delivery systems

Subcutaneous injections

Self-administered subcutaneous injection using a syringe has traditionally been the mainstay of insulin therapy. Injections have been made more convenient and less unpleasant by features such as disposable plastic syringes and ultrafine, lubricated needles. Technical problems with modern syringes are now very uncommon.

> Disposable plastic insulin syringes may be used several times (by the same individual)

It is no longer considered necessary to clean the injection site with alcohol before injecting (although the site should be clean), or to draw back on the plunger (to check that a vein hasn't been entered), or to compress the preferred site

Table 11.2
Recommended procedure for insulin injection.

1. Shake vial gently and invert.
2. Draw air (equivalent to injection volume) into syringe.
3. Pierce vial cap.
4. Expel air and draw insulin into syringe up to required mark on syringe.
5. Inject syringe contents at 90° to skin surface.

routinely. Too shallow an injection will be delivered intradermally, which can be painful and may cause local atrophy (evident as pitting), while too deep an injection may be delivered intramuscularly. The recommended procedure for subcutaneous insulin injection is outlined in Table 11.2.

Anatomical injection sites

Traditionally, patients are advised to vary the location of their injection site (Figure 11.7). This helps to avoid local reactions to insulin, although these are now infrequently encountered in patients with type 2 diabetes.

Allergy

Local allergic reactions are uncommon with modern insulin preparations; transient tender nodules developing at the injection site are suggestive, but generalized allergic reactions are rare.

Lipohypertrophy

Localized areas of lipohypertrophy, although comfortable for injections, are thought to cause erratic absorption of insulin at the site. The hypertrophy is attributed to the trophic effects of insulin on fat metabolism. Avoidance of the area may lead to regression; liposuction has also been used.

Lipoatrophy

Lipoatrophy has been rare since the introduction of highly purified insulins and human insulins. Its incidence may be reduced by injection of highly purified short-acting insulin around the edge of the lesion.

Patients may occasionally complain of recurrent minor local bleeding or bruising, but this rarely presents any cause for serious concern.

Pen injector devices

These continue to increase in popularity and are suitable for most insulin-treated patients. So-called pen injectors are self-contained devices which obviate the need to draw insulin into a syringe from the vial. They use replaceable

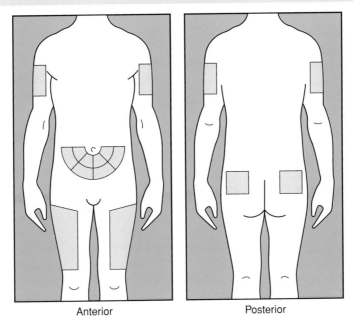

Anterior   Posterior

Figure 11.7

Recommended sites for subcutaneous insulin injection. Reproduced with permission from Krentz AJ. *Churchill's Pocketbook of Diabetes*. Edinburgh: Churchill Livingstone, 2000.

insulin cartridges and the mechanized dosage selection facilitates more accurate dispensing of injection volumes. Errors arising from air bubbles are also eliminated if the needle is cleared by expelling two to four units before use. The required dose is dialled and then injected by depressing a plunger. Pens can be very useful for the visually impaired (magnifiers are available) and patients with arthritis or other physical problems interfering with their manual dexterity. They can also improve compliance – particularly in children and adolescents. In fact, few patients now elect to use a conventional syringe.

A selection of pen designs incorporating different features to appeal to different patients is available (no extra charge) and patients should be allowed to choose the one that suits them best. Options include preloaded, entirely disposable one-piece pens containing 300 ml of 100-unit insulin and an integral needle, and reusable pens which can take cartridges containing either 1.5 ml or 3 ml of 100-unit

insulin. The latter require disposable needles. The maximum single dose delivered by the current pen injectors ranges from 36 to 100 units. Pens may be used to give boluses of short- or rapid-acting insulin more conveniently before meals (this is more common among type 1 patients) or to deliver premixed (biphasic) insulins – used by about 75% of type 2 patients in the UK – more conveniently twice-daily. The Autopen will accept animal insulin cartridges. While, overall, glycaemic control is not necessarily improved with pen injector use, these tools have several definite advantages over conventional syringes:

- more accurate dosing
- portability
- ease of use (especially with impaired dexterity or vision)
- more convenient.

Other modes of delivery

Other modes of insulin delivery, either infrequently used or currently at an experimental stage, include the following:

Jet injectors

Jet injectors are designed to eject a gaseous stream at high pressure. The stream contains tiny particles of insulin which penetrate the skin. The procedure may be uncomfortable and insulin delivery erratic, and the principal indication, true needle-phobia, is rare.

Nasal insulin

Nasal insulin delivery is still at the experimental stage. Subsequent bioavailability seems low. Absorption is rapid, but the use of absorption enhancers may damage the nasal mucosa.

Pulmonary insulin

Pulmonary delivery is currently in phase III clinical trials. The lungs have a large surface area, making them an attractive site for insulin delivery by aerosol. Preprandial doses administered by a breath-activated device are under evaluation. Combined with a long-acting basal insulin or with oral antidiabetic agents, this approach is attractive for selected patients with type 2 diabetes.

Continuous subcutaneous infusion

Continuous subcutaneous insulin infusion is a specialized insulin delivery technique suitable for intensive therapy but offered by relatively few centres; it currently has a limited role for patients with type 2 diabetes. Type 2 patients wanting excellent glycaemic control during pregnancy are potential candidates. The apparatus now comprises convenient, miniature, programmable pumps (produced by Minimed and Diestronics).

Unwanted effects of insulin therapy

A significant proportion of patients with type 2 diabetes require insulin therapy in the long-term because oral agents are unable to provide adequate glycaemic control – so-called 'secondary failure' (chapter 9). Reservations about insulin therapy in patients with type 2 diabetes, particularly elderly patients with cardiovascular complications, have focused on the risks of hypoglycaemia and weight gain. Theoretical concerns about promotion of atherosclerosis have also exercised clinicians for decades, but without any definitive outcome.

Weight gain

Weight gain is a common consequence of initiating insulin (and sulphonylurea) treatment in patients with type 2 diabetes. Over the course of the United Kingdom Prospective Diabetes Study, the gain in additional weight (beyond that observed in patients treated with diet alone) was more than doubled in the insulin-treated group compared with the glibenclamide group (4.0 vs 1.7 kg). Reduced urinary glucose loss is a likely explanation, coupled with the general anabolic effects of insulin. Dietary counter-measures may be partially effective, particularly when combined with an exercise programme, and weight gain is not inevitable, but certainly can detract from the sense of achievement for some patients; it is almost universally cited as undesirable. Also, greater obesity exacerbates insulin resistance and certain cardiovascular risk factors. Weight gain tends to plateau after a few months, however, and there is evidence that combination therapy with insulin and metformin can limit weight gain (page 173).

Hypoglycaemia

Hypoglycaemia occurs with considerably lower frequency in type 2 diabetes than in type 1, but may be of paramount importance in the elderly, socially isolated, demented or otherwise infirm type 2 patient. The United Kingdom Prospective Diabetes Study associated insulin treatment with an average of 1.8 episodes of severe hypoglycaemia per year (severe hypoglycaemia being defined as hypoglycaemia requiring the assistance of another person or medical attention). Increased duration of insulin therapy increases the risk of hypoglycaemia. Concomitant use of oral antidiabetic agents may increase the risk of hypoglycaemia.

> Severe hypoglycaemia is relatively uncommon in insulin-treated patients with type 2 diabetes compared to those with type 1 diabetes

Causes of iatrogenic hypoglycaemia

Iatrogenic hypoglycaemia either results from a mismatch between the supply of glucose for metabolic requirements (eg due to a missed meal) and the rate of glucose use (eg an increase during or following physical exercise), or a relative excess of insulin leading to a fall in the circulating glucose concentration. There are other causes in insulin-treated patients, but their influence varies from patient to patient and most are considered uncommon or rare in patients with type 2 disease. Some may, however, assume greater importance with the increasing incidence of type 2 diabetes in the young. These include:

- *Changes in insulin pharmacokinetics* – Pharmacokinetics are commonly affected by exercise, which enhances insulin absorption in the exercising limb, and renal impairment, which is also relatively common in type 2 patients (chapter 6). Less significant influences are a change in insulin species from, for example, bovine to human (this is more of a problem in type 1 patients) and a change in anatomical injection site (which is rarely clinically significant).

- *Changes in insulin sensitivity* – Insulin sensitivity will increase with marked weight loss and the withdrawal of certain drugs that induce insulin resistance (eg the corticosteroids). It will also increase with hypopituitarism or Addison's disease, but both conditions are rare. Hypothyroidism is a more common condition, but a rare cause of hypoglycaemia in insulin-treated patients.

Much more rarely (especially in type 2 diabetes), malabsorption syndromes, gastroparesis due to autonomic neuropathy, and eating disorders such as anorexia and bulimia, have all been associated with the development of hypoglycaemia in insulin-treated patients.

Relative severity of iatrogenic hypoglycaemia

Cerebral function is critically dependent on an adequate supply of glucose from the circulation. Glucose is transported into the brain across the blood–brain barrier by a facilitative glucose transporter protein. The most serious consequence of acute hypoglycaemia is cerebral dysfunction with the risk of:

- injury (to self or others)
- generalized epileptic seizures
- coma.

Cognitive impairment progresses ultimately to loss of consciousness as plasma glucose levels fall. Seizures and transient focal neurological deficits may occur with severe neuroglycopenia. Prolonged severe hypoglycaemic coma, often exacerbated by excessive alcohol consumption, may lead to cerebral oedema and permanent brain damage. The effects of recurrent hypoglycaemia on cerebral function in middle-aged and elderly patients are not particularly well documented.

Clinically, hypoglycaemia induced by exogenous insulin is similar to sulphonylurea-induced hypoglycaemia (page 133) and may be graded as follows:

- *Grade 1* – biochemical hypoglycaemia (eg plasma glucose <3.0 mmol/l [54 mg/dl]) in the absence of symptoms
- *Grade 2* – mildly symptomatic (successfully treated by the patient)
- *Grade 3* – severe (the assistance of another person is required)
- *Grade 4* – very severe (causing coma or convulsions).

Note that biochemical definitions of hypoglycaemia may differ according to the circumstances of the patient and may be modulated by previous episodes of hypoglycaemia. The physiological response to acute hypoglycaemia comprises:

- suppression of endogenous insulin secretion
- activation of a hierarchy of counter-regulatory hormone responses.

Counter-regulatory hormone responses to hypoglycaemia

Most of the data concerning counter-regulatory hormone responses to acute hypoglycaemia have been derived from healthy subjects and patients with type 1 diabetes; more studies are required in patients with type 2 diabetes. However, long-duration insulin therapy in patients with type 2 disease is associated with an increased risk of hypoglycaemia; progressive insulin deficiency is thought to result in a situation similar to that in patients with type 1 diabetes, ie profoundly impaired insulin secretion. Patients with type 2 diabetes who progress rapidly to a need for insulin are more likely to be affected. As the plasma glucose concentration falls below certain thresholds, hormones which antagonize insulin's actions are secreted in the following sequence: glucagon, catecholamines, cortisol, and growth hormone.

Catecholamine secretion occurs in the setting of generalized sympathetic nervous system activation. Glucagon and catecholamines are the principal hormones protecting against acute hypoglycaemia. They stimulate glycogenolysis and gluconeogenesis, thereby increasing hepatic glucose production (chapter 2); enhanced hormone-stimulated lipolysis may also contribute to recovery from hypoglycaemia through stimulatory effects on gluconeogenesis. If healthy subjects are given carefully controlled doses of insulin, the secretion of these two hormones occurs at arterial plasma glucose levels of approximately 3.8 mmol/l; cortisol secretion occurs at lower levels. If the response of either glucagon or catecholamines is inadequate, the other will usually compensate. Deficiency of both hormones will result in severe hypoglycaemia.

> Failure of counter-regulatory hormone responses predisposes to severe recurrent hypoglycaemia

Cortisol and growth hormone play a less important role during acute hypoglycaemia, and are more important in the later recovery of glucose levels.

Antecedent hypoglycaemia can alter the glycaemic threshold for counter-regulatory hormone secretion; scrupulous avoidance of hypoglycaemia may restore symptoms. Clinical studies have shown that intensive insulin therapy leads to symptoms which develop at lower plasma glucose levels, resulting in less time between the onset of symptoms and the development of severe neuroglycopenia. Biochemical evidence of recurrent hypoglycaemia, if well documented, is therefore a contraindication to intensive insulin therapy and a dose reduction should be considered. Non-diabetic patients with chronic recurrent hypoglycaemia due to insulinomas may also lose the typical symptoms and signs of hypoglycaemia.

Warning symptoms of hypoglycaemia

The symptoms and signs of acute hypoglycaemia are conveniently divided into two main categories (Table 11.3): autonomic (or adrenergic) if they arise from activation of the sympathoadrenal system; and neuroglycopenic if they result from inadequate cerebral glucose delivery. Under experimental conditions, adrenergic activation occurs at a higher plasma glucose concentration than that at which cerebral function becomes impaired (about 2.7 mmol/l). Thus, the patient is alerted to the falling plasma glucose concentration by adrenergic activation and is usually able to take corrective action. If the warning symptoms are deficient or their perception is impaired, eg by certain drugs or alcohol, then the patient may become irrational and aggressive due to the onset of neuroglycopenia. Prompt assistance from another party may then be required to avert loss of consciousness and more serious sequelae.

> Severe hypoglycaemia carries risk of coma, convulsions, injury and (albeit rarely) even death

Risk factors for severe hypoglycaemia

Insulin treatment of long duration (ie five years or more) is often associated with defective

Table 11.3

Autonomic, neuroglycopenic and non-specific symptoms and signs in acute hypoglycaemia. Sourced from Hepburn DA *et al. Diabetes Care* 1991; **14:** 949-57.

Autonomic (adrenergic)	Neuroglycopenic	Non-specific
Tremor	Impaired concentration	Hunger
Sweating	Confusion	Weakness
Anxiety	Irrational, uncharacteristic or inappropriate behaviour	Blurred vision
Pallor	Difficulty in speaking	
Nausea	Non-co-operation or aggression	
Tachycardia	Drowsiness, progressing to coma	
Palpitations	Focal neurological signs including transient hemiplegia	
Shivering	Focal or generalized convulsions	
Increased pulse pressure	Permanent neurological damage if prolonged, severe hypoglycaemia	

glucagon responses to hypoglycaemia in patients with type 1 diabetes. In addition, intensive insulin therapy (aiming for sustained near-normoglycaemia) can lead to the loss of the normal autonomic hypoglycaemia warning symptoms, giving rise to a high risk of recurrent severe hypoglycaemia. Factors predisposing to severe hypoglycaemia include:

- a history of severe hypoglycaemia
- a history of symptomatic unawareness of hypoglycaemia
- intensive insulin therapy regimens aiming for near-normoglycaemia (eg during pregnancy)
- glycated haemoglobin within the non-diabetic range
- long-duration insulin treatment
- excessive or inappropriate alcohol consumption.

(It should be noted that this list is derived mainly from studies in type 1 patients.)

Driving and insulin treatment

Patients who have lost their warning symptoms for hypoglycaemia should not drive motor vehicles. The fact that hypoglycaemia while driving could have serious consequences should be explained to the patient, preferably in writing. This advice should also be recorded in

the patient's case notes; fatalities have occurred. In the UK, patients should be reminded that it is their legal responsibility to inform the driving licensing authority if:

- treatment with hypoglycaemic potential, including insulin, is commenced (patients should be advised not to drive until their glycaemic control is acceptable)
- significant tissue complications – eg acute or chronic visual impairment, severe peripheral neuropathy, ischaemic heart disease, cerebrovascular disease – develop. Expert advice is required if night vision is affected by extensive retinal photocoagulation (chapter 6).
- hypoglycaemia unawareness occurs.

In these circumstances, a report from the responsible clinician will usually be requested by the licensing authority. If a patient is involved in a road traffic accident in which hypoglycaemia is thought to have been contributory, the police will usually notify the licensing authority and the patient's licence (usually renewed every three years if insulin-treated) is likely to be withdrawn until there is convincing evidence that the risks have become acceptable. General precautions for driving on insulin treatment are listed in Table 11.4. The regulations concerning public service and heavy goods vehicles differ, of course, and vary from

Table 11.4
Advice for insulin-treated diabetic drivers.

- A supply of readily accessible glucose tablets (or a suitable alternative) must always be carried in the car
- Plan each journey
- Make provisions for unexpected delays
- Check blood glucose before, and periodically during, long journeys
- Take regular breaks on long journeys and avoid fatigue
- Have regular meals and snacks at the designated times
- If hypoglycaemia develops, stop the car at the earliest safe opportunity, switch off the engine, remove the ignition key and vacate the driver's seat (take care on busy roads)
- Always carry an identity card or bracelet confirming your diagnosis
- Never drink alcohol before driving

country to country. In the UK, taxi licences are granted by the local authority, and insulin treatment not necessarily disallowed, as long as glycaemic control is deemed satisfactory. Certain professions, such as the armed forces, often exclude insulin-treated patients, however, which can lead to conflicts of interest and encourage some patients to avoid insulin treatment longer than is advisable. The regulations are flexible in many cases, though, subject to regular, satisfactory medical reports. A commitment to frequent self-monitoring is required.

> Patients who have lost their hypoglycaemic warning symptoms must not drive motor vehicles

Recreational implications for insulin treatment

Certain sports, such as scuba diving, carry predictable risks for patients at risk of hypoglycaemia. It is important to note that

post-exercise hypoglycaemia can occur several hours after the event, which can lead to diagnostic difficulties if appropriate enquiries are not made. Patients may find that they have to reduce their insulin dose substantially before rigorous exercise; this should always be planned. Conversely, patients with minimal endogenous insulin secretion may need to consume additional carbohydrate both before and during exercise. Insulin sensitivity tends to improve rapidly with aerobic exercise (page 121), but the effect is lost rapidly if the exercise programme is interrupted for more than a few days.

Long-haul travel

Adjustment of insulin dosing during long-distance travel is often relatively easy for patients with type 2 diabetes, particularly if a twice-daily regimen is applied and some endogenous insulin secretion present. Plans should be discussed with the diabetes care team ahead of travel, and the relevant airline informed. Insulin should not be stowed in the hold (freezing will denature it), nor should it be exposed to extreme heat, such as direct sunlight.

> Insulin treatment has implications for driving, certain occupations and some recreational activities

Meticulous glucose control

Meticulous avoidance of low glucose levels – ie those <4.0 mmol/l – may restore the warning symptoms of hypoglycaemia in some insulin-treated patients. The use of rapid-acting insulin analogues is being explored, but it is often difficult to decide whether improvements in glycaemic control are attributable to altered pharmacokinetics or education and greater input from the diabetes care team. Although the loss of warning symptoms has been described as a form of acquired autonomic dysfunction, it is generally accepted that classic diabetic autonomic neuropathy *per se* is not responsible in most cases.

Nocturnal hypoglycaemia

The frequent occurrence of nocturnal hypoglycaemia – which may affect more than 50% of patients and often goes unrecognized – is an important cause of hypoglycaemic unawareness. Conventional strategies to minimize nocturnal hypoglycaemia include:

- reducing the dose of evening intermediate insulin
- moving the time of the evening injection of intermediate insulin to 2200 hours
- eating a snack containing 10–20 g carbohydrate before bed
- avoiding excessive alcohol consumption.

The contribution of the evening dose of short-acting insulin to the problem of hypoglycaemia at 0200–0300 hours may well have been underestimated in the past and recent evidence points to a lower rate of nocturnal hypoglycaemia when the insulin analogues lispro or insulin aspart are used in place of the soluble short-acting preparation. Since lispro and aspart have a shorter duration of action their effects will dissipate earlier in the evening, resulting in lower plasma insulin concentrations in the early hours of sleep.

In addition, studies in children have shown that the physiological responses to hypoglycaemia are impaired during stages 3–4 (the slow-wave) of sleep.

> Evening doses of conventional short-acting insulins may contribute to nocturnal hypoglycaemia in some patients

Insulin species and hypoglycaemia risk

In the UK there has been intense debate about the effect of insulin species on the warning symptoms of hypoglycaemia. A minority of patients with type 1 diabetes complained that their symptoms reduced in intensity when they changed from animal to human sequence insulin. It is recognized that a change in species may necessitate changes in dosage, and minor differences in pharmacokinetics and, in some patients with diabetes of long duration, the presence of high titres of anti-insulin antibodies is thought to be responsible. This is particularly true for patients changing from bovine to the less immunogenic porcine or human insulin preparations. Whether there is any effect of species *per se* on the symptom complex of hypoglycaemia remains less certain, with most studies showing no appreciable difference. Alternative causes of hypoglycaemia must always be excluded (page 165) and the great majority of patients in the UK and elsewhere are now treated with human sequence insulin.

Treatment of insulin-induced hypoglycaemia

Insulin-treated patients are advised to carry dextrose tablets at all times, but surveys indicate that a high proportion do not comply; periodic reiteration of the advice is required. At the onset of symptoms patients should take either:

- two to four dextrose tablets
- two teaspoonfuls (10 g) of sugar, honey or jam (ideally in water)
- a small glass of a carbonated, sugar-containing soft drink.

If there is no improvement within five to 10 minutes, the treatment should be repeated. If the next meal is not imminent, a snack (eg biscuit, sandwich, piece of fruit) should be eaten to maintain blood glucose levels. Over-treatment ('emptying the fridge') should be avoided if possible.

Where the hypoglycaemia is more severe (grade 3 or 4; page 165), a friend, colleague or relative may notice its development before the patients themselves. A subtle change in appearance or behaviour may prompt another person to encourage oral carbohydrate consumption. Unfortunately, cognitive dysfunction may lead to a negative or even hostile response. As the level of consciousness falls, it becomes hazardous to try to forcibly administer carbohydrate by mouth. Alternatives then include:

- *Buccal glucose gel* – proprietary thick glucose gels (eg Hypostop), or honey, can be smeared on the buccal mucosa; efficacy is variable.

- *iv glucose* – 25 ml of 50% dextrose or 100 ml of 20% dextrose may be administered into a large vein, ideally after cannulation. Paramedical expertise is required – extravasation of hypertonic 50% dextrose can cause tissue necrosis and thrombophlebitis may also complicate iv delivery – but this technique will usually lead to restoration of consciousness within a few minutes.

- *Glucagon* – parenteral glucagon is not recommended for type 2 patients because there may be sufficient remaining β-cells to respond with increased insulin secretion.

Recovery from hypoglycaemia may be delayed if:

- the hypoglycaemia has been very prolonged or severe
- an alternative cause for impairment of consciousness (eg stroke, drug overdose) co-exists (the hypoglycaemia may cause falls and head injury)
- the patient is post-ictal (convulsion caused by severe hypoglycaemia).

If cerebral oedema is suspected, adjunctive treatment, ie iv dexamethasone (4–6 mg, six-hourly) or mannitol, is usually administered in an intensive care setting. However, evidence for the efficacy of these drugs, or for other measures such as controlled hyperventilation, is scarce. Cranial CT imaging should be performed.

> Hypertonic 50% dextrose must be administered into a large vein in order to avoid extravasation

Special situations

Surgery

Insulin-treated patients require careful monitoring to avoid hypo- and hyperglycaemia during surgery or other invasive procedures that have required them to be 'nil-by-mouth'. An iv infusion and dextrose is usually recommended. Subcutaneous insulin is recommenced with the first meal after the procedure. Some patients treated with oral antidiabetic drugs (especially long-acting sulphonylureas and metformin) are best converted to insulin temporarily ahead of

Table 11.5
Dextrose and insulin infusions* for control of perioperative diabetes.

- Glucose is administered via a drip counter at a rate of 100 ml/hour of 10% dextrose (containing an appropriate amount of potassium).

- Short-acting ('soluble') insulin (50 units) is added to 50 ml saline (0.9%) in a 50 ml syringe and delivered via a variable rate electromechanical pump (with built-in battery supply).

- Insulin (approximately 1 unit/ml) is co-infused via a Y-connector at a variable rate, with the aim of maintaining blood glucose concentrations at approximately 5–10 mmol/l.

  Sample regimen:

Infusion rate (units/hour)	Blood glucose (mmol/l)
0	0–3.9[†]
1	4.0–6.9
2	7.0–9.9
3	10.0–14.9
4	≥15.0[†]

[†]Call medical staff to review. Recheck blood glucose and treat hypoglycaemia if necessary.

- Starting infusion rate is 2 units/hour. Rate is then increased or reduced on the basis of hourly blood glucose measurements.

- Advantage = Adjustable ratio of insulin to glucose.

- Disadvantage = Risk of both hypo- and hyperglycaemia if infusion rate incorrect or delivery interrupted.

*Note that insulin requirements are variable and that the infusion rates suggested are just a guide.

major surgery. This is usually done as part of inpatient treatment (Table 11.5). The management of type 2 diabetes during surgery is outlined in Table 11.6. Note that patients with type 2 disease are more likely to require surgery than non-diabetic individuals – for diabetic foot complications, for example. They may also have complications (eg nephropathy, autonomic neuropathy) which can adversely affect outcome. Poor metabolic control impedes wound healing in general and exacerbates plasma electrolyte disturbances, and the hormonal response to surgical stress can lead to major metabolic decompensation.

Table 11.6
Management of diabetes during surgery and other invasive procedures.

Measures are required to (a) avoid hypoglycaemia and (b) maintain good metabolic control:

- Liaison with the anaesthetist is recommended.
- Metabolic control should be optimized in good time if possible (this may require temporary insulin treatment for some patients otherwise not on insulin).
- The patient should be placed near the start of a morning list on the day of operation, if possible.
- During emergency surgery, any major metabolic disturbance should be corrected as far as possible. The effects of previously administered antidiabetic therapy necessitate even more frequent monitoring and use of dextrose and insulin as indicated.
- Electrolyte disturbances should be corrected before surgery wherever possible.

Diet- or tablet-treated diabetes:
In well-controlled patients undergoing minor procedures such as endoscopy, avoidance of glucose- and lactate-containing iv fluids, and missing out their short-acting sulphonylurea dose on the morning of surgery may be sufficient. In any case:

- Blood glucose levels should be monitored every one to two hours pre- and postoperatively.
- Longer-acting sulphonylureas (eg chlorpropamide, glibenclamide) should be discontinued several days before surgery since they may cause serious and prolonged postoperative hypoglycaemia; these should be temporarily replaced by insulin or short-acting agents (eg tolbutamide).
- Metformin should also be avoided perioperatively and at the time of radiological contrast investigations because of the risk of lactic acidosis. If renal function is normal (metformin is contraindicated if renal impairment is present), then discontinuation of the drug on the evening before the procedure should allow sufficient elimination.
- Management of major surgery should follow that for insulin-treated patients.

Insulin-treated patients:

- For all but the most trivial procedures, patients should be stabilized pre-operatively with iv dextrose and insulin infusion as outlined in Table 11.5.
- Plasma electrolytes should be checked frequently and the amount of potassium adjusted accordingly.
- Subcutaneous insulin should be restarted with an appropriate meal. When it is reinstated, the initial injection should include a short-acting insulin and the iv infusion should be terminated 30–60 minutes later to minimize the risk of transient insulinopenia.
- Other special situations include acute myocardial infarction (chapter 7), open heart surgery with cardiopulmonary bypass (which requires considerably more insulin to compensate for the glucose-containing fluids used in the procedure), and labour (which should be managed with dextrose–insulin infusion in insulin-treated patients). Insulin requirements fall rapidly back to pre-pregnancy levels after placenta delivery and insulin may no longer be required in women with gestational diabetes or diabetes previously managed with diet or oral agents. NB Dexamethasone and β-agonists may cause metabolic decompensation.

Hormonal stress response to intercurrent illness

Transient insulin resistance may arise in the course of intercurrent illnesses, such as severe sepsis. Temporary increases in insulin dosage, sometimes necessitating a change to iv or multiple subcutaneous doses, are required. Insulin may also become temporarily necessary during illness in patients previously well-controlled by oral antidiabetic agents; re-introduction of oral therapy may be possible following recovery.

Anti-insulin antibodies

The role of acquired anti-insulin antibodies, once thought to be an important mechanism of insulin resistance, has faded with the introduction of modern, less antigenic insulin preparations.

Renal failure

Care is required with insulin treatment in patients with progressive renal impairment. Decreased insulin degradation by the failing kidneys, reduced renal gluconeogenesis, and anorexia with decreased calorie intake may all contribute. Reductions in insulin dosage, sometimes substantial, may be required.

> Progressive renal failure may necessitate a reduction in insulin dose

Some patients with end-stage renal failure on continuous ambulatory peritoneal dialysis (page 86) inject their insulin into the dialysate bags to deliver it intraperitoneally. Insulin requirements vary widely from patient to patient, partly dependent on the strength of the dialysate used; hypertonic solutions can contain high concentrations of glucose.

Transient deterioration of retinopathy

Transient deterioration in pre-existing retinopathy may follow rapid improvement in glycaemic control, for example when insulin treatment is commenced. This phenomenon has mainly been observed in trials in patients with type 1 diabetes, but may also occur in some type 2 patients. Careful surveillance and explanation of this apparent paradox is required. The long-term prognosis is generally much better with improved glycaemic control.

Insulin neuritis

An analogous complication is so-called insulin neuritis in which acute symptomatic neuropathy develops following the institution of insulin treatment; uncommon.

Patient acceptability

Clinical studies suggest that insulin therapy can be successful if patients are selected appropriately and prepared carefully. Twice-daily isophane or pre-mixed insulins are used routinely in many centres; pen injectors are suitable for most patients and may increase acceptability by increasing convenience. Morbidly obese patients inadequately controlled with oral agents remain a particularly difficult therapeutic problem. Some centres use a combination of oral antidiabetic agents and bedtime insulin. Patient acceptance of insulin can be facilitated by a positive attitude from the diabetes care team and discussion of the possibility of subsequent insulin treatment early in the course of the disease. Some studies suggest that quality of life is not necessarily impaired by the additional complexity of insulin treatment. Indeed, the sense of wellbeing experienced by patients who improve on insulin after months or years of hyperglycaemia can be rewarding for both patients and healthcare professionals alike. Adequate support from a multidisciplinary diabetes care team is an important component of safe and effective insulin therapy.

Combination therapy with oral agents

Sulphonylureas with insulin

No clear long-term benefits of such combined therapy have yet emerged, but this approach has enthusiastic support and is gaining popularity. Several studies (generally relatively small-scale and of limited duration) have suggested that concomitant treatment with insulin and a sulphonylurea may allow a reduction in insulin dose of up to 50%. Typically, isophane insulin is administered at bedtime, with sulphonylureas taken during the day. The aim is to control fasting plasma glucose concentration with the bedtime insulin by suppressing hepatic glucose production. Clearly, given the mode of action of sulphonylureas (page 130), this approach is dependent on partial residual β-cell function and its use in the longer term not yet clear. Since β-cell function seems to deteriorate inexorably in most patients with type 2 diabetes, it is likely that the sulphonylureas will eventually lose their effect; full replacement therapy with insulin would then be required.

Metformin with insulin

There is increasing evidence that metformin may help to avert weight gain when patients with type 2 diabetes are transferred to insulin. A recent randomized trial showed that metformin and insulin (at bedtime) were associated with better glycaemic control and the lowest risk of hypoglycaemia during the first year of therapy than other regimens, including twice-daily insulin. Patients assigned to this combination used more insulin to attain fasting blood glucose targets, possibly gaining the confidence to increase insulin dose due to the low risk of hypoglycaemia. Some centres now routinely continue metformin in overweight patients when insulin is introduced, but further studies are required.

> Metformin may help to limit the weight gain associated with insulin treatment in some patients with type 2 diabetes

Thiazolidinediones with insulin

There is accumulating evidence that these insulin-sensitizing drugs may allow the insulin dose to be reduced; reductions >50% were reported in trials of obese insulin-treated

patients after the addition of troglitazone. Substantial dose reductions with concomitant improvements in glycaemic control have since been observed with rosiglitazone and pioglitazone. In the US, but not in Europe (because of concerns about cardiovascular side-effects), pioglitazone is licensed for use in combination with insulin. Weight gain (part of which is likely to be fluid retention) is not eliminated by combining insulin with a thiazolidinedione; both groups have the potential to cause weight gain as monotherapy.

> Combination therapy with insulin and a thiazolidinedione may allow the insulin dose to be reduced

Discontinuation of insulin therapy

In some situations it may be appropriate to discontinue insulin treatment. Certain elderly or infirm patients, once-obese patients who have slimmed through dietary and exercise measures, and patients who took insulin because of a concurrent condition that has subsequently resolved, may all benefit from discontinuation. The essential criterion is that the patient has endogenous insulin secretion sufficient to permit control with oral agents or even diet alone, but certain other criteria should also be satisfied:

- There should be no history of ketosis. An exception is ketosis that was clearly associated with a severe acute illness such as major sepsis (which can sometimes precipitate ketosis in patients with type 2 diabetes).

- The patient should not have been underweight at diagnosis (this usually indicates marked insulin deficiency).

- Serum markers of autoimmune type 1 diabetes (eg islet cell antibodies) should be absent.

Patients with secondary forms of diabetes (chapter 3) represent a heterogeneous group. A history of diabetes complicating chronic pancreatitis will point to the need for insulin treatment due to severe β-cell destruction, for example. On the other hand, temporary steroid-induced diabetes may not require insulin, provided the steroid dose can be lowered sufficiently.

Demonstration of the previous inadequacy of oral agents (so-called primary or secondary failure) usually means that insulin treatment should continue. The need for small doses of insulin (eg <20 units/day) is not always a reliable guide to the success of oral agents because insulin requirements vary considerably between patients. In any case, very careful expert supervision is needed when insulin is withdrawn.

> Insulin dose cannot be reliably equated with need for insulin treatment

Transfer back to oral agents requires reconsideration of the potential risks and benefits. Measurement of plasma (or urinary) C-peptide, which is co-secreted with insulin on an equimolar basis, provides a measure of endogenous insulin reserve. Stimulation tests (eg peak C-peptide response six minutes after a 1 mg iv injection of glucagon) have been used in clinical trials to improve the accuracy of

classification. These are rarely used in routine clinical practice, where the decision to use insulin treatment rests principally on clinical judgement.

Further reading

Evans A, Krentz AJ. Benefits and risks of transfer from oral agents to insulin in type 2 diabetes. In: Krentz AJ (Ed). *Drug treatment of type 2 diabetes*. Auckland, ADIS International 2000; 85-101.

Edelman SV, Henry RR. Insulin therapy for normalizing glycosylated hemoglobin in type II diabetes. Application, benefits and risks. *Diabetes Rev* 1995; **3**: 308-34.

Galloway JA. Treatment of NIDDM with insulin agonists or substitutes. *Diabetes Care* 1990; **13**: 1209-39.

Hayward RA, Manning WG, Kaplan SH *et al.* Starting insulin therapy in patients with type 2 diabetes. *JAMA* 1997; **278**: 1663-9.

Hermann LS. Optimising therapy for insulin-treated type 2 diabetes mellitus. *Drugs Aging* 2000; **17**: 283-94.

Riddle MC. Learning to use troglitazone. *Diabetes Care* 1998; **21**: 1389-90.

Selam JL. Implantable insulin pumps. *Lancet* 1999; **354**: 178-9.

Turner RC, Cull CA, Frighi V *et al.* Glycemic control with diet, sulphonylurea, metformin, or insulin in patients with type 2 diabetes mellitus (UKPDS 49). *JAMA* 1999; **281**: 2005-12.

United Kingdom Prospective Diabetes Study Group. United Kingdom Prospective Diabetes Study (UKPDS) 13: relative efficacy of randomly allocated diet, sulphonylurea, insulin, or metformin in patients with newly diagnosed non-insulin dependent diabetes followed for three years. *Br Med J* 1995; **310**: 83-8.

Yki-Jarvinen H, Ryysy L, Nikkila K *et al.* Comparison of bedtime insulin regimens in patients with type 2 diabetes mellitus. A randomized controlled trial. *Ann Intern Med* 1999; **130**: 389-96.

1) Identifying individuals at increased risk of type 2 diabetes

Type 2 diabetes should be suspected in individuals with:

Obesity
Abdominal obesity
First-degree relative with type 2 diabetes
History of gestational diabetes and/or large babies
Previous glucose intolerance and/or hyperinsulinaemia
Ethnic predisposition
Dyslipidaemia
Hypertension
Low birth weight
Microalbuminuria
Atherothrombotic symptoms
High parity
Diabetogenic drug therapy
Recurrent infections
Old age

2) Diagnosis of type 2 diabetes*

A) With symptoms**
i)   random venous plasma glucose $\geq$11.1 mmol/l ($\geq$200 mg/dl)
     or
ii) fasting *plasma* glucose $\geq$7.0 mmol/l ($\geq$126 mg/dl) or fasting *blood* glucose $\geq$ 6.1 mmol/l ($\geq$110 mg/dl)
     or
iii) 75 g OGTT[†], two-hour *plasma* glucose $\geq$11.1 mmol/l ($\geq$200mg/dl)

B) Without symptoms
Measurement of i), ii), or iii) (above) on two separate occasions. If fasting or random values are equivocal, a two-hour value after a 75 g OGTT[†] should be used

*Diagnosis is normally based on two separate measurements of plasma or blood glucose. It should normally be confirmed by at least one plasma or blood glucose measurement made by a recognized clinical chemistry laboratory
**Polyuria or polydipsia, plus visual disturbance, fatigue, unexplained weight loss, recurrent infection, macrovascular complications, retinopathy, nephropathy, or neuropathy
[†]OGTT = oral glucose tolerance test

3) Diagnostic glucose concentrations for type 2 diabetes, impaired glucose tolerance and impaired fasting glucose

	Glucose concentration, mmol/l (mg/dl)			
	Whole blood		Plasma	
	Venous	Capillary	Venous	Capillary
Diabetes mellitus				
Fasting	$\geq$6.1 ($\geq$110)	$\geq$6.1 ($\geq$110)	$\geq$7.0 ($\geq$126)	$\geq$7.0 ($\geq$126)
Two hours post-glucose load*	$\geq$10.0 ($\geq$180)	$\geq$11.1 ($\geq$200)	$\geq$11.1 ($\geq$200)	$\geq$12.2 ($\geq$220)
Impaired glucose tolerance (IGT)				
Two hours post- glucose load*	$\geq$6.7 ($\geq$120) & <10.0 (<180)	$\geq$7.8 ($\geq$140) & <11.1 (<200)	$\geq$7.8 ($\geq$140) & <11.1 (<200)	$\geq$8.9 ($\geq$160) & <12.2 (<220)
Impaired fasting glucose (IFG)				
Fasting	$\geq$5.6 ($\geq$100) & <6.1 (<110)	$\geq$5.6 ($\geq$100) & <6.1 (<110)	$\geq$6.1 ($\geq$110) & <7.0 (<140)	$\geq$6.1 ($\geq$110) & <7.0 (<126)

*Two hours after a 75 g oral glucose load, conducted after an overnight fast

4) 75 g oral glucose tolerance test

Procedure

- Patient asked to withhold food after last meal of previous day (nothing to eat or drink from midnight, except water, until test).

- Morning medications should be deferred until after test.

- Patient should arrive at least 30 minutes in advance of test, preferably by transport (ie with minimal physical exertion).

- Start test at 0800–0900 hours.

- Insert venous line (unless capillary test, eg finger prick, is to be performed).

- Take pre-test blood sample (approximately 15–30 minutes before test; this sample is not usually used for measurement, but serves to verify that patient was stable when compared with next 'time zero' sample). Collect blood into fluoride-oxalate tube (unless immediate capillary measurement being performed).

- Take 'time zero' blood sample.

- Within about five minutes, patient consumes 75 g anhydrous ᴅ-glucose dissolved in about 300 ml water.

- Take blood samples at ½, 1, 1½ and 2 hours.

- Remove venous line.

- A simplified approach involves the measurement of glucose in the fasting state (time zero) and two hours after the glucose challenge (since these are the values used for diagnostic purposes).

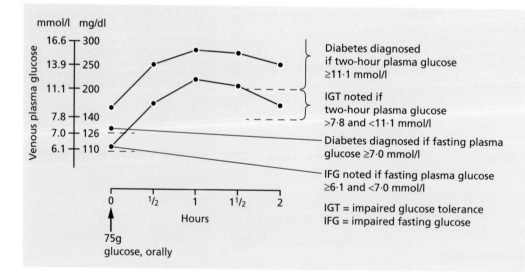

page 176

5) HbA$_{1c}$

HbA$_{1c}$ (glycated haemoglobin A$_{1c}$) is a measure of the non-enzymatic attachment of *glucose* to the terminal valine of the β chain of haemoglobin. HbA$_{1c}$ is expressed as a percentage of the haemoglobin that is glycated (normally about 4–6%). HbA$_{1c}$ has largely replaced HbA$_1$, which is a measure of *all sugars* attached to the terminal β chain of haemoglobin. HbA$_{1c}$ is the largest component (60–80%) of HbA$_1$. Values for HbA$_{1c}$ are therefore about 1–2% (absolute units) lower than HbA$_1$. Since the lifespan of an erythrocyte is about 120 days, HbA$_{1c}$ gives an

indication of average glycaemia over half of this period, ie over 60 days. However, more recent changes in glycaemia will have a slightly greater impact on the extent of glycation, so HbA$_{1c}$ provides a more useful indication of glycaemia over the 40–60 days (six to eight weeks) preceding the assay.

Guidelines for optimal glycaemic control suggest aiming for an HbA$_{1c}$ value of ≤ 6.5% (European Policy Group), or <7% (American Diabetes Association), based on a non-diabetic reference range of 4–6%.

6) Ideal targets for metabolic control

	European Diabetes Policy Group	American Diabetes Association
HbA$_{1c}$ %	≤6.5	<7.0
Fasting plasma glucose		
mmol/l	≤6.0	–
mg/dl	<110	–
Preprandial blood glucose		
mmol/l	-	4.5–6.7
mg/dl	-	80–120
Fasting total cholesterol		
mmol/l	<4.8	–
mg/dl	<185	–
Fasting triglycerides		
mmol/l	<1.7	<2.2
mg/dl	<150	<200
Blood pressure		
mmHg	<140/85	<130/85
Body mass index		
kg/m²	18.5–25	
Waist:hip ratio	Men <0.95 Women <0.80	

7) Starting therapy with oral antidiabetic agents

Agent	Recommended daily dose (mg)[a]	Duration of action[†]	Starting dose (mg)[‡]	Exclusions and contraindications	Side-effects and adverse events	Precautions[§]
α-glucosidase inhibitors (slow rate of carbohydrate digestion[a])						
Acarbose	150–300	Short	50	Intestinal diseases, severe kidney disease	Gastrointestinal intolerance	Check LFT for high dose
Miglitol	75–300	Short	25 (td; take with each main meal)			? check creatinine
Voglibose	1.5–15	Short	0.5			? check LFT
Sulphonylureas[b] (increase insulin secretion)						
Chlorpropamide	100–500	Long	100 od	Choice of agent restricted by severe liver or kidney disease, or porphyria	Hypoglycaemic episodes, sensitivity reactions, weight gain	Interactions with other protein-bound drugs
Glibenclamide[c]	2.5–15	Intermediate–long	2.5 od			
Gliclazide[d]	40–320	Intermediate	40 od[d]			
Glimepiride	1–6	Intermediate	1 od			
Glipizide[e]	2.5–20	Short–intermediate[e]	2.5 od or bd			
Gliquidone	15–180	Short–intermediate	15 od or bd			
Tolazamide	100–1000	Short–intermediate	100 od or bd			
Tolbutamide	500–2000	Short	500 od or bd			
Meglitinide non-sulphonylurea 'prandial' insulin releasers (increase insulin secretion)						
Repaglinide	1–16	Very short	0.5 bd or td, before main meals	Liver or severe kidney disease	As for sulphonylureas	Drug interactions
Nateglinide	180–360	Very short	60 td before main meals			
Biguanides (counter insulin resistance)						
Metformin	500–3000	Short–intermediate	500 od or bd, 850 od, with meals	Kidney, liver, cardiac or any hypoxic disease	Gastrointestinal, risk of lactic acidosis	Check creatinine; vitamin B_{12} or haemoglobin
Thiazolidinediones (improve insulin sensitivity)						
Rosiglitazone	2–8	Intermediate	2 od or bd	Cardiac failure, oedema, anaemia, liver disease	Oedema, anaemia, weight gain	Check LFT, haemoglobin
Pioglitazone	15–45	Intermediate	15 bd			
Sulphonylurea–metformin fixed dose combinations (increase insulin secretion and counter insulin resistance)						
Glibenclamide–metformin	1.25:250–10:2000	Intermediate	1.25:250 od or bd before or with meals	As for sulphonylureas and metformin	As for sulphonylureas and metformin	As for sulphonylureas and metformin

Maximum recommended daily dose can vary between countries; [†] long = >24 hours; intermediate = 12–24 hours; short = <12 hours; very short = < 5 hours; [‡] od = once daily; bd = twice daily; td = three times daily; titrate up dosage slowly; [§] glycaemic control should be monitored throughout and rigorously during titration phase with all antidiabetic drugs; [a] meals should be rich in complex carbohydrate; [b] take with first main meal; large doses of intermediate-acting agents can usually be divided and taken before each of the two main meals, preferably breakfast and lunch; [c] glibenclamide = glyburide; maximum dose 20 mg in some countries; [d] modified-release formulation of gliclazide (Diamicron MR) – daily dose 30–120 mg; [e] extended-release formulation of glipizide (Glucotrol XL) – intermediate duration; LFT = liver function test, eg alanine transaminase

8) Insulins available in the UK

Name	Manufacturer	Species	Vial or cartridge	Onset, peak and duration of action (hours)
Rapid-acting insulins				
NovoRapid (aspart)	Novo Nordisk	Human	Vial, preloaded pen and cartridge	
Humalog (lispro)	Lilly	Human	Vial and cartridge	
Short-acting insulins				
Actrapid	Novo Nordisk	Human	Vial, preloaded pen, cartridge	
Humaject S	Lilly	Human	Preloaded pen	
Human Velosulin	Novo	Nordisk Human	Vial	
Humulin S	Lilly	Human	Vial and cartridge	
Hypurin Bovine Neutral	CP Pharmaceuticals	Beef	Vial and cartridge	
Hypurin Porcine Neutral	CP Pharmaceuticals	Pork	Vial and cartridge	
Insuman rapid*	Aventis Pharma	Human	Cartridge and vial	
Pork Actrapid	Novo Nordisk	Pork	Vial	
Intermediate- and long-acting insulins				
Humaject I	Lilly	Human	Preloaded pen	
Human Insulatard ge	Novo Nordisk	Human	Vial, preloaded pen, cartridge	
Humulin I	Lilly	Human	Vial and cartridge	
Humulin Lente	Lilly	Human	Vial	
Humulin ZN	Lilly	Human	Vial	
Hypurin Bovine Isophane	CP Pharmaceuticals	Beef	Vial and cartridge	
Hypurin Bovine Lente	CP Pharmaceuticals	Beef	Vial	
Hypurin Bovine PZI	CP Pharmaceuticals	Beef	Vial	
Hypurin Porcine Isophane	CP Pharmaceuticals	Pork	Vial and cartridge	
Insuman Basal*	Aventis Pharma	Human	Vial and cartridge	
Lentard MC	Novo Nordisk	Pork and beef	Vial	
Human Monotard	Novo Nordisk	Human	Vial	
Pork Insulatard	Novo Nordisk	Pork	Vial	
Human Ultratard	Novo Nordisk	Human	Vial	
Pre-mixed insulins				
Humaject M1-3	Lilly	Human	Preloaded pen	
Humaject M4	Lilly	Human	Preloaded pen	
Humalog Mix 25, pen	Lilly	Human	Cartridge, preloaded pen	
Human Mixtard 30/50	Novo Nordisk	Human	Vial	
Human Mixtard 10-50 pen	Novo Nordisk	Human	Preloaded pen	
Humulin M1-M5†	Lilly	Human	Vial and cartridge	
Hypurin Porcine 30/70 mix	CP Pharmaceuticals	Pork	Vial and cartridge	
Insuman 15–50*	Aventis Pharma	Human	Vial and cartridge	
Human Mixtard 10-50	Novo Nordisk	Human	Cartridge	
Pork Mixtard 30	Novo Nordisk	Pork	Vial	

Chart axis: Onset, peak and duration of action (hours): 0 2 4 6 8 10 12 14 16 18 20 22 24 26 28 30 32 34

Times shown for onset and duration are approximate and may vary from person to person. Onset = the time taken for the insulin to start having an effect. Reproduced from the July/August 2000 *Balance*, with permission from Diabetes UK, the charity for people with diabetes (www.diabetes.org.uk).

* In 2001, Aventis introduced Optiset prefilled disposable pen versions of these insulins.

† Humulin M1 and M4 are to be withdrawn, as are the 1.5ml cartridges of Humulin I, Humulin S, Humulin M3 and Humulin M5.

9) Synopsis of antidiabetic agents

	Insulin	Sulphonylureas and meglitinides	Metformin	α-glucosidase inhibitors	Thiazolidinediones
Basal glucose	↓↓	→	→	– or →	↓ [a]
Postprandial glucose	↓↓	→	→	→	↓ [a]
Insulin concentration	↑↑	↑	– or ↓	–	– or →
Body weight	↑	↑	– or ↓	–	– or ↑
Free fatty acids	↓	– or ↓	– or ↓	–	↓
Triglyceride	–	–	– or ↓	–	– or →
Total cholesterol	–	–	– or ↓	–	– or ↑
Safety risks	Hypo [b]	Hypo [b]	LA [c]	–	? [d]
Tolerability	Inject		GI [e]	GI [e]	–
Exclude/caution	–	Liver/renal [f]	Renal/liver/hypoxia [c]	GI [g]	Cardiac/liver [d]
Monitor [h]	–	– [f]	Creatinine, B_{12} [i]	LFT [j]	LFT, Hb [k]

↑ = increase; ↓ = decrease; – = no significant change
[a] Blood glucose-lowering efficacy may be better in combination therapy
[b] Hypoglycaemia
[c] Lactic acidosis is a rare risk: patients with impaired renal or liver function or predisposition to hypoxia are excluded
[d] Safety issues may include fluid retention, haemodilution, anaemia and oedema. Patients with cardiac and liver disease are excluded
[e] Gastrointestinal disturbances, especially if dosage is increased too rapidly
[f] If liver or renal disease, select agent with appropriate pharmacokinetics and monitor accordingly
[g] Exclude patients with established gastrointestinal diseases
[h] Monitor glycaemic control for all antidiabetic drug treatments
[i] Monitor creatinine and vitamin B_{12}
[j] Monitor liver function test, eg alanine transaminase, with high-dose acabose or voglibose
[k] Initial rigorous monitoring of liver function test and check haemoglobin

10) Body mass index (BMI)

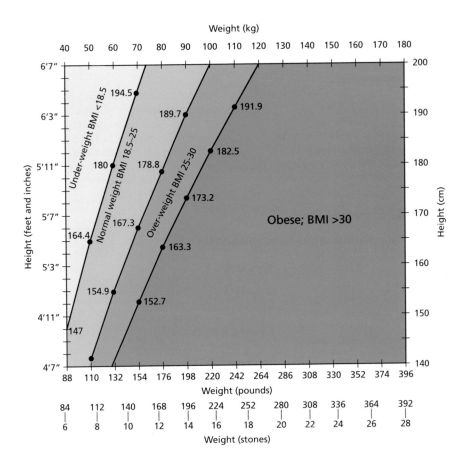

11) Hypoglycaemic emergency

Sulphonylurea- or repaglinide-induced:
If mild, oral carbohydrate, such as two to four dextrose tablets, or two teaspoons of sucrose in water or milk. If severe (ie coma), *admit to hospital as an emergency*. NB – chlorpropamide and glibenclamide carry the highest risks of severe hypoglycaemia (although all secretagogues have this potential).

Insulin-induced:
If mild, as above.
If no improvement, repeat in five to 10 minutes. Severe hypoglycaemia may require iv dextrose (25 ml 50% into a large vein). Intramuscular (im) glucagon may be given by relatives or paramedics to type 1 patients.

Failure to respond necessitates emergency hospital admission.
Alternative causes for coma, such as stroke or drug overdose, should be considered.

Note:
Metformin, acarbose, voglibose, miglitol and the thiazolidinediones (rosiglitazone, pioglitazone) do not usually cause hypoglycaemia as monotherapy. If acarbose contributes to hypoglycaemia (eg in combination with a sulphonylurea), oral dextrose, rather than sucrose, should be given (because of delayed intestinal digestion).

12) Laboratory data: normal values* and conversions

Measurement	Value units	Other value units
Haematology		
Erythrocyte count		
male	4.5–6.5 million/cu mm	$(x10^{12}/l)$
female	3.9–5.6 million/cu mm	$(x\ 10^{12}/l)$
Haematocrit		
male	40–54% (ml/dl)	
female	37–47% (ml/dl)	
Haemoglobin		
male	13.5–18.0 g/dl	2.09–2.79 mmol/l
female	11.5–16.0 g/dl	1.78–2.48 mmol/l
Mean corpuscular volume (MCV)	80–100 cu μm	
Mean corpuscular haemoglobin (MCH)	27–32 pg	
Mean corpuscular haemoglobin concentration (MCHC)	32–36 g/dl	
Platelets	150–500 x 10^9/l	
Reticulocyte count	0.1–2.0/100 erythrocytes	
White cell count	4.0–11.0 x 10^9/l	
Cerebrospinal fluid		
Cells	0–5 white cells/cu mm	
Glucose	2.8–4.4 mmol/l	50–80 mg/dl
Protein	0.15–0.45 g/l	
Urine		
Microalbuminuria	30–300 mg/day	
Proteinuria	>300 mg/day	
Albumin:creatinine ratio	male <2.5 mg/mmol female <3.5 mg/mmol	

* Values commonly recognized as being within a 'normal range' – consult your local laboratory for precise reference ranges.

12) Laboratory data: normal values* and conversions (contd.)

Measurement	Value units	(Conversion)	Other value units
Blood			
Albumin	35–50 g/l	(÷10)	3.5–5.0 g/dl
Amylase	90–300 units/l		
Anion gap [Na⁺] – [Cl⁻ + HCO₃⁻]	7–15 mmol/l		
Aspartate transaminase (AST, SGOT)	5–35 units/l[a] (at 37°C)		
Alanine transaminase (ALT, SGPT)	5–35 units/l[a] (at 37°C)		
Bicarbonate	24–30 mmol/l		
Bilirubin – total	5–19 µmol/l	(x0.06)	0.3–1.1 mg/dl
– conjugated	1.7–6.8 µmol/l	(x0.06)	0.1–0.4 mg/dl
C-peptide (fasting)	0.2–0.8 nmol/l	(÷0.33)	0.6–2.4 ng/ml
Chloride	95–105 mmol/l		
Calcium	2.25–2.75 mmol/l	(x4)	9–11 mg/dl
Cholesterol	3.1–5.7 mmol/l	(x39)	120–220 mg/dl
Creatinine	60–133 µmol/l	(÷88.4)	0.67–1.5 mg/dl
Cortisol (morning)	150–700 nmol/l	(÷27.6)	5–25 µg/dl
Catecholamines – total	<7000 pmol/l	(÷5.9)	<1100 ng/l
– adrenaline (epinephrine)	<1300 pmol/l	(÷5.4)	<200 ng/l
– noradrenaline (norepinephrine)	<5700 pmol/l	(÷5.9)	<900 ng/l
Fatty acids (non-esterified)	0.3–0.6 mmol/l		
Glucose (fasting venous plasma)	3–6 mmol/l	(x18)	54–108 mg/dl
Glucagon (fasting)	<50 pmol/l	(x3.4)	<170 pg/ml
Glycated haemoglobin A₁c (HbA₁c)	4–6 %		
Gases – pO₂	10–13.3 kPa		75–100 mmHg
– pCO₂	4.7–6.0 kPa		35–45 mmHg
Insulin (fasting)	15–130 pmol/l	(÷6.6)	2–20 µunit/ml
Lactate (fasting)	0.5–2.0 mmol/l	(x9)	4.5–18 mg/dl
Magnesium	0.7–1.1 mmol/l	(x2.6)	1.8–3.0 mg/dl
Ketones (β-hydroxybutyrate, acetoacetate, acetone)	0.05–0.2 mmol/l		
Globulin	20–35 g/l	(÷10)	2.0–3.5 mg/dl
Growth hormone (morning)	<2.0 munits/l	(x2.5)	<5.0 ng/ml
Lipoproteins – LDL-cholesterol	1.5–4 mmol/l	(x39)	60–155 mg/dl
– HDL-cholesterol	1–2 mmol/l	(x39)	40–80 mg/dl
Osmolarity	280–305 mOsmol/l		
Oestradiol (luteal)	150–1100 pmol/l	(÷3.67)	40–300 pg/ml
Oestrone (luteal)	90–460 pmol/l	(÷3.69)	25–125 pg/ml
Phosphate	0.8–1.5 mmol/l	(x3)	2.5–4.5 mg/dl
Potassium	3.5–5.0 mmol/l		
Progesterone (luteal)	15–80 nmol/l	(÷3.18)	5–25 ng/ml
Proinsulin (fasting)	<30 pmol/l	(x9)	<300 pg/ml
Prolactin (female)	<500 munits/l	(÷20)	<25 ng/ml
Protein (total)	60–80 g/l	(÷10)	6–8 g/dl
Pyruvate (fasting)	0.03–0.1 mmol/l	(÷1.13)	0.3–0.9 mg/dl
Sodium	135–145 mmol/l		
Testosterone (male)	10–42 nmol/l	(÷3.5)	3–12 ng/ml
Testosterone (female)	0.5–2.5 nmol/l	(÷3.5)	0.2–0.5 ng/ml
Thyroid stimulating hormone	0.5–6.0 munits/l		

* Values commonly recognized as being within a 'normal range' – consult your local laboratory for precise reference ranges.
[a] There are substantial variations in normal ranges between laboratories.

12) Laboratory data: normal values* and conversions (contd.)

Measurement	Value units	(Conversion)	Other value units
Thyroxine (T_4)	70–140 nmol/l	(÷12.9)	5–10 µg/dl
Thyroxine (free)	10–25 pmol/l	(÷12.9)	0.7–2.0 ng/dl
Triiodothyronine	1–3 nmol/l	(÷0.015)	65–200 ng/dl
Triglyceride (fasting)	0.4–1.7 mmol/l	(x89)	35–150 mg/dl
Urea nitrogen	2.9–8.2 mmol/l	(x2.8)	8–23 mg/dl
Uric acid	0.18–0.48 mmol/l	(x17)	3–8 mg/dl

* Values commonly recognized as being within a 'normal range' – consult your local laboratory for precise reference ranges.
[a] There are substantial variations in normal ranges between laboratories.

Index

Page numbers in *italics* refer to information that is shown only in a table or diagram.

Social Research

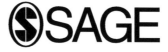

Social Research

A Practical Introduction

Bruce Curtis and Cate Curtis

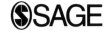

Los Angeles | London | New Delhi
Singapore | Washington DC

SAGE Publications Ltd
1 Oliver's Yard
55 City Road
London EC1Y 1SP

SAGE Publications Inc.
2455 Teller Road
Thousand Oaks, California 91320

SAGE Publications India Pvt Ltd
B 1/I 1 Mohan Cooperative Industrial Area
Mathura Road, Post Bag 7
New Delhi 110 044

SAGE Publications Asia-Pacific Pte Ltd
33 Pekin Street #02-01
Far East Square
Singapore 048763

Library of Congress Control Number: 2011924088

British Library Cataloguing in Publication data

A catalogue record for this book is available from the British Library

ISBN 978-1-84787-474-0
ISBN 978-1-84787-475-7 (pbk)

Typeset by C&M Digitals (P) Ltd, Chennai, India
Printed and bound in Great Britain by TJ International Ltd, Padstow, Cornwall
Printed on paper from sustainable resources

To our parents, Mary Anderson, Peter Curtis, Edmond Knops
and Jeanne Knops.
And Winnie.

CONTENTS

ABOUT THE AUTHORS

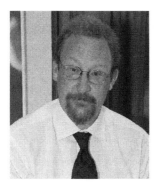

Bruce Curtis is a Senior Lecturer in the Sociology Department at the University of Auckland, New Zealand. He teaches in the areas of social research, the sociology of work and leisure, and sociology of the media. His research interests include academic life; Marxist value analysis; sociology of organisations and work; research methods and new technologies. In addition to these areas, he has published in the areas of gambling, and the sociology of New Zealand. Previous books include *Gambling in New Zealand* and he is one of the editors of *Being Sociological* (Palgrave).

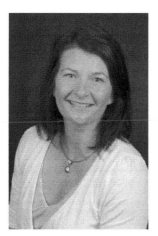

Cate Curtis is a Senior Lecturer in the School of Psychology at the University of Waikato, New Zealand, teaching in the social and community psychology programme. She has experience in research both in academic and with private research organisations, following extensive experience working with social agencies. She has particular interests in social factors in mental health and wellbeing particularly with regard to young women. Previous publications have mainly been in the area of suicidal behaviour, including economic influences and sexual abuse. She is also one of the authors of *The Social Psychology of Everyday Life* (Palgrave).

LIST OF FIGURES

LIST OF TABLES

ACKNOWLEDGEMENTS

We'll keep it short but sweet: we're very grateful to Chris Rojek, Jai Seaman, Katherine Haw, the anonymous reviewer(s) and our extremely thorough copy editor Sarah Bury.

ONE
INTRODUCTION

CONTENTS LIST

Key words: data collection – case-centric – variable-centric – analytical induction – hypothesis-testing – epistemology – ethics – reliability – validity – preparation – proposal preparation

SUMMARY

An outline of the main concepts underlying social research, specifically: (i) case-centric or variable-centric research; (ii) analytical induction or hypothesis-testing; (iii) epistemological positions in the social sciences; (iv) issues of reliability and validity; and (v) fixed or fluid analytical framings or research, as well as an overview of ethical considerations and the precursors to research.

This textbook is intended for readers who are emergent researchers: undergraduate students, in particular students in the later stages of their degrees who are located in the social sciences, including sociology, social psychology, social anthropology, education, nursing or social work programmes. These programmes and disciplines have an interest in the empirical investigation of the social world, and in training their students how to do so. We have selected eleven research approaches that we think will be useful to emergent researchers in their future studies and employment. Taken collectively, the eleven approaches provide an overview of how social scientists do research. We have designed the textbook to be read in its entirety (of course!), but we have also tried to make each of the chapters self-contained. In each chapter we have tried to combine a how-to-do, methods-oriented, or practical element with a discussion of conceptual underpinnings and epistemology (we will discuss epistemology below).

This chapter deals with all the normal stuff that introductory chapters do. We outline the main concepts used: (1) case-centric or variable-centric research, (2) analytical induction or hypothesis-testing, (3) we reference three epistemological positions in the social sciences, (4) issues of reliability and validity, and (5) fixed or fluid analytical framings or research. This introductory chapter also follows the outline used in the others. There are sections on: *Doing data collection and analysis, Some issues in research, Putting the approach in context* and *Conclusion.* We discuss the main concepts used in the appropriate sections.

We also consider this chapter as a substantive one. It includes material about ethical considerations in research and some suggestions about things you might want to think about before starting research (precursors to research).

In accordance with our efforts to produce a book that is both a practical guide and discusses underlying concepts (both *how* and *why*) we have included two types of key point summaries: practice points and conceptual concerns. These briefly sum up or reiterate what we consider to be essential issues for the users of this book to grasp, as below.

PRACTICE POINT 1

This textbook is intended for students in the second or third years of under-graduate degrees in the social sciences.

DOING DATA COLLECTION AND ANALYSIS

In this section we discuss the origins of our approach to the book, and how this informs the book's structure. We introduce the key concepts which are used throughout, such as case-centric/variable-centric and analytical induction/ hypothesis-testing. We also compare these concepts to the classic social research binary: qualitative/quantitative.

Origins of the approach

It is our impression that most textbooks on research or methods give one-sided accounts of either how-to-do stuff (methods) or theories of knowledge (episte-mology). If we push this idea further, we discover that research approaches that are fairly standardised also tend to be thoroughly positivistic in their orientation – such as survey research (see Chapter 6) or content analysis (see Chapter 9) – and have textbooks that gloss issues of epistemology. Those approaches that are very unstandardised are either lacking textbooks or have discussions about abstracted ideas that never touch on the humdrum how-to-do and method (see Chapter 11, semiotic analysis).

Jacques Derrida (1930–2004) said:

> I have tried to mark the ways in which, for example, deconstructive questions cannot give rise to methods, that is to technical procedures that can be transposed by analogy – this is what is called a teaching, a knowledge, applications – but these rules are taken up in a text which is in each time a unique element and which does not let itself be turned totally into a method. (Derrida, 1995: 200)

Derrida was an important social theorist. His argument was that deconstructive questioning (which we address in the chapter on semiotic analysis) was a meth-odology, a logic of doing research that could not be transformed into a method (a set of replicable techniques) because of the unique nature of the texts he stud-ied. We disagree, in so far as we think it is possible to discuss the procedures of semiotic analysis in a coherent way. Thus, we have stressed the need for emer-gent researchers to be familiar with a linguistic grammar, the analytical tools of semiotics. It is of the same importance as knowing about probability and statisti-cal analysis is for readers contemplating survey research (see Chapter 6).

Overall we have strived to find a balance between the standardised how-to-do accounts and more abstracted debates about epistemology. This has meant that our 'template' for chapters has had to be flexible. At times we have extended debates about fairly abstract issues because we think them pertinent to contextualising research. At other times we have endeavoured to distil a series of how-to-do procedures in the absence of such accounts.

Structure of the book

Every chapter discusses a specific research approach and contains a discussion of the key concepts of case-centric/variable-centric and analytical induction/hypothesis-testing as noted above. We also discuss reliability and validity, and the fixedness or fluidity of the approach throughout. These concepts are introduced further below. They tend to nest together, though there are some exceptions. For example, case-centric approaches, such as in-depth interviewing (see Chapter 2), tend to be fluid in their framing and use analytical induction, while the reverse is usually true for variable-centric approaches such as surveys.

This book is also structured around the degree of interaction required in the approach discussed, from the more to less interactive. For example, in-depth interviewing is focused on the interaction between the researcher and the person being interviewed (the research participant). Chapters 3–5 are similar in this regard. Chapter 6 on survey research, usually involves interaction, but at a shallow level – the participant merely responds to questions with little opportunity to add information. Experimental research, discussed in Chapter 7, certainly involves interaction between researcher and participant, but in contrast to the desire for collaboration between researcher and participant, which is a feature of in-depth interviewing, life history, and ethnographic approaches, this is much less intimate, more formulaic and prescribed by a set of protocols. The experimenter seeks to tightly control the interaction, directing the participant (or subject) to behave in a certain way, sometimes with the subject not even knowing the purpose of the research. Unobtrusive research (Chapter 8) seeks to avoid direct interaction, and where there is interaction it is minimised in the interests of avoiding any collaboration whatsoever. The remaining chapters are not interactive and do not involve other people at all.

Defining social research

social science

noun [mass noun]: the scientific study of human society and social relationships.

[count noun]: a subject within the field of social science, such as economics or politics. (*Oxford Dictionary of English*)

The term 'social research' refers to research conducted by social scientists, for example, anthropologists, geographers, historians, social psychologists and sociologists, as well as scientists in allied fields interested in human society, such as law and medicine. The idea that human society could be studied 'scientifically' developed throughout the western world during the nineteenth century, largely as a result of successes of the natural sciences, such as biology and physics. If the application of scientific methods to the natural order increased knowledge and enabled us to create new technologies, might not the application of the scientific method to human beings enable us to understand ourselves?

Social scientists employ a range of methods in order to analyse a vast range of social phenomena. As will be discussed in the following chapters, the choice of method often depends on what the researcher intends to explore. For example, a researcher may be interested in why people drink alcohol. Variable-centric methods, such as surveys, can help to describe issues statistically: how many people drink, how drinking varies across different demographic groups, whether people are influenced by the drinking behaviour of friends or family, and so forth. On the other hand, these methods can not answer questions such as why someone started to drink, what they think about drinking, why some people may have influenced their attitude to drinking but others didn't, and other complex questions. For this level of detail, case-centric research methods, such as in-depth interviews, are more helpful. However, case-centric research methods can only tell us about the beliefs of the research participants, not the wider population. We will return to these issues later.

Case-centric or variable-centric research

Most textbooks and accounts of research make a distinction between qualitative and quantitative forms of doing research. This is a longstanding division that has its origins in the debates between the supporters of a positivistic social science and its radical, feminist and Marxist critics. These debates culminated in the 'science wars', regarding the status of feminist and radical scholarship in the 1970s (Oakley, 1998) and more recently of postmodernity (Matthewman and Hoey, 2006). What remains of these historical debates (that is if the positivists lost, then no one got round to telling them – see Chapters 6, 7 and 9) is a sometimes useful template that portrays 'qualitative' and 'quantitative' research as a series of binary oppositions (i.e., either/or assumptions) (Table 1.1).

The points in Table 1.1 are by no means all-inclusive. However, they provide a useful starting point for discussion about the context of research. Whether research is regarded as an example of good science or not is ultimately determined by its context. For example, if a researcher conducts a piece of qualitative research that eschews traditional measures of validity and reliability, she or he will find it near impossible to get published in many top-ranked academic journals. This is regardless of any intrinsic worth in the research. Autoethnographers (see Chapter 12) regularly complain about the difficulty of getting their autobiographical research published in 'mainstream' journals, yet many consider themselves to be social scientists (Anderson, 2006).

Charles Ragin has published a fascinating series of monographs about research approaches which transcend the qualitative/quantitative divide. In *Constructing social research: The unity and diversity of method* (1994), he talks about case-centric and variable-centric approaches as a better symbolic and analytical marker than the oppositions of qualitative versus quantitative research. Elsewhere he also champions a comparative approach that combines the best features of each (Ragin, 1987, 2008; Ragin and Becker, 1992).

We have divided the research approaches used in this textbook into case-centric and variable-centric ones. We hope we have not overly bowdlerised Ragin's account. We have done so because this seems a better schema. In our opinion most of the research approaches we cover have moments of both qualitative *and* quantitative research. For example, survey research (Chapter 6) is surely the epitome of quantitative research and does indeed produce an analysis that may be strictly numerical. But the design of questions is largely a qualitative process.

Cases and variables are close synonyms for 'examples' and 'characteristics', as used in Table 1.1. Every piece of research has both cases and variables. In this textbook possible cases include: people as research participants, their life histories, their autobiographies, texts in the form of writing or images or objects, material traces, focus groups, communities, and more. Further, a single case can 'nest' other cases, if the research becomes more detailed. For example, a focus group (Chapter 5) can be thought of as a single case, if we wish to

TABLE 1.1   Key elements of qualitative research and quantitative research

	Qualitative research	Quantitative research
1.	Uses writing.	Uses numbers.
2.	Data takes the form of words, texts, images, material traces, narratives of all kinds; in fact, almost anything.	Data take the form of counts, correlations and other statistical formulae.
3.	Is used to study the multiple characteristics of a few (or singular) examples of something. Usually ($n < 50$).	Is used to study the limited characteristics of many examples of something. Usually ($n > 50$).
4.	Emphasises the richness of accounts (using as many characteristics as possible in the description).	Emphasises the parsimony of accounts (using as few characteristics as possible in the analysis).
5.	The researcher adopts a subjective stance. The aim is to interpret or reinterpret events.	The researcher adopts an objective stance. The aim is to control for and discount subjective understandings.

count the group as a collective (as in one focus group), or several cases, if we wish to count the number of participants in the group (that is, typically six to nine people).

The range of variables or characteristics is, if anything, even wider than the possible type and number of cases. Variables are the characteristics or features that are used to describe a case. They are always associated with a single value, in each particular case. Oftentimes in interactive research (where the researcher interacts directly with people) the variables are questions. For example, 'What colour is your hair?' Values are the descriptors that make variables measurable. For example, 'hair colour' might be a variable used to describe some features of appearance. We might determine that there are 19 possible values for the variable 'hair colour'. Any case may be assigned only one value for the variable: flaxen blond, yellow blond, platinum blond, sandy blond, golden blond, strawberry blond, dirty blond, ash blond, auburn, brunette, dark brown, chestnut brown, medium brown, medium golden brown, light golden brown, light ash brown, lightest brown, black, and the best one, red.

The distinction between case-centric and variable-centric research highlights what it is that the researcher starts with, or grabs his/her attention, or initiates the research process. Case-centric research starts with a case. The traditional example of case-centric research is the anthropological ethnography (Chapter 4) in which the researcher (a western anthropologist) lives among indigenous peoples for a sustained period and in doing so details their daily lives, rituals and customs. There isn't so much traditional anthropology done in the twenty-first century – the villagers around the world are not so keen – but there is a huge amount of other case-centric research undertaken by social scientists.

The main features of case-centric approaches are that the researcher:

- begins with a *case* that is somehow defined by a spatial, temporal or conceptual boundary (e.g., a village in Wales, an occupation, TV game shows of the 1990s, military uniforms of the Cold War) and
- must then discover the most significant variables and values to describe the case or commonalities between cases (what makes them unique or alike).

Variable-centric research works in the opposite direction. The researcher begins with some ideas about variables, normally about the relationship between variables, and then seeks a sufficient number of cases to explore this relationship. The easiest to grasp of the variable-centric approaches is survey research (Chapter 6). Here the researcher may start with an idea about the relationship between a couple of variables, for example 'educational achievement' and 'income'. She/he may believe that higher levels of educational achievement are associated with higher levels of income. Once the survey researcher has:

(1) determined how she/he is going to test her/his hypothesis by developing appropriate *variables* and values for her/his questionnaire, the next task is

(2) to find sufficient cases (survey respondents) of the right type to complete the survey.

There is one more dimension to the case-centric versus variable-centric divide. That is, case-centric research usually combines a single or few cases with many variables and values, while variable research is the opposite – few variables with many cases. This reflects the differing focuses of research. Research on cases tends to be in-depth, seeking richness and completeness, and therefore requiring a diversity of variables and values. For example, what would be the minimum number of variables and values a researcher would need to describe the unique properties of the students in any of your tutorials? We imagine it would be many hundreds. In contrast, variable-centric research tends to focus on a restricted number of variables, or propositions about variables, and to seek out as many appropriate cases as possible.

CONCEPTUAL CONCERN 1

We have divided the research used in this textbook into case-centric and variable-centric approaches. Case-centric research has a single or few cases and many variables and values. Variable-centric research has few variables and values and many cases.

We use the terms case-centric and case-first, variable-centric and variable-first interchangeably. What we want to emphasise (after Ragin) is that case-first research centres on finding the best variables/values to describe the case(s), while variable-first research centres on finding the right number and types of case. Our breakdown of case-centric and variable-centric research approaches is shown in Table 1.2.

We discuss six case-centric approaches and five variable-centric ones. We note that unobtrusive research is only weakly variable-centric. It does not fit cleanly into our schema. This is because the approach is commonly undertaken as a supplementary form of research and may rely on fortuitous or found data (see Chapter 8). Conversely, focus group research is only weakly case-centric because it is often used in hypothesis-testing, especially as a preliminary to survey research (see Chapter 5). Semiotic analysis is another slightly uncomfortable fit in terms of our terminology. Here we have dropped the term 'research' in favour of 'analysis'. This reflects that semioticians tend to rely on found data (in the form of signs) rather than engage in coherent search and data collection strategies. A discussion of data collection pertaining to signs or texts (i.e., written, visual or material objects that can be 'read')

TABLE 1.2 Case-centric and variable-centric approaches

Approach (in order of chapters)	Case-centric or variable-centric	Notes
In-depth interview research	A case-centric approach	
Life history research	A case-centric approach	Often single-case research
Ethnographic research	A case-centric approach	Often single-case research
Focus group research	A case-centric approach	Weakly case-centric; often used to test-hypotheses or as preliminary research
Survey research	A variable-centric approach	
Experimental research	A variable-centric approach	
Unobtrusive research	A variable-centric approach	Weakly variable-centric; often a supplemental approach; data sometimes found rather than collected
Content research	A variable-centric approach	
Secondary research	A variable-centric approach	
Semiotic analysis	A case-centric approach	Often single-case research; data (signs) tend to be found rather than collected
Autoethnographic research	A case-centric approach	Often single-case research

is covered in the chapters on content research (Chapter 9) and secondary research (Chapter 10).

Analytical induction or hypothesis-testing

The case-first versus variable-first schema has a further advantage over the qualitative versus quantitative variant in that it provides a better base for understanding the two logical processes of doing research that we use in this textbook: (1) analytical induction and (2) hypothesis-testing. We argue that case-centric approaches tend to favour analytical induction and variable-centric ones – forms of hypothesis-testing.

CONCEPTUAL CONCERN 2

We have divided the logical processes of doing research into: (1) analytical induction and (2) hypothesis-testing. Analytical induction is used to develop new theory. Hypothesis-testing is used to assess existing theory.

We have tried to emphasise that case-first research centres on finding the best variables/values to describe the case(s), while variable-first research centres on finding the right number and types of case. This means that researchers who start with exploring a case do so with something of a blank slate. This is not to say that they have forgotten all that they know of anthropology, or psychology, or sociology, etc., but it does mean that they enter the field with a lot to learn. Often this is called an inductive approach. Inductive means reaching a conclusion based on observation. Some textbooks describe inductive research as a bottom-up approach. The researcher builds up a new theory from observations and then develops propositions and hypotheses about them. In other words, beginning with a case (or a limited number of cases), the researcher has to determine what are the key variables and associated values and what are the significant relationships between them. Howard Becker (1993, 1998, 2009) has done much to refine and explain the research process of induction. He uses the term analytical induction – which we also prefer. Key techniques used in analytical induction include grounded theory and thematic analysis – see the next chapter.

In contrast, hypothesis-testing is a top-down approach to theory and research. It is a deductive way of doing research. A deductive approach means finding the solution to a problem based on evidence. A more formal name for this approach to research is 'hypothetico-deductive reasoning' (Blaikie, 2007). The researcher begins with a developed problem, in the form of a hypothesis about the relationship between some variables, and seeks a solution by testing this theory across a number of cases.

We discuss the logic of analytical induction and hypothesis-testing throughout this textbook. Table 1.3 contains the main differences in the logic of research. It is important to stress that this distillation to two logical approaches is not universally accepted. Blaikie (2007), for instance has four logics or research strategies: induction, deduction, abduction, retroduction, and also some combinations. Such fine-grained discussion of the logics of research is primarily philosophical in character and does tend to see the procedures of research methods as overly determined by epistemology (see below).

SOME ISSUES IN RESEARCH

In the following section we discuss epistemology, explaining the three positions used in this book to discuss the approaches: positivism, social realism and social

TABLE 1.3   Key elements of analytical induction and hypothesis-testing

	Analytical induction	*Hypothesis-testing*
1.	Inductive: bottom-up in building theory.	Deductive: top-down in testing theory.
2.	Begins with a case(s) and seeks to understand the key variables and values needed to describe the case.	Begins with a theory or hypothesis about the relationship between variables and seeks to test this proposition across a range of cases.
3.	Has a limited number of cases explored in-depth through multiple variables.	Has a restricted number of variables tested across many cases.
4.	Emphasises the richness of accounts (using as many variables as possible in the description of the case(s)).	Emphasises the parsimony of accounts (using as few variables as possible in the hypothesis-testing).
5.	Describes a single-case or relatively few cases in-depth.	Measures the covariance of or correlation between different sets of variables across a large number of cases.

constructivism. We also discuss reliability and validity – the key means of evaluating research. We finish with a discussion of ethics, from the perspective of why ethical issues are given priority in research, and as a practical guide to ethical research.

Epistemology

Epistemology refers to the theory of knowledge that informs how research is shaped in its broadest sense. It is primarily a philosophical debate. Eskola (1998) describes the three most important epistemological positions in the social sciences. These three can be thought of, as Eskola notes, as differing attitudes to observation and the possibilities for science. We label them: (1) positivism, (2) social realism and (3) social constructivism.

> Let's illustrate these ways of thinking with the help of a story of three baseball umpires who are discussing how each one of them whistles a foul ball. The one who believes in the possibility of describing the world objectively says: 'I whistle the ball foul when it is a foul ball.' The subjectivist who understands the constructive, observer- and instrument-dependent nature of knowledge confesses: 'I whistle a foul ball when it seems to me that it is a foul ball.' The third umpire, for whom the world is socially constructed, says: 'The ball is foul when I whistle it a foul ball.' (Eskola, 1998:14, cited by Engeström, 2000: 302, also see Sarbin and Kitsuse, 1994)

In Eskola's metaphor, the baseball umpires are, of course, researchers, and the 'foul balls' are social phenomenon.

As an aside, in preparing to write this section, we made an interesting discovery. We had two versions of this story, one of which cites an article written in 1979, which in turn cites an article written in 1976. The other version, written more recently, does not credit a previous source, giving the impression that they came up with the analogy. So an ironically pertinent question arises – whose knowledge (or intellectual property) was this story originally and how was the story in the most recent version constructed?

PRACTICE POINT 2

Epistemology refers to the theory of knowledge that informs how research is shaped in its broadest sense. This textbook discusses research approaches in terms of three epistemological positions: (1) positivism, (2) social realism and (3) social constructivism.

The three epistemological positions outlined in this textbook have differing approaches to doing social science and what might be considered scientific. In each case these are political as well as philosophical positions:

1. **Positivism** ('I whistle the ball foul when it is a foul ball'): Positivists accept as true a social reality that exists independently of our perceptions of it. The ball is foul, and this is an observable fact. As a result, they have the greatest confidence in the ability of social scientists to reveal the truth. Positivists stress the techniques of observation and measurement and the potential for scientists to form objective/unbiased understandings of the social world. For them, good science is objective science, and the methods of doing research are largely about eliminating a subjective stance or bias on the part of the researcher and the research participants. This is an important – but tacit – 'political' agenda and as a result positivism is commonly accused of ignoring issues like power, subjectivity (meaning) and cultural relativism. For example, positivists are unlikely to accept as 'good science' any research approaches that rely on single case studies (e.g., life history, ethnography, semiotic and autoethnographic research) because they 'lack' the number of cases needed to test for positivistic measures of reliability and validity.

2. **Social realism** ('I whistle a foul ball when it seems to me that it is a foul ball'): Social realists also believe in an external and measurable social reality, but one that exists through the mediation of our perceptions of it and our actions. Social realists argue that revealing the social world is far more problematic than suggested by positivists. For social realists, doing science is a legitimate

goal, but it is understood as a project that is limited by factors that social scientists have great difficulty in controlling for or being objective about. Where positivists strive for objectivity, social realists emphasise subjectivity – perspective – and the appreciation of factors like power, meaning and the need for researcher reflexivity (self-awareness). Any search for truth is always clouded by, among other things, the ways in which researchers and institutions impose bias. Controlling for institutional and researcher bias becomes an important component of socialist realist efforts at doing science, whereas positivists, in their narrow focus on methods, tend to discount these political underpinnings of science. Social realists tend to make explicit the political assumption about epistemology and how it impacts method. This textbook or, more properly, both its authors are oriented to a social realist position. We believe that social realism is the mainstream position within the social sciences today.

3. **Social constructivism** ('The ball is foul when I whistle it a foul ball'): Social constructivists take the political-philosophical criticism of positivism further than their social realist colleagues, to the point where it challenges the notion of science as a legitimate concept. They don't accept social reality as an independent phenomenon, or a straightforward idea of truth or of science. They have no faith in science as a project that generates anything resembling universal rules or laws. In this epistemology it is impossible to differentiate truth-claims based in science, or folklore, or common sense, or metaphysics, because individuals or actors actively create the social world and all potential measures of that social world. They argue that it is impossible to have a scientific stance – meaning an objective position outside the data and its analysis (if you are a positivist), or to control/filter the subject effects of power, meaning and bias (if you are a social realist). This does raise the issue of whether social constructivists can be considered social scientists at all. We have given them the benefit of the doubt, in so far as the radical imagining of what a constructivist science might look like is worth exploring (see Table 1.4).

Reliability and validity

Doing good science is about rigour of the research, and its two most important measures are reliability and validity. Reliability measures the extent to which the analysis of data yields reliable results that can be repeated or reproduced at different times or by different researchers. Validity measures the extent to which the research is accurate and the extent to which truth-claims can be made, based on the research – i.e., that it measures what is intended.

For example, we may decide to measure intelligence by having students sit exams. If the same students get good results every time they sit exams, we can say that the results are reliable. However, the reason they get good results might be because the markers are very generous, therefore the results would

TABLE 1.4 Prevailing epistemologies of research approaches

Approach	Case-centric or variable-centric	Prevailing epistemology
In-depth interview research	A case-centric approach	Social realism/social constructivism
Life history research	A case-centric approach	Social realism
Ethnographic research	A case-centric approach	Social realism/social constructivism
Focus group research	A case-centric approach	Social realism/positivism
Survey research	A variable-centric approach	Positivism/social realism
Experimental research	A variable-centric approach	Positivism
Unobtrusive research	A variable-centric approach	Positivism/social realism
Content research	A variable-centric approach	Positivism/social realism
Secondary research	A variable-centric approach	Social realism
Semiotic analysis	A case-centric approach	Social realism/social constructivism
Autoethnographic research	A case-centric approach	Social realism/social constructivism

not be valid. We think we're measuring intelligence, but we're actually measuring marker generosity.

Sometimes distinguishing the two can be confusing. A common way to tell them apart is to think of the researcher as an archer, shooting arrows at a target. When the archer gets her/his arrows near the target's bulls-eye, then the results are valid (accurate). When the archer gets a good cluster, then the results are reliable (repeatable). The most rigorous research is both reliable and valid (Figure 1.1).

However, the standards and measures of reliability and validity are very much influenced by the epistemological position that has shaped the research (or, more pertinently, has shaped the opinions of potential journal editors). Positivists have the clearest and most developed measures of reliability and validity. This reflects their dominance in the hard sciences, the longstanding desire of social scientists to emulate 'real' scientists, and that positivists have the narrowest range of variables or research findings to measure.

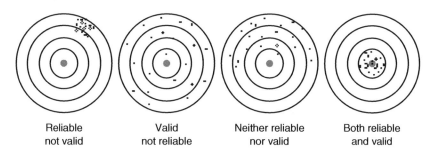

| Reliable
not valid | Valid
not reliable | Neither reliable
nor valid | Both reliable
and valid |

FIGURE 1.1 Validity and reliability illustrated by the archery metaphor

---

PRACTICE POINT 3

Reliability refers to the extent to which the analysis of data yields results that can be repeated or reproduced at different times or by different researchers. Validity refers to the extent to which truth-claims can be made, based on the research – it is dependent on the research measuring the appropriate phenomenon.

Where research involves data collection and analysis that cannot be reduced to numbers, measures of rigour are far more problematic. Thus, case-centric research carries a double burden: (1) it tends to undertake analysis that is not reducible to numbers (qualitative research, in other words), and (2) it lacks a number of cases that might facilitate measures of covariance or correlation. Single-case research is even more problematic (and disturbing for positivists). Nevertheless, social realist and social constructivist researchers continue to challenge positivism in this area, and come up with innovative attempts at new measures of reliability and validity. For example, we draw attention to the work of Robert Yin (2003), who suggests that a case protocol can assist reliability in case-centric research, including single-case research (see Chapter 3 on life history research and Chapter 12, on autoethnographic research).

Ethical considerations

A key concern that contributed to the decrease in popularity of some research approaches in the social sciences, notably unobtrusive approaches (particularly observation) and experiments, is that of ethics, especially with regard to informed consent. Most chapters of this book deal with ethical issues specific to the approach discussed. In this section we deal with general considerations.

The most important aspect of ethically appropriate research is *voluntary informed consent*. It is generally considered to be an essential requirement of ethical research, in the context of minimising the risk of harm (and, a cynic might say, the risk of lawsuits). Let's briefly look at the three words that make up this important term:

- **Voluntary:** referring to the recruitment of participants, this includes the notion of free will – that it is just as easy for a potential participant to decline to take part as it is for them to agree. This is most easily effected by making information available to appropriate people via some form of advertising, rather than directly approaching them.

- **Informed:** simply providing potential participants with enough information about what will be asked of them, so that they can make an informed decision about taking part (often via a written participant information sheet).

- **Consent:** a formal process in which the participant affirms, usually in writing, that they have been provided with all the information they require and are agreeing to take part of their own free will. A standard form is usually provided to all participants for this purpose.

The process of gaining informed consent usually has several steps:

1. **Recruitment of participants:** This necessitates the development and distribution of recruitment materials, such as flyers or posters, to stimulate potential participants' interest and to provide them with the contact details of the researcher(s). Once contact is made by the possible participant, the next step is usually …

2. **Provision of a participant information sheet (PIS):** As the name suggests, the PIS contains all the information a possible participant needs in order to be able to make an informed decision about participation, such as: what is involved; where the research will take place; how long it will take; who has reviewed the research for ethical appropriateness and how to contact them; and a statement about the ability to change one's mind after volunteering, to refuse to answer questions, to withdraw data, and so forth. If the possible participant makes contact at this point to volunteer to take part, this is followed with a …

3. **Formal consent process:** Usually at the beginning of an experiment, interview, focus group, or whatever the case may be, the researcher restates the key points covered in the PIS, asks the participant if she/he has any questions (and answers any such questions) then asks the participant to sign a form attesting to the fact that she/he has been provided with all the information she/he requires and agrees to take part.

Gaining informed consent is not always practicable, especially where deception is used, as in experiments (see Chapter 7) and unobtrusive research (see Chapter 8). Yet, as Page (2000) notes, ethical and good practice guidelines have increasingly frequently stipulated that 'good' research is '*with participants*' who are collaborators rather than '*on subjects*'. While we contend that it is almost always naive to suggest that research participants have equal power in the research relationship so that the process is truly one of joint collaboration, it must certainly be acknowledged that ethical review boards and publishers of academic works alike expect an explicit discussion of informed consent processes and the role of participants in the research.

After the issue of consent, the next most important consideration is the risk of discomfort or harm.

Ethical issues: risk of harm

Often the risk of harm to participants will be negligible – though one can never be certain that a participant has not had a negative personal experience related to the research topic (and so revisiting that experience could cause discomfort). In some cases, though, the research clearly carries with it a risk of emotional discomfort, for example, if the topic is domestic violence or any one of the other myriad sources of trauma that exist in modern society, and the participants are survivors. There are several steps that can be taken to minimise risk. These can include:

- Specifying a minimum age for participants, in the hopes that maturity will increase coping skills (in any case, it is common to exclude people aged under 16 for reasons of power differences between researcher and participant, unless there are good reasons for not doing so).

- Specifying a minimum amount of elapsed time between the last experience and the research participation. For example, one of the authors has conducted interviews with survivors of suicidal behaviour and specified that at least one year should have elapsed since the last suicidal episode. By doing so, it was hoped that participants would have moved beyond suicidality and therefore be at less risk, and also that greater emotional (and temporal) distance would allow for greater or easier reflection and discussion.

- Explicitly discussing the potential for distress with possible participants during the recruitment process, including in the participant information sheet and any other written material, and asking participants to consider this carefully before volunteering.

- Suggesting that because it is a sensitive topic, they may like to plan something for immediately after the research takes place, such as visiting a friend or undertaking another enjoyable activity.

- Reminding participants of this possibility before commencing the interview or other research and giving them the opportunity to decline to be interviewed (and perhaps including a statement about this in the consent form, such as 'I am aware of the potential for the interview topic to cause distress and have considered this before consenting to take part').

- Inviting participants to bring a support person with them.

- Providing participants with a list of appropriate services and contact details, and perhaps forewarning these agencies of the research.

None of these steps guarantees that participants will not experience distress and researchers must consider how they would deal with this, should the situation occur. We will return to this topic below.

Lastly, ethics committee and review boards will often want to be assured of the *value* of the research. That is, will it make some useful contribution to knowledge? A director of a private research organisation that one of the authors briefly worked for used to rail against ethics committee and the amount of his valuable time taken up in preparing responses to such questions, but researchers should bear in mind that they are asking participants to give up *their* valuable time, and ethically, there should be some purpose to this beyond satisfying a researcher's curiosity or providing amusement (Ring, 1967). This may be of particular concern for some sectors of the population who are frequently asked to take part in research. For example, Maori, the indigenous people of New Zealand, are rumoured to be one of the most researched people in the world. Over recent years it has become difficult to recruit Maori participants in research, especially for non-Maori researchers, in part due to the prioritisation of the state in addressing gaps in well-being between Maori and other New Zealanders. This has required much research on Maori, supposedly to inform policy, but often with little apparent benefit: '"Research" is probably one of the dirtiest words in the indigenous world's vocabulary' (Tuhiwai Smith, 1999: 1). As a result, ethics applications in New Zealand need to clearly demonstrate cognisance of these issues and explicitly state the relevance of research to Maori.

Averting/dealing with discomfort

From time to time researchers may have to deal with a participant at risk of or becoming emotionally distressed. Paying attention to non-verbal cues is an important warning system. Most of us would readily pick up on these cues if they occurred while talking to a friend, but they may be missed in research situation because of a focus on the research process itself, or not being familiar with the participant's mannerisms. For example, drumming fingers on the table-top or rapid tapping of toes or other fiddling can indicate that the participant is becoming agitated, while hesitancy, a change in voice tone, speed or volume, and avoiding eye contact may indicate emotional distress. It's often fairly easy to prevent an uncomfortable situation developing by saying something like, 'If you feel you don't want to talk about that for a while, that's fine', 'Let's take a breather for a few minutes', or 'We can come back to this topic later, if you prefer'.

However, sometimes cues are not readily perceived or distress develops very rapidly. In such cases, it is best to immediately stop the interview (or experiment, etc.). Unless you are an experienced counsellor or therapist, you should attempt to minimise further discussion of the topic that has caused distress. Instead, express your sympathy and ask the participant what can be done to improve the situation: 'I'm sorry this has upset you. Let's stop the interview/experiment/discussion. Is there someone I can call?' You may wish to follow up with a phone call, email or note, reiterating your sympathy, though it should not be necessary to take the blame for the person's distress, providing they were given appropriate information about the topic beforehand. This can be distressing for the researcher also. If you have taken reasonable precautions to prevent distress occurring, as discussed above, you should not be afraid to debrief with a supervisor, colleague or friend.

Ethical issues: deception

Deception in research often applies to pretending that an experiment is about something different from what appears to be the case. Here we also use the term to refer to pretending that an experiment is a naturally-occurring, real-life event; for example, pretending that a deliberately planted letter has been accidentally dropped to see whether someone will post, ignore, or discard it.

Newman and Krzystofiak (1979) asked whether deception is ever warranted, in the context of deception, as it usually applies to unobtrusive research – a lack of awareness that one is engaging in research. They found that the answer to this question is yes, in some circumstances. This is illustrated by their own research. Their study of employment discrimination compared two methods: unobtrusive observation of employment decisions and a self-report survey of employment practices. Strikingly different results were obtained: when employers were unaware that they were taking part in a study, employment decisions tended to be made on the basis of the race of the applicant; when employers were aware of their participation, race did not play a part in decision-making. Newman and Krzystofiak argued that because we seek to present ourselves in a positive manner, self-reports may be 'distorted'. Therefore, deception may be required in order to produce accurate results. However, they cite three criteria for consideration, as discussed by Kelman (1972):

- the degree of deception involved balanced by the probability of harmful consequences,

- the importance of the research topic, and

- the availability of other data collection strategies that are both capable of producing similar information and are deception-free.

CONCEPTUAL CONCERN 3

Concerns about ethical issues had a major impact on the practice of unobtrusive approaches. Concern focused on the informed consent of participants and the use of deception. These concerns have also arisen with regard to experiments (see Chapter 7).

Ethical issues: debriefing

Researchers – especially psychologists – have been criticised for consent and deception issues, particularly with regard to experiments (see Chapter 7). Informed consent has also been an issue for anthropologists (particularly regarding observation in ethnographic research – see Chapter 4). However, with experiments, these issues are often ameliorated by debriefing at the end of the experiment: telling participants what the experiment was really about, talking through their experiences and minimising the risk of any ill effects caused by the deception. Similarly, though distress may occur in interviews or focus groups, there are strategies available for minimising this through a well-handled debriefing (see Chapter 2). This is rarely possible with unobtrusive approaches (see Chapter 8).

Ethical issues: where to from here?

Ethical conduct is a very real concern for social science researchers, and rightly so. However, with careful planning, research on most topics can safely be carried out. Specific issues likely to arise with the use of different approaches are discussed further in the following chapters, in particular with regard to interviews, experimental research and unobtrusive research.

PUTTING THE APPROACH IN CONTEXT

In this section we focus on the framing of research, using a 'fixed or fluid' binary. This is followed by a practical guide to getting started with research; developing the research topic, preparing a proposal and ethics application; sampling and recruitment of participants, and so forth.

Fixed or fluid framings or research

Ragin (1994) identifies three analytical framings of research, of which we use only two: fixed and fluid. Fixed and fluid framings relate primarily to the fixedness or fluidity of the sequence of steps or procedures that make up any research project. A fluid framing means that the researcher is free to revisit and significantly modify early stages of research. This can include the overall focus of the research. A fixed framing means that the researcher must adhere to a sequence of procedures. Earlier stages may not be revisited. Hence, survey research is very fixed (Chapter 6). For example, once participants have filled in the questionnaire it is normally impossible to add new questions. In contrast, autoethnographic research is highly fluid (Chapter 12). The researcher can revisit any aspect of the research at any moment, including in the process of writing a journal article! The main impacts on analytical framings are:

1. **The size and complexity of the research**: Small research projects that can be accomplished by a lone scholar also tend to be more fluid. This is an issue of management, of time and other resources – the lone scholar may more easily be able to revise the research process. Larger research projects, especially using research teams, are more likely to have fixed analytical frames because this simplifies issues of management. For example, research assistants can be given clear instructions at the start of the project.

2. **The interactive or non-interactive aspect of research:** Interactive research means the creation of data at the point of its collection. Interactive research requires exchanges between researcher and research participants (people) in the process of collecting data. For example, in-depth interviewing (Chapter 2), life history research (Chapter 3), ethnographic research (Chapter 4), focus groups (Chapter 5) and surveys (Chapter 6) create situations, encounters and pose questions that would not exist otherwise. For example, unless a researcher is posing questions, most people don't spend their days telling strangers about their preferences for public transport, etc. Interaction often creates an incentive for fluid framings – in part because researchers want to respond and make changes in the face of interaction with participants. However, this isn't always the prevailing driver.

3. **The analytical inductive versus hypothesis-testing elements of research:** Research that seeks to build *new* theory and broadly uses induction (Becker, 1993) tends to have a fluid framing. In contrast, hypothesis-testing (finding the solution to an established 'problem') is closely aligned with a fixed framing.

4. **It is always a combination of the above:** As Table 1.5 suggests, whether the analytical framing of a piece of research is fluid or fixed is always the result of a combination of factors:

TABLE 1.5 Analytical framing of research approaches

Approach	Case-centric or variable-centric	Analytical frame
In-depth interview research	A case-centric approach	Fluid
Life history research	A case-centric approach	Fluid
Ethnographic research	A case-centric approach	Fluid
Focus group research	A case-centric approach	Fixed, especially if focusing on hypothesis-testing
Survey research	A variable-centric approach	Fixed
Experimental research	A variable-centric approach	Fixed
Unobtrusive research	A variable-centric approach	Fixed, especially if focusing on hypothesis-testing
Content research	A variable-centric approach	Fixed, with partial exception of very small-scale research
Secondary research	A variable-centric approach	Fluid; this is unusual for a hypothesis-testing approach, mainly because it is non-interactive
Semiotic analysis	A case-centric approach	Fluid
Autoethnographic research	A case-centric approach	Fluid

PRACTICE POINT 4

A fluid analytical framing means that the researcher is free to revisit and significantly modify earlier stages of research. This can include the overall focus of the research. A fixed analytical framing means that the researcher must adhere to a sequence of procedures.

Precursors to research

Most empirical research will follow the same set of procedures:

1. Developing the research topic.
2. Preparing a proposal and ethics application.
3. Sampling and recruiting participants.
4. Collecting and managing data.
5. Transcribing.
6. Analysing data.
7. Disseminating the findings.

We will deal with the first three of these in this section, as they are fairly standard across approaches. The remainder are discussed in specific chapters, as appropriate.

Developing the research topic

The initial idea for a piece of research can come from any one of many sources, such as a personal experience of the researcher or an opportunity to be paid to work on a project, or it may be limited by the availability of supervisors and their interests. In any case, the basic steps of developing the research topic are the same:

1. Start asking questions – of yourself, colleagues, supervisors, etc. – begin narrowing down your general area of interest into a specific area of enquiry (sometimes referred to as a conceptual variable).
2. Search the literature – find out what is already known, and what is not.
3. Narrow your initial ideas down to an idea that can be studied. Begin shaping the idea into an operational research question(s): a manageable area of enquiry.

CONCEPTUAL CONCERN 4

An operational definition transforms the research topic from the abstract (conceptual) to the specific (operational).

During this process, be critical and analyse your observations (whether they are your personal observations, something you have read about, or something someone has told you). As you find out more, for example by a literature review, be open to revising your initial thoughts – or finding out that the question that you thought was original has already been answered.

Preparing a research proposal

In some situations, beginning researchers may not find it necessary to prepare a research proposal, for example, if they are taking part in a class research project. However, preparing a proposal, serves several valuable purposes that will often be essential:

- Clarification of the research aims – a well-written proposal must clearly state the aims of the research and how they will be achieved. In order to be sure that these aims will be met, researchers must engage in ...

- Clarification of the process – exactly how will the research be carried out?

- Preparation of a document that can be used to provide necessary information to:

    o possible supervisors

    o collaborators

    o administrators involved in university enrolments

    o ethics committees or institution review boards

    o scholarship and other funding providers.

The length of the proposal will vary according to its purpose. For example, an initial proposal whose purpose is to provide a background document for discussion with possible research supervisors may be less than a page. A proposal to accompany an ethics application will probably run to between three and ten pages, depending on the nature and complexity of the research and the requirements of the committee. A proposal to accompany a university enrolment may be a page or less for enrolment in a graduate dissertation, or 50 pages for confirmation of full enrolment in a doctoral programme, depending on the requirements of the institution. In all of these varied situations it will be expected that the proposal will include:

- Background information on the topic, including some discussion of existing research and what the proposed new research will add to this body of knowledge (the aims of the research).

- Discussion of the research methods to be used and the rationale for choosing the method. (Include the practicalities of the research, such as where interviews will take place, how long they are expected to take, how you will record what is said, whether participants will be provided with a transcript and offered the opportunity to comment on it.)

- A timeframe for the project, including dates for beginning work on the project in general, submission of the ethics application, beginning of recruitment of participants, beginning of data collection, end of data collection, beginning of analysis, completion of analysis, end dates for writing up of various sections or chapters of the resulting document (report, dissertation or thesis) and completion of the complete final version.

In our experience, the time required for recruitment and analysis are often underestimated by students. Recruitment, in particular, can involve waiting for responses to advertisements, letters of invitation, etc. Fortunately, some of the writing can be begun at this point, particularly the introduction and literature review and the basic elements of the method (obviously you won't be able to discuss the participants, but you should be able to discuss the methods used, and the underlying methodology).

Recruiting participants

It used to be that the most common source of research participants for psychologists and some other social scientists (whether conducting their first piece of research or their fiftieth) were students. This has at least two inherent limitations. First, students may be different from the broader population in important ways and this can impact on the results. They are likely to be better educated than the general population and they may have biases about the value or nature of the research. Second, as a group they may be more or less appropriate as a source of recruitment. For example, because of their relative youth they may be less able to talk about experiences normally associated with older sections of the population, such as employment or child-rearing, or, indeed, aging. Consider, then, how you can most readily access the particular population you're interested in and what recruitment tools can facilitate this, such as flyers, posters, newspaper advertisements. The following chapters include discussions of the recruitment issues specific to the approaches.

CONCLUSION

We hope at this point that you have an understanding of what to expect from this textbook, and of the core concepts that underpin it. We've also introduced key terms that will be used throughout the book and that structure each chapter. These include case-centric (beginning by determining what the case(s) will be as the primary consideration, e.g., who will be interviewed as participants) and variable-centric research (beginning by determining what the variables will be, e.g., the questions that will be asked in a survey); and analytical induction (the process of developing a new theory or revising an existing one, from the data gathered) and hypothesis-testing (testing a hypothesis derived from an existing theory). We've discussed three epistemological positions in the social sciences – positivism, social realism and social constructivism – issues of reliability and validity, and fixed or fluid analytical framings or research. You'll see how these can be applied to the individual approaches as you continue, which should take care of any remaining 'fuzziness'.

As you read through the book you will see that we have endeavoured to discuss the advantages and disadvantages of each approach, along with the types of research question best suited to each approach. Where appropriate, we've included recent and current developments, such as the use of new technologies. Though as researchers ourselves we have our personal preferences, we believe that all of these approaches are useful to emergent researchers. We hope you also enjoy this book.

FURTHER READINGS

As noted above, Charles Ragin has published a fascinating series of monographs about research approaches which transcend the qualitative/quantitative divide. His *Constructing social research: The unity and diversity of method* (1994) was important in shaping this textbook and our teaching. A second edition was published in 2011, just as we were finishing this textbook, but at the time of writing was not yet in our library. We are sure it will be of great use. Similarly, Howard Becker's *Tricks of the trade: How to think about your research while you're doing it* (1998) is an inspirational account of doing research. It is both sophisticated and clear.

Brinkmann and Kvale (2008) provide a useful discussion of the concepts underlying ethical research that we consider valuable to all emerging researchers, and those interested in case-centric approaches in particular.

We have found the *Sage benchmarks in social research methods* series to be extremely valuable and commend them to students seeking an in-depth understanding of a particular topic.

REFERENCES

Anderson, L. 2006. Analytic autoethnography. *Journal of Contemporary Ethnography*, 35, 373–395.

Becker, H. S. 1993. How I learned what a crock was. *Journal of Contemporary Ethnography*, 22, 28–35.

Becker, H. S. 1998. *Tricks of the trade: How to think about your research while you're doing it*. Chicago: University of Chicago Press.

Becker, H. S. 2009. The life history and scientific mosaic. In: Harrison, B. (ed.), *Life story research*. London: Sage.

Blaikie, N. 2007. *Approaches to social enquiry: Advancing knowledge*. Cambridge: Polity Press.

Brinkmann, S. & Kvale, S. 2008. Ethics in qualitative psychological research. In: Willig, C. & Stainton-Rogers, W. (eds.), *The Sage handbook of qualitative research in psychology.* London: Sage.

Derrida, J. 1995. *Points … : Interviews, 1974–1994,* Stanford, CA: Stanford University Press.

Engeström, Y. 2000. Activity theory and the social construction of knowledge: A story of four umpires. *Organization,* 7, 301–310.

Eskola, A. 1998. From small group research to conversation analysis. In: Lahikainen, A. R. & Pirttilä-Backman, A.-M. (eds.), *Social interaction.* Helsinki: Otava (in Finnish).

Kelman, H. D. 1972. The rights of the subject in social research: An analysis in terms of relative power and legitimacy. *American Psychologist,* 27, 989–1016.

Matthewman, S. & Hoey, D. 2006. What happened to postmodernism? *Sociology,* 40, 529–547.

Newman, J. & Krzystofiak, F. 1979. Self-reports versus unobtrusive measures: Balancing method variance and ethical concerns in employment discrimination research. *Journal of Applied Psychology,* 64, 82–85.

Oakley, A. 1998. Gender, methodology and people's ways of knowing: Some problems with feminism and the paradigm debate in social science. *Sociology,* 32, 707–731.

Page, S. 2000. Community research: The lost art of unobtrusive methods. *Journal of Applied Social Psychology,* 30, 2126–2136.

Ragin, C. 1987. *The comparative method: Moving beyond qualitative and quantitative strategies.* Berkeley, CA: University of California Press.

Ragin, C. 1994. *Constructing social research: The unity and diversity of method.* Thousand Oaks, CA: Pine Forge Press.

Ragin, C. 2008. *Redesigning social inquiry: Fuzzy sets and beyond.* Chicago: University of Chicago Press.

Ragin, C. & Becker, H. S. 1992. *What is a case? Exploring the foundations of social Inquiry.* Berkeley, CA: University of California Press.

Ring, K. 1967. Experimental social psychology: Some sober questions about some frivolous values. *Journal of Experimental Social Psychology,* 3, 113–123.

Sarbin, T. R. & Kitsuse, J. I. 1994. *Constructing the social.* London: Sage.

Tuhiwai Smith, L. 1999. *Decolonizing methodologies: Research and indigenous peoples.* London: Zed Books.

Yin, R. K. 2003. *Case study research: Design and methods.* London: Sage.

TWO

IN-DEPTH INTERVIEWING – THE INTERACTIVE BASE

CONTENTS LIST

Key words: interviewing – in-depth interviewing – survey interviewing – interview guide – sampling – recruitment – analytical induction – grounded theory – thematic analysis – interview technique – transcription

---

SUMMARY

The processes of data collection and analysis using in-depth interviews, in comparison to other case-centric approaches, including the practicalities of in-depth interviewing: (i) developing an interview guide; (ii) recruitment of participants; (iii) data collection; and (iv) management and analytical induction, as well as conceptual issues such as epistemology and the use of technical equipment (e.g., NVivo).

In this chapter we discuss the processes of data collection and analysis using interviews. We shall focus on in-depth interviews, in which the quality of the interaction between the interviewer and research participant is paramount. Though survey interviewing is touched on here, the in-depth approach to interviews contrasts with survey research in many respects – in particular, the amount of interaction involved and therefore the degree to which interviewing actually occurs as well as the framing of the approaches. Surveys are therefore discussed separately and in detail in Chapter 6.

The distinctions between in-depth interviewing and other case-centric approaches will be explored. This is followed by a discussion of the practicalities of in-depth interviewing, including developing an interview guide, recruiting participants, collecting and managing data, and taking an analytical inductive approach, including grounded theory and thematic analysis. The following section includes conceptual issues such as epistemology. Lastly, we discuss the use of technical equipment.

DOING DATA COLLECTION, ANALYSIS AND PRESENTATION

In-depth interviews have also been described as focused interviews, non-directive interviews, open-ended interviews and active interviews. Such interviews are developed through the use of schedules which contain the questions or topics – which may be thought of as variables – though it is vital to note that these questions are flexible, in accordance with this case-centric and fluid approach. In contrast, surveys are characterised by the questionnaire, which is often self-administered. This is possible because the survey is a variable-centric approach in which the questions (variables) are tightly defined and fixed.

CONCEPTUAL CONCERN 1

The in-depth interview is a case-centric approach, in which the framing is fluid. This allows for revision of the variables (interview topics/questions) as the research progresses.

What is an in-depth interview?

An interview is a way of gathering data from one person at a time. Interview approaches are often defined in terms of structure: they can be structured, semi-structured, or unstructured. These terms translate to the fixed/fluid dichotomy used throughout this book. The distinction between fixed and fluid framings has been introduced in the previous chapter. By way of a reminder, fluid framing means that the relationship between ideas and data is very likely to change during the research. Therefore flexibility to modify variables is necessary. With in-depth interviews, the variables are the questions that are asked of the people being interviewed (the research participants). Interviews may contain a mix of open-ended and closed questions (though the latter will probably be restricted to demographic data such as age) or no formal questions at all (in which case it would be 'unstructured' and completely fluid).

In contrast to the survey approach, in-depth interviews will not be highly structured (fixed) in terms of the questions asked as this will restrict the depth of data gathered.

PRACTICE POINT 1

In-depth interviews predominantly use open questions in an interactive process between a researcher and a participant.

How is an in-depth interview different from a questionnaire-based interview?

Both in-depth interviews and questionnaire-based interviews have individual people as cases and questions as variables. But that is largely where the similarity ends.

As mentioned above, in-depth interviews are case-centric, which means that the key requirement is to determine what (or in this approach, whom) the cases will be – they come first. The interviews are characterised by the use of open variables, questions such as 'What do you think about … ?'. These questions can be adjusted to suit the situation. Indeed, there may not be any prepared questions at all. Instead, the interviewer may have a list of topics to discuss, but broach these topics in whatever way seems most appropriate at the time. In-depth interviews are of most value in exploring an issue about which little is known, or to get a detailed picture of what people think. In-depth interviews may be used after a survey has been completed to elaborate survey findings.

- Example in-depth interview question (variable): What are the positives and negatives about being a university student?

- Example in-depth interview answer (value): 'I'm really enjoying being able to focus on a topic that I'm passionate about, and hopefully to be able to make a career out of it … I find juggling my study and work commitments really difficult, as well as trying to have a social life; it can get a bit overwhelming, especially at exam time …'

In contrast, questionnaire-based interviews, used in surveys, are variable-centric – the key concern is to determine the variables. Because the questions (variables) are closed, it is vital to get them right as there is little, if any, opportunity to elaborate or change them once data collection has begun (though a pilot survey may be completed to 'test' the survey before commencing data collection proper, and a draft questionnaire may also be evaluated via focus group; see Chapter 5). This is partly because the data generated is to be analysed statistically, and this requires precise answers and large numbers of participants. Therefore, the answer options (values) as well as the questions themselves are predetermined. These types of interviews are particularly useful for obtaining numeric information about a precise topic.

- Example survey question (variable): How strongly do you agree or disagree with the following statement: 'I enjoy being a university student'?

- Example survey answer options (values):

  1. Strongly agree.

  2. Agree.

  3. Neither agree nor disagree.

  4. Disagree.

  5. Strongly disagree.

Questionnaires are increasingly completed without any interaction between a participant and an interviewer at all. For example, many questionnaires are administered by asking potential participants to complete an electronic survey via a link in an email.

How is an interview different from a focus group?

The number of people participating in the interview is the most salient difference. However, a focus group is more than 'an interview with more people'. The quality and quantity of data may be different too as the group dimension adds other factors, for better or worse (see Chapter 5).

How is an interview different from a discussion?

Even an unstructured interview will usually have some guiding themes or topics to be addressed – that is, an agenda. There will also have been some formalities to go through, such as an ethics process, and introducing the topic, talking about follow-up, etc. As noted by Kvale (2007: xvii), 'The interview is a specific form of conversation where knowledge is produced through the interaction between an interviewer and an interviewee'. However, this interpretation of the interview, with explicit acknowledgement of interaction, is the result of a process of evolution, as will be discussed below. Earlier writers on the topic (and some contemporary ones) have tended to overlook this aspect: 'An in-depth interview is like the half of a very good conversation when we are listening. The focus is on the "other person's own meaning contexts" (Schutz, 1967: 113)' (Liamputtong and Ezzy, 2005: 58). This view does not acknowledge the fact that interaction between the interviewer and participant may result in the participant thinking about aspects of the topic not previously considered, thereby producing new knowledge.

Origins of the approach

Interviews take place in many contexts and we will all have been interviewed, whether as participants in research, prospective employees, patients in health facilities or witnesses in police investigations. Interviews, in the broad sense of conversations with the purpose of obtaining knowledge, have taken place since ancient times, for example Socrates' conversations with Sophists (Liamputtong, 2009). Research interviews in the social sciences date back at least a century (e.g., Booth, 1902–03), although they are often viewed as an aspect of a broader methodological category such as life history, ethnography or survey, rather than as a method itself (Platt, 2001). The 1930s saw interviews being combined with observations and experimental tasks by developmental psychologist Piaget as the basis for his theory of child development, although Platt (2001) points to one of the first social science methods textbooks, by Odum and Jocher (1929), as containing an early description of the interview. The development of the 'focused interview' by Merton and Kendall in the 1940s was a key progression in the interviewing method (Merton and Kendall, 1946). In the original concept of the focused interview, a 'stimulus' such as a film – the 'focus'– is presented before the interview itself begins, and it is this focus item which is the basis for the interview content (Merton and Kendall were interested in the impact of the media on mass communication). However, Merton and Kendall also promoted the use of the non-directive approach and specificity (discussed later in this section). The use of a stimulus to the discussion has parallels with the currently increasing use of visual methods, which will be discussed later with regard to the use of new technology. Further developments of the approach largely came about as a result of epidemiological concerns, discussed below.

The practicalities: what are the advantages of in-depth interviews?

Surveys and focus groups are the interview's close cousins. In comparison to focus groups, interviews can be easier to manage, as the interviewer can focus on one person and will not have to contend with group dynamics. This also potentially allows for easier rapport-building, so the participant may be more willing to discuss personal material, and there is more time to pursue interesting areas (without other participants interrupting). Building rapport is discussed in detail in the next chapter.

As discussed elsewhere, in comparison to questionnaires, it is possible to gather rich information – to follow-up on interesting points, to include material that the participant brings up that you may not have anticipated, to go into greater detail. Questions, themes or topics can be added or adapted as you progress through a series of interviews – or in the course of a single interview.

CONCEPTUAL CONCERN 2

In-depth interviews allow for 'rich' or 'thick' data to be gathered with detailed descriptions.

What are the disadvantages?

If you have built a good rapport, the participant may reveal quite sensitive information. While this may be desirable, it may also create an extra burden: to ensure that the participant remains comfortable during and after the interview and has any appropriate follow-up. Sometimes it is challenging to keep the interview on track: the participants may want to tell you things that are not really relevant. The richness of the resultant data (particularly in comparison to variable-centric methods such as the survey) may seem overwhelming for the beginning researcher, though this can be reduced by the adoption of good data management practices from the first interview. We will discuss data management below.

Preparing and undertaking a 'typical' set of interviews

Although in-depth interviews are fluid in terms of framing, most research using this method will follow the same set of procedures:

1. Developing the research topic.

2. Seeking ethics approval.

3. Sampling and recruiting participants.

4. Collecting and managing data.

5. Analysing data.

We have discussed general research procedures in detail in Chapter 1, especially points 1 and 2. In this chapter we build on this general material and focus specifically on its application to in-depth interviews. The practicalities of collecting, managing and analysing data are given particular attention.

Developing the research topic

Begin narrowing down your general area of interest into a specific area of enquiry, for example, from 'student life' to 'how do students cope with the transition from secondary education to university?', then into a research question(s): a manageable area of enquiry such as 'How do first year students' experiences differ depending on whether they live on-campus, with their parents, or go flatting?'

Consider how others have approached the topic. If you're interested in new students, you should consider others' definition of new students – should you only include students who have started university straight from secondary school, or should you also include those who've had a gap year? It might seem to make more sense to exclude those who've had a gap year on the grounds that they'll have more 'life experience' and therefore more internal resources to cope with the changes and stresses of student life. But on the other hand, if most of the previous research has included all students enrolling at university for the first time, then you won't be able to directly compare your results.

Seeking ethics approval

The importance of appropriate ethics processes has been discussed in Chapter 1. Generally speaking, the ethics process involved in interviewing is straightforward, although particular consideration may need to be given if the topic is of a sensitive nature and/or the participants are vulnerable in some way.

Ethics applications for interviews will usually need to include a list of questions or topics to be discussed. This is known as the interview guide. This should allow the committee/board to determine the risk of harm to the participants but reassure them as to the value of the research and the appropriateness of the approach.

Developing the interview guide

Questions will be predominantly open-ended, that is, encouraging an answer that takes at least a sentence, rather than a simple categorical answer such as 'yes' or 'no'. Often, rather than precise questions, a series of themes to be discussed will be prepared, which can be adapted to suit the individual participant. When beginning your interviewing career, and until you have developed confidence, you may find it best to have actual questions which you can refer to if you get 'stuck'. This will ensure you cover all the topics you had intended to ask about, and you can still adapt these as required. However, for unstructured interviews, the interviewer may simply begin by talking about the purpose and aims of the research, or by asking one very broad question or by making a general statement. For example, 'So, to begin, can you tell me about your experience of using mental health services?' The interviewer can then leave the participant to talk about whatever seems relevant to them. The interviewer's main role in this case is to ask for clarification or elaboration when required. This is often called *probing* (e.g., 'Can you tell me a bit more about that?' 'What was that like?' 'Can I check, you said x happened; how did you feel about that?') and ensures that the participant does not wander too far off topic. An example of the different

TABLE 2.1 Interview type and level of structure

Interview type	Structural Format
Structured	Question: 'Please rate x mental health service on a scale of 1 to 5.'
Semi-structured	Theme: 'Could you tell me about the positive and negative aspects of x mental health service?'
Unstructured	Topic: 'I'm interested in your experiences of mental health services.'

approaches to structure is shown in Table 2.1; this topic is also discussed in Chapter 3 on life history research.

Sampling and recruiting participants

In-depth interviews are a case-centric approach. This means that accessing the cases is a crucial step. That is, accessing the appropriate cases can make or break the research; the variables, though of course necessary, can be changed. With in-depth interviews, the cases are the people who are interviewed, usually referred to as the participants. It is worth making a distinction here between the *participants* in in-depth interviews (and other case-centric approaches), the *respondents* in surveys and the *subjects* in experiments. These distinctions can be linked to the prevailing epistemology of the approach, particularly in regards to views of collaboration between the researcher and the researched. These issues are returned to below.

PRACTICE POINT 2

Interviews are a case-centric approach. This means that the primary concern is recruiting a suitable number of appropriate cases – participants. The variables – questions – can be modified to suit each case.

As discussed in the previous chapter, recruitment of participants can take some time, and it is worth paying some attention to the development of 'tools' to maximise recruitment. If you're interested in the experiences of first-year students, then advertising via flyers on notice-boards around the university should be fairly straightforward, especially if you are able to offer an incentive for participation, such as a raffle draw. On the other hand, if you're interested in people's experiences of mental health services, you'll need to consider other means, such as placing posters and/or flyers in the reception areas of social service agencies and health professionals as well as in more 'public' places, such as supermarkets, bearing in mind that people with experience of mental illness may not necessarily be engaged with support services.

PRACTICE POINT 3

It is usually well worth putting some effort into the development of appropriate recruitment tools, including developing relationships with appropriate groups or services who may be interested in the research as well as posters, flyers or letters of invitation to participate.

Aside from the practicality of recruitment processes, two conceptual issues require consideration, both related to sampling: generalisability and size.

As will be discussed in detail in later chapters, variable-centric approaches are much concerned with generalisability: the notion that the findings from the sample who took part in the research (e.g., the people who responded to a survey (Chapter 6) or were subjected to an experiment (Chapter 7)) should be able to be generalised to, or be representative of, the population at large. In contrast, case-centric approaches are more concerned with specificity: whether the results describe the findings from a specific group of participants in a detailed and 'rich' manner (Flick, 2006).

CONCEPTUAL CONCERN 3

Case-centric approaches are more concerned with specificity than gener-alisability: do the results describe the findings from this specific group of participants in a detailed and 'rich' manner?

Case-centric samples are characterised by *purposive sampling* and *data satura-tion*. The aim of in-depth interviewing is to understand a topic deeply. Therefore, the key is to select information-rich cases (Patton, 2002). A crucial point is to recruit participants strategically – participants who will be able to contribute meaningfully to the research. For example, if you are conducting research into the experiences of first-year university students, there will be little point in interview-ing people who have never been university students. This is known as purposive sampling. It is conceptually the opposite of the representative sample that is required to make statistical comparisons – usually a key element of variable-centric approaches. It is very closely linked to theoretical sampling, which is a strategy to facilitate theory construction and requires that data collection be controlled by emerging theory (Flick, 2006), that is, participants are recruited according to the new insights they may be expected to bring to the developing theory.

PRACTICE POINT 4

The number of participants in an interview-based study is usually small and is recruited purposefully rather than randomly.

In case-centric research, there is no set formula to determine sample size. Instead, data saturation is used to determine when sufficient data has been gathered – when sampling can stop. Data saturation can be said to have occurred when no new information is gleaned by further interviews – participants report similar experiences, beliefs or understandings to those reported by previous participants. Of course, in order to determine if data saturation has been reached, the researcher must engage in preliminary analysis while collecting data. The concept of data saturation is linked to, but is not the same as, grounded theory (discussed below).

PRACTICE POINT 5

The size of an interview sample cannot easily be determined ahead of time; it requires revision of the data as it is collected, to determine when 'data saturation' is reached. Saturation is also discussed in Chapter 3 on life history research.

Collecting data: beginning the interview

Many interviewers will feel a little nervous at the beginning of an interview, especially if they have not met the participant before. It may be helpful to remember that:

- The participant is probably new to the process as well, and so is likely to be as nervous as you are. Therefore, they are probably not likely to notice your state due to focusing on their own!

- There are steps you can take to reduce the nervousness of both parties. These include engaging in general small talk, offering something to eat or drink, and attending to one's body language: take a few (surreptitious) deep breaths, uncross arms and legs, sit back and adopt a relaxed facial expression. Faking an emotion can fool us into feeling it, and the people around us are likely to follow (Duclos et al., 1989).

- The initial process of beginning the interview can follow a series of well-defined steps, as outlined below. In addition, Chapter 3 (Life Histories) includes a detailed discussion of building rapport:

1. Introduce yourself and any other researchers or assistants. Do what you can to assist the participant to feel at ease, as above.

2. Explain the broad purpose of the research, stressing that the aim is to get as much information on peoples' perspectives as possible; there are no correct or incorrect answers – you wish to hear what they think.

3. Explain what will happen afterwards, for example, if there will be a follow-up interview; if you will provide a transcript for them to read and comment on, and if so, a deadline for responding and what will happen if they don't respond (usually that it will be assumed that they are happy with the transcript as it stands); guarantees and/or constraints about the anonymity of information provided; whether you'll provide a copy or a summary of your report/thesis/article. Most of this information will have been contained in the participant information sheet.

4. Give the participant an information sheet (even if they have previously been sent out), read through the key points and invite questions.

5. Once the participant appears to be comfortable and to have asked all questions they may have, you may ask for the consent form to be signed.

6. Before beginning the interview, check that any recording devices you intend to use are working. We strongly advise that you take notes of key points as a back-up and listen to the recording as soon as possible to ensure the whole interview is recorded audibly.

Collecting data: during the interview

It is important not to lead the participant to the answers you anticipate. Do not pre-empt statements, for example, by saying 'You must have felt pleased/embarrassed/sad' or 'So you would agree that ...'. Remember that it is the participant who has the knowledge (if you already had the knowledge, you wouldn't need to be doing the interview!), although there may well be an element of co-creation of knowledge (discussed below).

Encourage the participant to continue talking about interesting material: 'That's really interesting', 'Then what happened?'.

Non-verbal cues and body language
Both the interviewer and participant will make use of non-verbal cues, consciously or not. These cues can be extremely useful – sometimes essential – sources of information.

One of the most important skills for beginning interviewers to learn is how to wait in the face of a participant's silence. It is tempting to suggest responses to fill in the silence. However, responses suggested by the interviewer may shift the thinking of the participant, disrupt their flow of thought or cause them to feel that they have not been giving the 'correct' answers. In this situation it is helpful to focus on the participant's body language. Do they appear to be thinking the question over (often signified by gazing up towards the left)? If so, let them continue. On the other hand, if they look puzzled or doubtful, consider rephrasing your last question or comment.

The interviewer's own body language can be a useful tool: a questioning look, a nod, a smile of understanding, to encourage a participant to continue speaking. However, it is the non-verbal cues used by the participant that have the power to completely change the meaning of the words spoken and thus the resulting data. Consider, for example, these two responses to the question 'What did you think of today's lecture?':

- Student 1: 'I loved it, it was really interesting', accompanied by a smile, nodding head and eye contact.

- Student 2: 'I loved it, it was really interesting', accompanied by a sneer, rolling of the eyes, and a snort of derision.

The non-verbal cues convey that Student 1 is sincere (or at least wants the person who asked the question to believe she is sincere) while Student 2 is being sarcastic and actually means the reverse of what she is saying.

Sometimes phrases are so frequently used to express sarcasm or other emotions that attention to non-verbal cues is not necessary. In New Zealand a popular advertising campaign used by a beer manufacturer, Tui, is based on the assumption of sarcasm that accompanies the phrase 'Yeah, right' (Figure 2.1).

Usually, though, when you read over a transcription there will be no way of telling from the words alone whether they are said sincerely or not. We strongly recommend that you note verbal cues such as sarcastic tone, strong emotion, or information emphasised by participant (e.g., by nodding or shaking of the head,

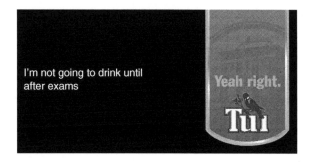

FIGURE 2.1 Assumed meanings in a billboard: 'Yeah right'
Reprinted with permission

raised voice) as the interview progresses. A typology for doing so is given in the section on transcribing, below.

Non-verbal cues can also be an extremely useful indicator that a participant is becoming distressed. Please see Chapter 1 for further discussion on averting and dealing with participant distress.

Collecting data: completing the interview

The beginning researcher may find the completion of the interview a little awkward, especially in unstructured interviews. On the one hand, you'll want to be sure the participant has said everything they consider relevant and not stop them too soon. On the other hand, despite your efforts at building rapport, developing a participatory environment etc., the participant may well consider you to be 'in charge' as the person who is gathering the information, and therefore will expect you to be the person to close the interview. You'll usually be able to tell that the participant is reaching the end of their 'story', because they will be pausing more and perhaps making comments like 'There was one other thing'. However, bear in mind that you may not have the opportunity to make contact with a participant later, so make sure you have all the information you need:

- Do you have sufficient detail?
- Are all themes or variables fully explored?

In our experience, participants are quite happy at this point for a researcher to say something like 'It seems like we're coming to the end of our discussion, but I just want to check my notes' and wait while the researcher checks their interview guide and notes. In general, participants seem to respond well to comments such as 'I'm sorry, I want to make sure I've got this right; you said …', 'Could you say a bit more about that?' or 'One topic we haven't talked about much is …'. And finally, 'It seems that we've covered the main things that I had in mind, but I want to be sure that you've told me everything that you think I should know. Is there anything else you'd like to say?'

Of course you'll thank participants for their time and contribution, and give them any donations, incentives or gifts you have arranged. You may also remind participants of any follow-up, such as how to contact you if they should wish to, arrangements for providing transcripts for checking, and so forth. If the interview was on a sensitive topic and/or the participant appeared to become uncomfortable, we recommend you engage in a debriefing process.

Debriefing
Debriefing involves talking participants through their interview experience and minimising the risk of any ill effects. If you knew ahead of time that the interview

topic carried with it a risk of discomfort, you may well have developed a strategy for dealing with this, as discussed in Chapter 1. If not, it's important to check with the participant that they are feeling ready to go on their way. For example: 'I realise this may have been/was a difficult issue to talk about. I really appreciate your contribution and hope that you're comfortable with it. What more can we do to complete this process?'.

Managing the data

The management of qualitative data occurs at several points of the data collection process:

1. During the initial data collection, that is, during the interview. As noted above, we recommend that you make notes during the interview, recording tone of voice, body language, and so forth.

2. During transcription, which is discussed immediately below. We recommend undertaking transcription as soon as possible after the interview, while the interview is fresh in your mind and you are readily able to add further remarks that may have been missed during initial note-taking.

3. During the journaling process. Journaling should also take place as soon as possible after each interview. We consider it to be an intermediary step between data collection and analysis. As such, it is discussed in detail in the section prior to data analysis.

Transcribing

Depending on the type of research you're doing, you may or may not want to fully transcribe the interview. If you're undertaking discourse analysis, or a narrative method, every 'um' and pause may be important. On the other hand, you may prefer to note key points as you go along, and flesh these out immediately after the interview, listening through the tape to make sure you haven't missed or misheard anything. However, for your first few interviews, it may be best to do full transcriptions until you are confident in your ability to recognise superfluous material (if there is any). We strongly suggest that you also record laughter, a sarcastic tone, body language that indicates that the participant is joking or being ironic, tearfulness, agitation, etc.

Gail Jefferson developed a set of transcribing conventions which are widely used (Jefferson, 1974). As discussed above, non-verbal cues can be as important as what a participant says. So can silences, changes in speech and 'non-speech' sounds. These conventions provide a form of short-hand to save

TABLE 2.2 Typology for recording cues

Sound	Symbol	Meaning
Pause/silence	(2.5)	Pause in the participant's speech, measured in tenths of seconds
Volume increase	BUT	Capitals indicate a rise in volume
Volume decrease	°but°	Degree signs indicate a decrease in volume
Emphasis	<u>but</u>	Underline shows emphasis and may be accompanied by non-verbal cue
Sound stretching	Bu::t	Colons indicate prolonging of sound (e.g., expressing doubt or thoughtfulness)
Unclear	(but)	Transcriber unsure of word
Inaudible	( )	Transcriber cannot hear what was said
Audible breathing	hh	Audible exhalation
'Non-speech' sound	((sigh))	Explanation of other sound made

transcribers from explaining every sound and pause. The most common of these are given in Table 2.2.

Journaling

Journaling, or memo-writing, serves three purposes:

1. It is an important aspect of case-centric research as it enhances the fluidity of the approaches. Through engaging with the data during the collection process, the researcher is able to determine if unexpected themes are emerging and adjust the interview schedule accordingly.

2. It allows the point of data saturation to be determined.

3. It is also essential to grounded theory in so far as it prompts the researcher to engage with and undertake preliminary data analysis during the data collection process.

Journal entries can include theoretical ideas and analytical insights, as well as notes on specific comments made by participants. They can take the form of notes or diagrams (or frequently both). Some researchers keep a separate journal for this purpose, though many will use a column alongside interview transcripts and for the coding of text (as in Table 2.3 in the section on data analysis below). We suggest both: preliminary notes alongside transcripts which are fleshed out in more detail in a journal, perhaps using diagrams in a separate document that brings together thoughts and insights from all transcripts.

PRACTICE POINT 6

Journal entries are an important tool and should be completed as soon as possible after an interview. They encourage the development of insights as well as
ideas about how the interview process can be improved. By facilitating the initial
interrogation of the data, the researcher can consider when data saturation has
been reached.

Analysing data

We use the term analytical induction (see Chapter 1) and inductive analysis
somewhat interchangeably. However, the former term is favoured in most of the
text we use in this chapter, so we will stick mainly with that. Analytical induction, thematic analysis and grounded theory are the processes most often used
in analysing in-depth interview data. Beginning researchers may come across
various terms, such as conversational analysis, discourse analysis and narrative
analysis, but all of these include processes of searching for patterns and/or
underlying meanings in the data. A detailed discussion of each is beyond the
scope of this chapter.

Analytical induction

Analytical induction is a process of identifying patterns and themes in the
data rather than deciding, prior to data collection or analysis, what the precise variables or data categories will be (Patton, 2002). The development of
variables occurs with analytical induction only after an interview has taken
place, rather than trying to fit participants' answers into a predetermined
frame. Analysis is *data-* (and case)-driven. Once data has been gathered, thematic analysis may be used to recognise, evaluate and describe patterns and
themes in the data (Braun and Clarke, 2006). We should note, however, that
it is possible to take a *theory*-driven approach to interviews, to search for
references to a particular notion that the researcher wishes to examine.
Indeed, the initial research topic will almost always have derived from a ker-
nel of a theory, even if it is as vague as 'Making the transition from secondary
school to university probably involves some challenges'. This idea will likely
have been followed up by reading on the topic to refine the research question
into something that can be operationalised (put into practice) and added to
the existing body of knowledge.

Liamputtong and Ezzy (2005) note that a number of famous researchers
describe such data analysis as 'calculated chaos' (Lofland and Lofland, 1971) and
that interpretation is an 'art that cannot be formalised' (Denzin, 1994).
Nevertheless they go on to write a chapter that attempts to formalise or sys-
tematise the fluid processes of case-centric research. Much of this process is

aimed at coding the data gathered in the field. This coding is an essential tool in transforming data into usable information. Coded interview transcripts are typically analysed through the processes of grounded theory and thematic analysis.

PRACTICE POINT 7

The coding of data into themes is an essential part of transforming data into usable information and is a building block of theory development.

Thematic analysis and grounded theory are key tools of analytical induction. They are often treated as the same thing in textbooks. However, according to Braun and Clarke (2006), thematic analysis does not require detailed theoretical knowledge of approaches such as grounded theory and discourse analysis. Rather, it can be used with different theoretical frameworks so may be more suited to beginning researchers (Braun and Clarke, 2006). Grounded theory (Glaser and Strauss, 1967; Strauss and Corbin, 1990) has become almost ubiquitous as *the* means of undertaking qualitative data analysis, although Braun and Clarke (2006: 81) argue that it is essentially used as 'Grounded theory "lite"', without a full commitment to theory development during the analytical process. They comment that this 'lite' version is indeed very much like thematic analysis. Though there are differences between thematic analysis and grounded theory, the methods are so similar and the terms are so often used interchangeably that we will not discuss the distinctions further here.

PRACTICE POINT 8

Thematic analysis and grounded theory are methods of analytical induction frequently used for in-depth interviews. Though there are differences between the two, they are very similar and the terms are used somewhat interchangeably.

Grounded theory and thematic analysis
The analysis of data collected in research is referred to as 'coding'. Three stages of data analysis are involved in grounded theory: open coding, axial coding and selective coding (discussed below). Theory develops and evolves during the research process due to the interplay between coded data and analysis phases. Codes may be thought of as a kind of shorthand linking values and variables.

- **Open coding:** Open coding is the process of selecting and naming categories from the analysis of the data. Open coding often involves the deconstruction of journal notes, interviews and observations into excerpts, phrases or key words. Variables involved in the research are identified, labelled and coded. This initial stage of data analysis aims to describe overall features of the research. For example, a core variable may be 'How do personal *commitments* impact upon first year university students'?. This could be coded (as seen in the diagram below) in terms of work, study, family and friends.

- **Axial coding**: In axial coding, data are put together in new ways – paying attention to the properties (values and variables) of the categories. This is achieved by utilising a system of coding that seeks to identify relationships between variables and values. The aim is to make explicit connections between categories. Axial coding involves explaining and understanding relationships between variables and codes in order to understand the phenomenon to which they relate.

- **Selective coding**: Selective coding involves the process of selecting and identifying the 'core' code from all those identified in open and axial coding. This core code is then related to all the other categories. This relationship building is the basis of generating new theory because it involves the integration of coded data (excerpts of interviews, phrases, etc.) in terms of their underlying commonalties and linkages.

Many researchers find it useful to draw up core codes, sub-codes and relationships in diagrams. Indeed, representing these relationships in some way is a key feature of grounded theory and Braun and Clarke's thematic map (Braun and Clarke, 2006). As well as providing a way of clarifying the codes, this structure is often translated into headings and sub-headings in resultant documents. Figure 2.2 illustrates codes that may arise from interviews with university students about the challenges of university life. Note that there are several sub-codes to the core

TABLE 2.3 Example interview transcript with notes and codes

Transcript	Notes	Codes
I'm really enjoying being able to focus on a topic that I'm passionate about, and	Excited	Following Passion
hopefully to be able to make a career out of it. It really feels like I'm doing something		Importance
constructive and important for my future. But what if I put in all this time and money and there's no job at the end, you know?	Frowns	
I find juggling my study and work commitments really difficult, as well as trying to have a social life; it can get a bit overwhelming, especially at exam time.		Commitments
There don't seem to be enough hours in the day (sigh). There's pressure from my parents to do well, and they don't understand that sometimes I need to cut loose in the weekend!		Others' expectations

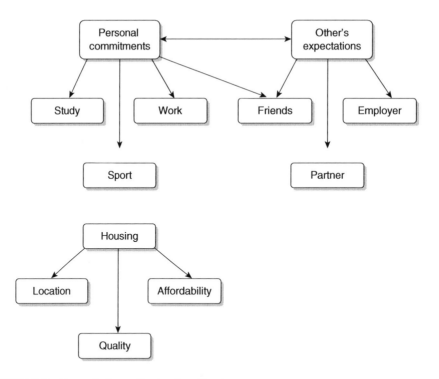

FIGURE 2.2 Example thematic structure 'tree'

code 'Personal commitments', and that this category is related to 'Others' expectations'. The 'friends' sub-code is included both in terms of personal commitments and others' expectations. The code 'housing' does not appear to be directly related to either of the other two core codes.

At this point it is necessary to distil the information in each collated sub-code into meaningful narratives, for example, discussing the combined participants' perspectives on balancing their various commitments.

SOME ISSUES IN RESEARCH

In this section we address some conceptual and epistemological issues, such as the researcher's role in creating data (not merely in collecting it) and practical resource issues.

Interviews as data sources and data creators

Various authors have discussed the ways in which the interview is similar to, and different from, a conversation. For example, '[An interview is] a pseudo-conversation ... it must have all the warmth and personality exchange of a conversation with the clarity and guidelines of scientific searching' (Goode and Hatt, 1952: 191, cited by Oakley, 1981: 33). Treating the interview as a social encounter during which knowledge is actively produced suggests that it is not a neutral, one-sided process. Each interview is dynamic, taking its own shape and content. This view of the interview clearly sits within the social constructivist position (see Chapter 1) – understanding *how* meaning unfolds is as important as *what* is said. This approach also reflects that of many feminist scholars (e.g., see Hesse-Beiber and Yaiser, 2004; Kitzinger, 1994; Oakley, 1981, 1998; Wilkinson, 2004). Compare Carl Rogers' classic work on the 'nondirective method' (1945). In contrast to Kvale's description of the interview as 'a form of conversation where knowledge is produced through the interaction' (2007: xvii), Rogers emphasises the need to 'place upon [oneself] the most unusual restraints and to develop a mode of discourse which is completely foreign to ordinary conversation' (Rogers, 1945: 279), merely reflecting what the other has said.

Rogers makes much of the nondirective technique as a means of avoiding bias (Rogers, 1945). However, recognition that the desire for neutrality is not only futile but counter-productive dates back at least to the 1950s, as noted by Oakley (1981: xx, and quoting Sellitz, Jahoda, Deutsch and Cook, 1965: 583): 'Much of what we call interviewer bias can more correctly be described as interviewer *differences*, which are inherent in the fact that interviewers are human beings and not machines and that they do not work identically.'

We have stated the importance of not leading the participant to a particular point of view and we stand by this statement. However, we also acknowledge that interview data are unlikely to be fully replicable. They may vary because both the interviewer and the participants will react to each other, as well as external factors, differently on different days. This brings us to the topic of epistemology (the study of the nature of knowledge).

Epistemological concerns and constraints

The epistemological underpinnings of the interview can be seen to have changed markedly. For several decades, the interview was seen as a neutral means of extracting information: the interviewer asks questions, the respondent or participant answers. The interviewer is to remain neutral. However, the perception of the *interviewer* as an active participant, a co-creator of knowledge, has increased (Holstein and Gubrium, 1997), as seen in the discussion above of the interview as a conversation.

Kvale (2007) discusses the interview as an inter-view, an exchange of views between two people conversing. This position is aligned with the social constructivist approach: knowledge is constructed through participant (and interviewer) discourse and the structure and effects of this discourse, or narrative, are of interest in their own right. Kvale argues that the positivist approach, with the emphasis on reliable, valid data based on unambiguous, value-neutral and objective facts, is incompatible with in-depth interviews. However, the positivist tradition can certainly be accommodated within a fixed interview framework (as discussed briefly above and in more detail in Chapter 6, Survey Research), and we know of both scholars and publishers who are concerned with issues such as inter-rater reliability in in-depth interviews, normally considered the domain of positivists (the concepts of reliability and validity and their application are discussed in detail in Chapters 6 (Survey Research), 7 (Experimental Research), 8 (Unobtrusive Research) and 9 (Content Research)).

We suggest that many researchers undertaking in-depth interviews take a social realist approach. They recognise that they, as participants in a discussion, may have a role to play in the creation of knowledge during the interview, in so far as the interview process may stimulate the participant to reflect on or articulate ideas for the first time or in a new way. However, the social realist believes that the participant comes to the interview with a set of beliefs, perceptions or understandings, and the interviewer seeks to draw these out. They may be subjective, but they are nonetheless 'real' to the participant.

We can also trace changing epistemologies through changing terms to describe those who provide research data: from 'subjects' (associated with the positivist approach and still frequently used by many conducting experiments), to 'respondents' (people whose role is merely to respond to questions), to 'participants', suggesting a more collaborative approach to the creation of data, as in the social constructivist view.

Resource issues

In-depth interviews are a time-consuming approach. We estimate that an 'average' interview process takes approximately 8–10 hours of work, when recruitment, the interview itself, transcribing and analysis are considered. This does not take into account the preliminary work of preparing a research plan, obtaining ethics approval and writing up outcomes such as a report, thesis or article. While an interview may take an hour or so to complete, plus possibly travel time, we recommend that no more than three be scheduled in a day, and preferably one or two. As noted above, it is best to undertake transcribing and journaling and/or preliminary analysis as soon as possible after the interview. In addition, interviewing is tiring work. However, other than time, the resources required may be minimal, perhaps not much more than the researcher's travel costs, perhaps a donation or incentive for participants and a small amount for stationery, assuming that the researcher already has access to a voice recorder and a computer.

PUTTING THE APPROACH IN CONTEXT

Though the conceptual underpinnings of the interview have evolved over time, it may appear that the process has changed very little. However, the development of various tools, such as cameras, has had some impact on interviewing, and has the potential to greatly enhance the richness of the data collected, while computer software developments can aid in data analysis.

Visual techniques: photo-elicitation and photo-voice

In this section we will normally discuss such things as the impacts of new technology on research. It is debatable whether the use of the camera fits within this category. Certainly, the use of the still camera as an aid to data collection is not new. Early examples include Bateson and Mead (1942), Mead (1963), Byers (1964), Becker (1974) and Bunster (1977) (we assume the dominance of people whose surname begins with B is a coincidence). However, in these early examples, the researchers photographed people in the course of anthropological and ethnographic research (see Chapter 4) and in some cases the photographs themselves formed part of the data (i.e., they were the research topic, rather than an aid to discussion, as is the case with photo-elicitation and photo-voice). Encouraging research *participants* to take photos of things the participants consider to be relevant to the research is a newer and, some would say, still under-utilised approach, although it has been made simpler and cheaper in recent years with the advent of first Polaroid and then digital photography.

Photo-elicitation requires an additional step in the research process: explaining to the participants what it is you want them to do, why and how. This will generally require a preliminary meeting and some careful consideration on the part of the researcher as to how to articulate these issues. This may include some discussion of ethical considerations, for example around taking photographs of other people, as well as explaining that the photos should in some way reflect their feelings or thoughts about the topic of interest.

The example below illustrates a successful piece of research using photo-elicitation.

PHOTO-ELICITATION IN A MENTAL HEALTH FACILITY

A graduate student supervised by one of the authors made good use of photo-elicitation in his Masters research, which explored mental health care in a community-based residential facility:

> When talking to Maui about his photographs, he pointed to one of a clock … the clock had run out of battery and stopped … Maui took a picture of it,

(Continued)

(Continued)

and reflected on the symbolic aspect of time standing still: 'Yeah, I sort of think that times go by and everyone has a purpose to fulfil but, and here for me time stops, I'm by myself. Sort of like that.' In Anthony [another research participant] and Maui's interviews there seemed to be a fundamental aspect of feeling alone and constrained to the individual lifestyle which the flat system at the complex promotes ... [Maui] did not consider taking any photographs outside his flat. This led to an interesting conversation about Maui's view of living at the complex and the fact that he spent a lot of time in the flat. 'Even if I know I can go anywhere whenever I want ... you can never sort of leave the place, you know ... you're always stuck in the system, you're always stuck on the drugs ... 'til maybe I die, medication and all that stuff, that's the future I see ...' (Lloret Andreasson, 2006)

Maui also took photographs of the flat evacuation plan, with the comment 'Looks sort of like a prison block to me!', and the view from his living room, explaining that 'This is what I see every day'. (Lloret Andreasson, 2006)

The photographs taken by Maui and the quotes that accompany them illustrate a key finding of the research – the sense that even though the research participants are living in the community, as opposed to an institution, they felt constrained by and apart from society.

Photo-voice takes photo-elicitation a step further by incorporating the photographs taken by research participants in the dissemination of findings. While this may simply involve including photographs in written publications, it may also take the form of a (semi-)public exhibition, often accompanied by printed relevant quotes. This can be a particularly powerful means of communicating issues to a broader audience.

We note that photo-elicitation is one of several forms of visual approaches. We will discuss photo-ethnography in Chapter 4. Other images may take the form of paintings and other media (Gillies et al., 2005). These forms may be particularly useful in research with people who have difficulty articulating their thoughts verbally. However, visual approaches may also pose additional ethical concerns (Lynn and Lea, 2005). For example, when preparing a photo-voice exhibition, it may not be possible to use all photographs. How should the photographs be chosen so that all participants' voices are represented equally? Should photographs that reveal a face or other identifying material be used?

CONCEPTUAL CONCERN 4

Visual methods provide opportunities for engaging powerfully with concepts that may be difficult to articulate, though some specific ethical concerns may need to be addressed.

Readers may also wish to read Chapter 5 (on focus groups) for further comments on the use of new technologies to gather data. These primarily include audio- and video-conferencing and the use of internet chat-rooms and message boards.

Computer-based data analysis

Although few researchers using variable-centric methods would consider doing analysis without the aid of a computer, the use of computer software to under-take analysis on case-centric data is reasonably uncommon. Such software has existed for some years. However, neither of the authors, nor most of the researchers they know, use it regularly even though it is certainly popular with some. This may in part be due to the fact that the initial set-up of programs like NVivo, which involves developing a coding 'tree' (similar to the thematic map in Figure 2.2 above), then uploading transcripts into the software followed by the coding of each piece of text, seems to offer little in terms of time-savings, though once this process has been undertaken it is very quick and easy to aggregate data by code. In addition, there is a temptation to quantify the data – to assume that if a particular code occurs frequently in the complete data set, then it must be more important than codes that occur less frequently. This, of course, is the antithesis of the purpose of case-centric research. Additionally, it can be difficult to retain the emphasis placed on specific items by the research participants, and therefore it is easy to lose the richness of the data. One way around this may be to be diligent in the use of Jefferson's (1974) typology.

PRACTICE POINT 9

Although setting up software may appear time-consuming at first, it does allow for very quick-and-easy aggregation of data by code which will be useful for large projects or those that may result in multiple outputs (presentations, reports, articles, etc.).

CONCLUSION

The history of the interview in the social sciences dates back at least a century (e.g., Booth, 1902–03), although it has often been as an aspect of a broader methodological approach, rather than as a method itself (Platt, 2001). The in-depth interview is a case-centric approach, in which the framing is fluid. This allows the potential for revision of the variables as the research progresses, though in-depth interviews are developed through the use of schedules which contain the questions or topics. When questions are used, they will be predomi-nantly open-ended, that is, encouraging an answer that takes at least a sentence, rather than a simple categorical answer such as 'yes' or 'no'. Often, rather than precise questions, a series of themes to be discussed will be prepared, which can be adapted to suit the individual participant.

Case-centric samples are characterised by purposive sampling and data saturation. The aim of in-depth interviewing is to understand a topic deeply. The key is therefore to select information-rich cases (Patton, 2002). A crucial point is to recruit participants strategically – i.e., participants who will be able to contribute meaningfully to the research. Data saturation can be said to have occurred when no new information is gleaned by further interviews and at this point sampling can stop. The forms of data analysis are more varied than with variable-centric research and the process may take longer to understand and develop than beginning researchers expect. However, analysis usually takes an inductive form, reviewing the data and developing theory while data collection takes place.

Many beginning researchers start their careers by asking themselves whether they are more comfortable with words or numbers, and on this basis choose in-depth interviews or the survey (or perhaps the experiment) as their primary research method. We consider this division somewhat simplistic and hope to demonstrate the usefulness of many other approaches. Nonetheless, the interview has long been the interactive base of social science and we expect this primary role to continue, even as it evolves.

FURTHER READINGS

Jennifer Platt (2001) provides an interesting history of the interview, although it is limited to the US context. She includes summaries of key writings, empirical practice and, to some extent, epistemology.

Uwe Flick (2006: Chapter 27) has written a useful overview of text interpretation which compares various methods – including text derived from interviews – based on various theoretical or epistemological positions (such as conversation, discourse and narrative analysis). He includes methods that may use text derived by other means, such as content analysis (see Chapter 10 for a further discussion of this approach).

Emerging researchers looking for a comprehensive but easy-to-read manual on interviewing should consider Steinar Kvale's *Doing interviews* (2007). As well as addressing the practicalities of planning, conducting and analysing interviews, he discusses ethics, epistemology and validity and reliability – a balance of the practical and the conceptual that is rarely achieved.

We recommend Reavey and Johnson's work on visual approaches to those interested in these techniques (Reavey and Johnson, 2008). Chapter 4 of this text (Ethnographic Research) also discusses the use of photography in case-centric research.

REFERENCES

Bateson, G. & Mead, M. 1942. *Balinese character.* New York: New York Academy of Sciences.
Becker, H. S. 1974. Photography and sociology. *Studies in the Anthropology of Visual Communication*, 1, 3–26.

Booth, C. 1902–03. *Life and labour of the people of London*. London: Macmillan.

Braun, V. & Clarke, V. 2006. Using thematic analysis in psychology. *Qualitative Research in Psychology*, 3, 77–101.

Bunster, X. 1977. Talking pictures: Field method and visual mode. *Signs*, 3, 278–293.

Byers, P. 1964. Still photography in the systematic recording and analysis of behavioral data. *Human Organization*, 23, 78–84.

Denzin, N. 1994. 'The art and politics of interpretation'. In: Denzin, N. K. & Lincoln, Y. S. (eds.) *Handbook of qualitative research*. Thousand Oaks, CA: SAGE.

Duclos, S. E., Laird, J. D., Schneider, E., Sexter, M., Stern, L. & Van lighten, O. 1989. Emotion-specific effects of facial expressions and postures on emotional experience. *Journal of Personality and Social Psychology*, 57, 100–108.

Flick, U. 2006. *An introduction to qualitative research*. London: Sage.

Gillies, V., Harden, A., Johnson, K., Reavey, P., Strange, V. & Willig, C. 2005. Painting pictures of embodied experience: The use of nonverbal data production for the study of embodiment. *Qualitative Research in Psychology*, 2, 199–212.

Glaser, B. & Strauss, A. L. 1967. *The discovery of grounded theory: Strategies for qualitative research*. New York: Aldine.

Goode, W. J. & Hatt, P. K. 1952. *Methods in social research*. New York: McGraw-Hill.

Hesse-beiber, S. & Yaiser, M. L. (eds.) 2004. *Feminist perspectives on social research*. New York: Oxford University Press.

Holstein, J. A. & Gubrium, J. F. 1997. The active interview. In: Silverman, D. (ed.), *Qualitative research: Theory, method and practice*. Thousand Oaks, CA: Sage.

Jefferson, G. 1974. Error correction as an interactional resource. *Language in Society*, 3, 181–199.

Kitiznger, J. 1994. The methodology of focus groups: The importance of interaction between research participants. *Sociology of Health and Illness*, 16, 103–121.

Kvale, S. 2007. *Doing interviews*. London: Sage.

Liamputtong, P. 2009. *Qualitative research methods*. Melbourne: Oxford University Press.

Liamputtong, P. & Ezzy, D. 2005. *Qualitative research methods* (2nd edn). Melbourne: Oxford University Press.

Lloret Andreasson, J. H. 2006. 'You're always stuck in the system': Mental health care in the community: A qualitative inquiry into individual treatment participation. Master of Social Science Thesis, University of Waikato, New Zealand.

Lofland, J. & Lofland, L. H. 1971. *Analyzing social settings: a guide to qualitative observation and analysis*. Belmont, CA: Wadsworth.

Lynn, N. & Lea, S. J. 2005. Through the looking glass: Considering the challenges visual methodologies raise for qualitative research. *Qualitative Research in Psychology*, 2, 213–225.

Mead, M. 1963. Anthropology and the camera. In: Morgan, W. D. (ed.), *The encyclopedia of photography*. New York: Greystone Press.

Merton, R. K. & Kendall, P. L. 1946. The focussed interview. *American Journal of Sociology*, 51, 541–557.

Oakley, A. 1981. Interviewing women: A contradiction in terms. In: Roberts, H. (ed.), *Doing feminist research*. London: Routledge and Kegan Paul.

Oakley, A. 1998. Gender, methodology and people's ways of knowing: Some problems with feminism and the paradigm debate in social science. *Sociology*, 32, 707–731.

Odum, H. W. & Jocher, K. 1929. *Introduction to social research*. New York: Howard Holt.

Patton, M. 2002. *Qualitative research and evaluation methods*. Thousand Oaks, CA: Sage.

Platt, J. 2001. The history of the interview. In: Gubrium, J. F. & Holstein, J. A. (eds.), *Handbook of interview research: Context and methods*. London: Sage.

Reavey, P. & Johnson, K. 2008. Visual approaches: Using and interpreting images. In: Willig, C. & Stainton-Rogers, W. (eds.), *The Sage handbook of qualitative research in psychology.* London: Sage.

Rogers, C. 1945. The nondirective method as a technique for social research. *The American Journal of Sociology*, 50, 279–283.

Schutz, A. 1967. *The phenomenology of the social world.* London: Heinemann Educational.

Sellitz, C., Jahoda, M., Deutsch, M. & Cook, S. W. 1965. *Research methods in social relations.* London. Methuen.

Strauss, A. L. & Corbin, J. 1990. *Basics of qualitative research: Grounded theory procedures and techniques.* Newbury Park, CA: Sage.

Wilkinson, S. 2004. Focus groups: A feminist method. In: Hesse-biber, S. N. & Yaiser, M. L. (eds.), *Feminist perspectives on social research.* New York: Oxford University Press.

THREE

LIFE HISTORIES – PRIVATE TROUBLES AND PUBLIC ISSUES

CONTENTS LIST

Key words: life history – oral history – memory – recall – triangulation – Becker – analytical induction – validity – reliability

SUMMARY

Building on Chapter 2, a focus on: (i) the practicalities of preparing for and undertaking semi-structured interviews; (ii) the epistemological challenges of case-centric research, particularly reliability and validity; (iii) building rapport; (iv) enhancing memory and recall; (v) analytical induction; (vi) a comparison of life history and oral history; and (vii) an introduction to triangulation.

Life history research neatly follows on from the previous chapter on in-depth interviewing due to the importance of interviewing in life history research. In this chapter we elaborate on some of the issues touched on with regard to interviewing that are of particular relevance to life history research. These include the practicalities of preparing for and undertaking semi-structured interviews; the epistemological challenges of case-centric research, particularly reliability and validity; building rapport; enhancing memory and recall; and looking at analytical induction – a process that builds theory (and present the classic example of Howard Becker's *How I learned what a crock was* (1993)).

We also introduce topics that are unique to life history research, such as the development of the approach, and we compare life history research with the oral history. In addition, we introduce for the first time some topics that are important to life history researchers and others, such as triangulation, which is the use of more than one method to increase or cross-check the data collected from another method.

DOING DATA COLLECTION AND ANALYSIS

The life history is not conventional social science 'data', although it has some of the features of that kind of fact, being an attempt to gather material useful in the formulation of general sociological theory. Nor is it a conventional autobiography, although it shares with autobiography its narrative form, its first-person point of view and its frankly subjective stance. It is certainly not fiction, although the best life history documents have a sensitivity and pace, a dramatic urgency, that any novelist would be glad to achieve. (Becker, 2009: 3)

Life history research is an approach that collects and analyses data sourced from semi-structured interviews with an individual about their biography. This interview material is typically subjected to triangulation – using secondary research

(Chapter 10) to help contextualise the life history. The prevailing focus of life history research is to describe 'social agency in action' and note its socio-structural limits (Rustin, 2009: 166). C. Wright Mills (1916–62), the radical sociologist and a champion of life history research, described this focus as distinguishing between private troubles and public issues (Mills, 1959).

PRACTICE POINT 1

Life history research is an approach that collects and analyses data sourced from (normally at least six) semi-structured interviews with an individual about their biography. This interview material is typically subjected to triangulation – using secondary research to help contextualise the life history.

Life history research is commonly (though not always) a single-case form of research. For example, Bertaux (1981) used about 60 life histories in his research into the French bakers' trade.

CONCEPTUAL CONCERNS 1

Life history research is a case-centric approach. The aim of a life history is to generate a biography and to explore individual choice and its constraints. However, the approach can use multiple cases, multiple life histories.

Origins of the approach

Life history research is an approach that has its origins in the consolidation of anthropology and sociology as academic disciplines. Sedgwick (1980: 1) notes that:

> [T]he life history method in American anthropology and sociology is nearly as old as the disciplines themselves. In the course of this history the method has gained prominence as the implicit core of cultural anthropology and has been used in sociology, along with participant observation, to make a major contribution to urban and community research. But in neither discipline has it achieved the status of a formal method.

Life history research is therefore both a longstanding approach and a somewhat marginalised one in terms of it lacking a standardised method. Harrison (2009: xxv) says:

> Despite … early exhortations to put lives to the forefront of sociology and the social sciences more generally, there were only piecemeal attempts to utilise approaches that

might do so; and the life history or life story methods developed slowly until the 1980s when interest in lives and in personal experience began to be taken seriously and practised more widely …

Sedgwick (1980) argues that despite its longevity, life history research has also been somewhat marginalised and, when used, has studied the lives of people considered marginal: native Americans, juvenile delinquents, black youth, members of the underclass. This marginalisation of the approach reflects the primary concern of anthropology and sociology (until fairly recently) with the social and cultural life of the mainstream rather than the margins, and – more importantly – with social structure rather than with individuals.

CONCEPTUAL CONCERNS 2

Life history research is both a longstanding approach and a somewhat marginalised one in terms of it lacking a standardised approach.

More generally, Harrison (2009) identifies trends in the development of life history research: an initial appreciation of individual lives, the Chicago School, the input of C. Wright Mills, and the rise of oral history. Alongside these four we add what Rustin (2009) calls the 'biographical turn in social science'. Arguably these five moments in the development of life history research reflect the more general ebb and flow of epistemological debate in the social sciences.

Epistemology refers to the theory of knowledge that informs how research is shaped in its broadest sense (see Chapter 1). Life history research is one of many approaches that flourished with the gradual decline of positivism. Life history research focuses on the individual and their life choices and constraints, whereas positivists downplay the uncertainties that other epistemologies raise about the impact of power, meaning and culture on doing science (some common social realist critiques) or more radical concerns about the logical impossibility of developing an objective scientific stance (the social constructivist critique of 'science'). These concerns – of power and subjectivity – are precisely those of life history researcher.

The development of life history research can be thought of as a series of epistemological challenges.

1. **An initial interest in life stories:** The notion that 'individual lives and lived experience' might be important to understanding the social world was most famously advanced by W. I. Thomas (1863–1947) and Florian Znaniecki (1882–1958) in the their study of *The Polish peasant in Europe and America* (Thomas and Znaniecki, 1918). Thomas and Znaniecki used the letters of

Polish migrants and a single detailed life history to capture life experiences and to generate theories about social dislocation and integration. Their approach was largely welcomed by leading scholars of the day, but was not incorporated into mainstream social science. The prevailing epistemology within anthropology and sociology was thoroughly positivist (Plummer, 2009). Positivists stress the techniques of observation and measurement and the potential for social scientists to form objective/unbiased understandings of the social world. Often their work is quantitative, i.e., numbers-based (see Chapter 1). In this context, the validity and reliability of Thomas and Znaniecki's work was held in some doubt. Their work was seen as an interesting extrapolation from scientifically untested data. The approach, including initial discussions about a form of analytical induction, was regarded as an interesting potential fillip to genuine scientific study.

2. **A home in urban studies**: A coherent focus on individual lives and lived experiences, often using forms of life history research, became a central part of the urban and community research associated with the 'Chicago School' in the interwar period (Becker, 2009). However, despite this prestigious institutional location, elsewhere the life history approach remained somewhat marginal to mainstream social science. This reflected the consolidation of a positivist epistemology at the time when anthropology and sociology departments were becoming more common across the UK and the USA. The new departments and academics seeking tenure, in particular sociologists, embraced positivist social sciences in part to demonstrate their scientific credibility.

3. **A social realist challenge to positivism – C. Wright Mills**: The stranglehold of positivist epistemology on the social sciences was increasingly challenged in the postwar period (after 1945). This challenge took many forms and had many proponents. C. Wright Mills was one of the most important. His book, *The sociological imagination* (Mills, 1959), provided a devastating critique of positivism as an increasingly sterile endeavour and introduced the distinction between 'private troubles and public issues' as a subject for research, including life history research. Mills was a social realist. Social realists argue that revealing the social world is far more problematic than suggested by positivists. For social realists, doing science is a legitimate goal, but it is understood as a project that is limited by factors that social scientists have great difficulty in controlling for or being objective about. Where positivists strive for objectivity, social realists emphasise subjectivity and the appreciation of factors like power, meaning, and the need for researcher reflexivity (or self-awareness). Mills built on the works of Thomas and Znaniecki (1918) and the Chicago School in arguing that the importance of developing a life history was not so much about describing a biography, rather it was about putting biography into context. This involved distinguishing between private troubles (individual problems) and public issues (socio-structural constraints). For example, the inability of someone

to get a job might be the result of private troubles (the individual is lazy, shiftless and idle), or it could be the result of public issues (the product of economic downturn, racism, sexism, forms of prejudice), or it could be some combination of both. Mills' focus on the individual was used to reveal the socio-structural limits of individual choice. At the same time, the use of life histories became more popular during the 1960s and 1970s. Many of these detailed studies focused on issues of poverty and working lives. Harrison notes Oscar Lewis's *Children of Sanchez* (1961), Studs Terkel's *Hard Times* (1986 [1970]) and *Working* (1974).

4. **A social constructivist challenge to social realism**: The challenge to positivism played out as a double movement or double critique. The social realist critique that positivists were overly narrow, numbers-focused and blind to power, meaning and culture was itself subjected to criticism by social constructivists. Social constructivists have little faith in science of any variant as a viable project that generates anything resembling universal rules, laws or theorems. According to this epistemology, it is impossible to differentiate truth-claims based in science, or folklore, or commonsense, or metaphysics, because individuals or actors actively create the social world and all potential measures of that social world (thereby making measures of reliability and validity redundant). We also discuss this double movement in more depth in Chapter 11 on semiotic analysis. In terms of life history research, Rustin (2009) identifies the 'biographical turn in social science' in the 1980s. This represented a new look at the nature of the individual and society.

   Rustin argues that this symbolised a turn from a study of culture to a study of biographies – most importantly of how biographies and individual subjectivities are made up. The biographical turn is a manifestation of a broader rejection of positivist and social realist social science that, among other things, begins with assumptions of *commonality* in human experience. Social constructivists tend to favour ideas of *exceptionality*. This 'turn' is analogous to the shift from structuralism to post-structuralism in semiotic analysis (see Chapter 11). Many social constructivists were drawn to autoethnography as a form of capturing biography and even community experiences (see Chapter 12, Autoethnographic Research).

5. **The rise and rise of oral history**: The slow and piecemeal consolidation of life history research was greatly advanced by the rise of oral histories as both a scholarly and popular undertaking from the 1980s. Oral histories were championed by academics interested in confronting social theories that focused only on social structure and tended to 'disappear' the individual. Oral history was championed by radical feminists and anti-racist and post-colonial scholars, as well as by Marxist scholars – most notably Bertaux (1981) and Bertaux and Bertaux-Wiam (1981).

Comparing life history research with oral history

Life history research overlaps with what many textbooks and writers call 'oral history' (Thomson, 2006). Indeed, oral history has eclipsed life history as a popular, as opposed to a scholarly, undertaking. However, there are important methodological differences between the academic and popular approaches. The main ones are:

1. Oral history centres on recalling events, situations and fragments of some-one's biography, whereas life history research has as its core the development of a chronology of an entire life.

2. Oral history privileges the role of memory and relies solely on the interview process to generate data, whereas life history typically uses forms of triangulation.

3. Oral history is focused on developing a biography or fragments of it, whereas life history (in both its Millsian and post-structuralist variants) is more concerned with contextualising and theorising biography: placing the life in context.

4. Oral history is atheoretical – the aim of an oral historian is to describe a life – whereas life history researchers are informed by social theory and use analytical induction.

PRACTICE POINT 2

Life history research is not oral history. There are important methodological differences between the academic and popular approaches. Most significantly, the aim of an oral historian is to describe a life. Life history researchers are informed by social theory and use analytical induction.

Pointers in doing a life history

There is a lot of useful material on conducting life history research to be found on the internet. The bulk of this material is popular rather than academically focused and is oriented to researchers/enthusiasts doing oral history. As noted above, oral history and life history are not one-and-the-same, although they share a common interest in documenting lived experience and use semi-structured interviews as the primary means of gathering data. We found the 'Step-by-step guide to oral history' website developed by Judith Moyer (1999) to be extremely useful. We have modified and in parts augmented Moyer's 'reminder list' to improve its relevance to life history researchers:

- Decide your research goals and determine if a life history will help you to reach them. This selection of a method is crucial to all research. Remember the aim of a life history is normally to generate a biography and to explore individual choice and its constraints.

- Conduct preliminary research using non-interview sources. For example, the more you know about the conditions and events that someone has experienced in their life, the better you can respond to and formulate questions.

- Contact potential interviewees, explain your project and ask for help. Researchers working in university contexts will inevitably require approval from their institutional ethics committee before starting to interview.

- Life history research generally involves between 6 and 20 hours of interviewing. This requires a big commitment from your interviewee – be sure you have secured that commitment before starting.

- Find and practise with the best audio or audio-visual recording gear you can get. Become completely familiar with this equipment.

- Compile a list of topics or questions. Most interviewing in life history research uses a semi-structured approach. This requires the use of open-ended questions and the exploration of themes (see Chapter 2).

- If you are a new researcher it is always useful to practise interviewing.

- Verify your appointment a day or two before the interview. On the day of the interview, give yourself extra time to get there.

- Interview and record in a quiet place.

- Make sure the interviewee understands the purpose of the interview and how you intend to use it. This is not a private conversation. If you have ethics approval, you will probably have consent forms for your interviewee to sign.

- Start each recording with a statement of who, what, when and where you are interviewing, and check the recording.

- Listen actively and intently.

- Speak one at a time.

- Allow silence. Give the interviewee time to think.

- Ask one question at a time.

- Follow up your current question thoroughly before moving to the next.

- Start with less probing questions. Ask more probing questions later in the interview.

- Wrap up the interview with lighter talk. Do not drop the interviewee abruptly after an intense interview.

- Be aware of and sensitive to the possibility that the interviewee may experience psychological discomfort.

- Limit interviews to about one to two hours in length, depending on the fatigue levels of you and your interviewee.

- In general, don't count on photos to structure your interview, but you can use them as initial prompts.

- Label and number all recordings immediately.

- After the interview, make notes about the interview. Your notes should include areas that you want to explore using non-interview sources (e.g., triangulation). For example, if the interviewee was divorced, it might be useful to check-up the prevailing divorce rates at the time. If the interviewee did not finish school, can you find out from secondary research (see Chapter 10) whether this was unusual or not at the time?

- Write a thank-you note after each interview. Use this opportunity to remind the interviewee when you will be seeing them next.

Building rapport

In Chapter 2 (In-Depth Interviewing) we stressed the importance of building rapport in interviewing. The benefits of building rapport with the interviewee or participant are:

- it encourages a respectful relationship with the participant

- it allows the interview to run more smoothly and efficiently

- it encourages a fuller discussion of topics

- it is easier to keep the interview on track or focused on particular subjects.

Of course, for you to have any hope of building rapport you have to be at ease. This requires that you have worked your way through the reminder list (see above), have familiarised yourself with your research focus, the interview topics, the recording technologies, and arrived on time, at the right location, looking fresh and appropriately dressed. These are the minimum criteria for a successful interview. Rapport builds on this.

Brown and Levinson (1978) suggested four strategies for building rapport in face-to-face interaction. This includes while you conduct the interview. In order to secure and maintain rapport, the researcher should consider the following:

1. **Seek agreement:** This involves initial safe talk about the weather, etc., as well as being seen to empathise with the interviewee when they are speaking (by nodding, smiling, etc.).

2. **Presuppose common ground**: This can involve the use of inconsequential gossip or using the pronoun 'we' rather than 'you' and 'I'.

3. **Avoid disagreement**: Never disagree outright. If you must vocalise a dissenting position, hedge and limit your disagreement.

4. **Joke**: The use of appropriate humour (and we stress *appropriate*) is arguably the most powerful way of building and maintaining rapport. This doesn't mean being a stand-up comedian or challenging your interviewee's preconceived notions about how a researcher acts. However, gentle, inclusive and sometimes self-deprecating humour can be very effective.

Leech (2002: 665) stresses the importance of rapport: 'Without rapport, even the best-phrased questions can fall flat and elicit brief, uninformative answers. Rapport means more than just putting people at ease. It means convincing people that you are listening, that you understand and are interested in what they are talking about, and that they should continue talking.' She goes on to note ways of enhancing rapport in semi-structured interviewing:

1. **Be neither dim nor an expert**: Leech recommends a middle road for the interviewer between presenting as slightly dim but agreeable or as an expert. Both extreme strategies can stop communication. On the one hand, because the interviewee/participant thinks they have to dumb-down their responses; on the other, because they are too intimidated to express an opinion. Leech (2002: 665) states: 'The interviewer should seem professional and generally knowledgeable, but less knowledgeable than the respondent on the particular topic of the interview.'

2. **Make the interview seem natural**: In most cases the interviewee will be more nervous than the interviewer. It is up to the interviewer to put the interviewee at ease. Appearing relaxed helps, as does creating the impression that it is normal for the interviewee to want to discuss their life.

3. **Respond and restate**: As the interview progresses it is a useful technique to respond to the interviewee by restating their responses. This shouldn't be overdone but can be used at the end of each section or topic of discussion. Restating the answers to questions (perhaps closely paraphrasing but not reinterpreting them!) demonstrates to the interviewee that active listening is taking place (the interviewer is paying attention) and allows for clarification and checking.

4. **Question order**: Start with non-threatening questions: name, age, place of birth, residences, etc. Sensitive questions should not be left to the end of an interview but should occur near the middle. This allows the interviewee to 'recover' by the end of the interview.

5. **Avoid presuming questions**: 'Presuming questions are presuming in the sense that they imply that the researcher already knows the answer – or at least part

of it. So one danger is that the respondent will bluff to save face and make something up' (Leech, 2002: 666).

6. **Use 'grand tour questions'**: These sort of questions (Leech cites Spradley, 1979) ask respondents to give a verbal tour of something they know well. For example 'Could you describe a typical day at work?' Leech notes that these questions put the respondent at ease but run the risk of generating averaged answers. That is, not all days at work are typical. When conducting interviews for life history research it is important that the respondent talks about both what was typical and what was not.

7. **Use floating prompts**: Prompts keep the conversation flowing and elucidate greater detail in response. Prompts are not scripted questions. They are usually informal responses like 'Really?', 'Yes!' or even a nod of the head. These verbal and non-verbal prompts are crucial because they call forth further response without necessarily providing direction to the respondent.

PRACTICE POINT 3

Building rapport is most important in life history research, in which the bulk of data is generated through a series of semi-structured interviews that may total 6–20 hours in length (per participant).

Memory and recall

The steps suggested (above) for improving rapport with the life history participant are fairly straightforward and unproblematic. The most difficult aspect is researchers coming to terms with their role in the interview process, presenting themselves in a particular way and then trying to modify that presentation. This 'presentation of self' does involve an element of acting. Improving the memory and recall of participants is equally important in collecting data but, it has to be acknowledged, is far more problematic, as reflected by ongoing debates into the psychology and neurology of cognition.

Most of the effort in improving memory and recall has come from police and counsellors interested in the participants as witnesses of a crime. This in itself may be contradictory to the ethos that permeates life history as an emancipatory or collaborative process (Blackman, 2009). Certainly, the presentation of self used by a police officer to interview a witness to a crime – an interrogation, for example – may be decidedly at odds with efforts at building rapport. Furthermore, the common police procedure of the 'cognitive interview' in which the participant/witness is questioned is highly iterative, repetitive and focused on the recall of a single incident, not in elucidating an account of a life lived. Nevertheless, we have tried to distil the most appropriate aspects of memory- and recall-enhancing techniques that are suitable for life historians:

1. **Conduct the interview in a quiet place**: Eliminating external stimuli is commonly regarded as improving recall.

2. **Learn as much about the conditions of the participant's life as you possibly can**: The more you know about what life was like in the time and place the participant is describing, the better it is in terms of asking questions and gaining an understanding.

3. **Set the parameters of discussion but let the participant speak freely**: For example, use phrases like 'Now I'd like to discuss your last years at school and how you found a job?' Follow this up with something like 'What stands out for you?'

4. **Combine open-ended and direct questions**: Give the interviewee/participant as much freedom as possible to describe their life, but also use direct questions: 'Why did you decide to marry in a church?', 'How much did your first car cost?', 'Were you happy being the shop-floor supervisor?'

5. **When you need to focus on something, focus intensely**: Often the most useful insights in a life history are the result of the interviewer following up a 'loose end' or something the interviewee has glossed over. Such loose ends aren't always immediately apparent. They may appear to the researcher in the process of writing up interview notes or after several interviews. Maybe the interviewee/participant seems reluctant to talk about something. If so, why? More importantly, is it possible to investigate this area of life? Then, how to do so sensitively? It is often worthwhile returning to an issue that has been previously discussed. This isn't necessarily or even commonly a burden on the participant as generally most participants in the life history process find it enjoyable and want to offer more detail and insights as they 'warm up' over time.

6. **Gently, gently, use the techniques of interrogation – Restatement**: Members of the police force, typically, are not blessed with the high empathic quotient that surely characterises the greatest interviewers and fieldworkers in the social sciences. Nor is police procedure much interested in empowerment as a potential outcome of research, and collaboration as a mutually beneficial process. Instead, police interviewing/interrogation relies on authority and the threat of legal sanction. Indeed, witnesses can expect a degree of intimidation and harassment not just as techniques for aiding memory and recall, but because police officers often also need to gauge the robustness of their witnesses under potential cross-examination. Not much of this is of use to life historians. However, police forces around the world have also developed the 'cognitive interview', a series of techniques used to aid recall. These can be of use, if applied sparingly and appropriately.

The cognitive interview is an iterative process that aids the recall of events by asking the participant to restate them in various ways (Dando et al., 2009; Memon and Bull, 1997). There are four main restatements:

(i) **Restatement of the physical and personal contexts that existed at the time of event:** The participant (not witness!) is asked to remember the context of events – 'Where did the event take place?', 'What did the room look like?', 'What was the lighting, sound and temperature like?', 'How did the you feel at the time?', 'Were you happy, sad, angry, excited, etc.?' The evidence suggests that sort of contextual element is very beneficial to recall.

(ii) **Restatement of the temporal order of events:** The participant is asked for an exact, precise, account of the event in terms of the order in which it took place.

(iii) **Restatement of the event from the perspective of any others involved:** The participant is asked to speculate on how others saw or felt about the events. For example, 'How did your children feel about moving to London?', 'What did your husband think of you changing jobs?'.

(iv) **Restatement of everything, including partial information:** The participant is asked to recall everything and anything associated with the event, even if it does not seem relevant.

PRACTICE POINT 4

Improving participant recall and memory has many benefits. Cognitive interviewing is a powerful technique for enhancing memory, but it must be used sparingly.

Analytical induction

In Chapter 1 we introduced two logical processes of doing research: analytical induction and hypothesis-testing. We suggested that case-centric approaches tended to favour analytical induction and variable-centric approaches hypothesis-testing. Ragin (1994) and Curtis (2007) suggest that there is a clear distinction between 'testing theory' or hypothesis-testing and developing new theory – what we call analytical induction. Furthermore, analytical induction is most closely associated with life history research and ethnographic research (see Chapter 4). These two approaches can be thought of as the natural home of analytical induction.

We described analytical induction as a process that builds theory by progressively redefining a hypothesis about a phenomenon to be explained by using data that have been collected (see Chapter 1 for another discussion). Analytical induction oscillates or bounces between two moments: (1) data about an event (or something analogous) is collected and analysed, (2) this data – we can now call it information – is compared with a proposition or hypothesis about the 'event'. If the data/information confirm the proposition, then the proposition is strengthened. If the data/information confound the proposition, then it (a working hypothesis) has to be redefined or abandoned. However, the process of analytical induction doesn't just oscillate between moments '1' (data collection and analysis) and '2' (comparing information and proposition), there is also a cumulative movement. Knowledge is accrued as a proposition or working hypothesis is redefined by data/information into a new theory. In this respect, the process of analytic induction looks like a spring or spiral: the start point of which is the naïve researcher, the outward curvilinear path the moments of research, and the end point is the researcher with greater knowledge or a new theory.

The logic of analytical induction differs from hypothesis-testing because the initial data collection is used to create a new hypothesis or proposition, rather than testing an existing one. In analytical induction, the working hypothesis is continuously compared against collected and analysed data. Analytical induction assumes that a fairly small number of confirmations is required to support a new theory. Bertaux (1981) tacitly discusses this principle in terms of the 'saturation of knowledge' (see below).

In his review of the life history approach, Sedgwick (1980: 31) also stresses the importance of analytical induction. He quotes Robinson (1951: 813) on the procedural elements of analytical induction. This is a useful reformulation. Again, Robinson describes analytical induction as a way of developing a new hypothesis and theory:

1. A rough definition of the phenomenon to be explained is formulated.

2. A hypothetical explanation of that phenomenon is formulated.

3. One case is studied in light of the hypothesis, with the object of determining whether or not the hypothesis fits the facts in that case.

4. If the hypothesis does not fit the facts, either the hypothesis is reformulated or the phenomenon to be explained is redefined so that the case is excluded.

5. Practical certainty may be attained after a small number of cases has been examined, but the discovery of negative cases disproves the explanation and requires reformulation.

6. This procedure of examining cases, redefining the phenomenon, and reformulating the process is continued until a universal relationship is established, each negative case calling for a redefinition or a reformulation.

Howard Becker (1993, 1998, 2009) has done much to refine and explain analytical induction, the approach we associate most with case-centric research in this textbook. Becker also demonstrates how analytical induction is a way of describing research in general. Below we reproduce an extract of Becker's famous account of how he used the iterative process of analytical induction (Becker, 1993). He is describing a piece of fieldwork based on semi-structured interviews and participant observation, so his means of data collection differ somewhat from those of the life historian. Nevertheless, we feel his account is compelling:

> We were going to study medical students and medical education but, to be truthful, I had very little idea of what I was going to do beyond 'hanging around with the students,' going to classes and whatever else presented itself …
>
> With no problem to orient myself to, no theoretically defined puzzle I was trying to solve, I concentrated on finding out what the hell was going on, who all these people were, what they were doing, what they were talking about, finding my way around and, most of all, getting to know the six students with whom I was going to spend the next six weeks …
>
> One morning, as we made rounds, we saw a very talkative patient, who had multiple complaints to tell the doctor about, all sorts of aches, pains and unusual events. I could see that no one was taking her very seriously and, on the way out, one of the students said, 'Boy, she's really a crock!' I understood this, in part, as shorthand for 'crock of shit.' It was obviously invidious. But what was he talking about?…
>
> [M]y discovery of what the word 'crock' meant was not a lightning bolt of intuition. On the contrary, it was guided by sociological theorizing every step of the way… [S]pecifically … the invidious distinctions students made between classes of patients would show what interests they were trying to maximize in that relationship, what they hoped to get out of it …
>
> I made this theoretical analysis in a flash and then came up with a profoundly theoretical question: 'What's a crock?' He looked at me as if to say that any damn fool would know that. … After fumbling for a while, he said it referred to someone with psychosomatic illness. That let him off the hook for the moment by partially satisfying my curiosity, though I still wanted to know what interest of his as a student was violated by a patient with psychosomatic illness …
>
> When I pursued that paradox, students told me that you might have a lot of patients like that later on, but you couldn't learn anything from seeing them here in [medical] school. … [C]rocks did not add to their knowledge of crockdom, its differential diagnosis or its treatment. A crock presented no medical puzzles to be solved [and therefore was a waste of the students' time]. (Becker, 1993: 28–35)

Life historians use semi-structured interviews and forms of triangulation (mainly secondary research, see Chapter 10) as forms of data collection and so the practice of analytical induction differs from the classic piece of ethnography described by Becker. Rather than come across a discovery of the word 'crock' in the field or while writing up field notes, as Becker the ethnographer did, the life historian will have similar moments of insight perhaps while conducting an interview, or when writing up the interview notes, or in the process of triangulation and cross-checking the interview-based data. The logic is identical in both approaches.

Triangulation

Triangulation is the use of more than one method to double- or cross-check the collected and/or partially analysed data from another method. The origins of life history research include it being used as a form of triangulation to enrich and potentially verify the findings of more positivistic research. Similarly, unobtrusive research (Chapter 8) has often been used opportunistically as a form of triangulation. However, life history research, as an approach in its own right, typically relies on triangulation, that is, non-interview-based sources. Indeed, the semi-structured interviews that are used to gather data on the biography of the participant should be thought of as running in parallel with the process of triangulation. Triangulation in this regard is secondary research (see Chapter 10).

The main aspects of triangulation in terms of conducting life history research are:

1. Triangulation is an integral component of life history research. It is impossible to imagine life history research without triangulation. This is because the approach does not rely solely on the recall and memory of the participant, nor does it attempt to present an unedited account of a life lived (see below). Rather, life history research attempts to contextualise a life and, even further, often seeks to show the limits of what the participant may have seen as 'free choice'. In this respect, the semi-structured interviews and 'triangulation' are parallel research processes. One process informs the other.

2. Despite and because of the points made in '1' (above), the researcher does not use triangulation to check up on the interview data. The life history developed by participants is considered to be authentic (see also, Chapter 12 on autoethnographic research). Rather, triangulation is used to inform the researcher. It is an aid to editorialising, to contextualising a life lived, and provides the basis for better informed interviewing.

3. Triangulation in life histories takes the form of secondary research (see Chapter 10). The most useful sources available to the researcher are publically available, usually annual, official or national statistics. These sources should allow life historians to find out things like: 'What was the divorce rate in the UK in 1974?', or 'What was the average life expectancy in Australia for people born in 1926?' Depending on the background of the participant being interviewed, researchers may also want to consult business histories, school histories, war histories, community histories and other biographies and autobiographies. As is always the case with secondary research, the first thing a researcher should do is ask his/her librarian for help.

4. If and when triangulation produces some disconnect with the interview data – memory and recall are at odds with official statistics, for example – this warrants a footnote in the account of the life history. It should be explored with the participant, but not used to overwrite the biographical account.

PRACTICE POINT 5

Triangulation is an integral component of life history research. It is impossible to imagine life history research without triangulation. This is because the approach does not rely solely on the recall and memory of the participant, nor does it attempt to present an unedited account of a life lived. Triangulation is used to inform the researcher. Triangulation in life histories takes the form of secondary research (see Chapter 10).

Naturalistic and edited forms of life history

In our discussion of the origins of life history research (see above) we favoured a research focus championed by C. Wright Mills (1959), in which individual life histories are used to explore the limits of individual choice or freedom and hence demonstrate the constraints of social structure (e.g., the impact of class, gender, ethnicity, sexuality, etc.). This focus requires the life historian to triangulate the interview-based data, to use the logical processes of analytical induction, and to act as an editor of the life history. The life historian as editor is dependent on the type of life history being produced. Cohen, Manion and Morrison (2007: 199) suggest three 'modes of presentation' for life histories:

1. **Naturalistic life history**: These are predominantly first-person ('I') accounts of a life. The life historian may provide an introduction, commentary and conclusion. Often these types of life history use footnotes and/or appendices to discuss important points. By and large, the body of the account is unedited.

2. **Thematically edited accounts**: The life historian plays an important role in sorting and developing themes in the life history. While the words of the participant are largely unedited, they are systematically reworked into themes that the life historian has decided as being the most significant or pertinent.

3. **Interpreted and edited accounts**: These are the most reworked accounts. The participant's words are used primarily to illustrate the points the life historian has identified as being of greatest significance. This mode of presentation requires the most work by the life historian, over and above the 6–20 hours of interviewing time, per participant, associated with more naturalistic accounts. It is likely that the life historian will spend significantly more time triangulating the interview-based data than in actual interviewing.

SOME ISSUES IN RESEARCH

In this section, we review the epistemological issues that are particularly relevant to life history research, notably validity and reliability, and discuss approaches for dealing with these.

Epistemology and claims for validity and reliability

Reliability and validity are the most important claims of research approaches that aim to be scientific. Research is only considered to be rigorous when it aligns with accepted standards of reliability and validity. However, issues of reliability and validity are somewhat problematic for practitioners of life history. As noted in Chapter 1: (1) reliability measures the extent to which the analysis of data yields results that can be repeated or reproduced at different times or by different researchers; while (2) validity measures the extent to which the research is accurate and the extent to which claims can be made based on the research.

The 'problem' with life histories is that shared by all case-centric approaches. The low number of cases, including single-case research (see Becker, 2009), means they are not amenable to the sorts of tests of reliability and validity that are associated with survey research (Chapter 6) and other forms of predominantly positivist social science. The approach by some practitioners of some case-centric approaches to positivist and social realist criticisms of rigour is to argue that they are no longer interested in that sort of science, or in doing science at all (see Chapter 11, Semiotic Analysis, and Chapter 12, Autoethnographic Research). This is largely a social constructivist response. But life histories are typically not of great interest to social constructivists and the majority of its practitioners are allied with a social realist epistemology, and hence have an interest in proving/improving reliability and validity. Keeping this in mind, there are five main responses by life historians to issues of rigour:

1. **Case protocols:** Yin (2003) suggests that a case protocol can assist reliability in case-centric research, including single-case research like life history. His rationale is that a case study protocol 'is a major way of increasing the *reliability* of case study and is intended to guide the investigator in carrying out data collection from a single-case study' (Yin, 2003: 67). The protocol provides a template for other researchers to repeat the study. The protocol requires researchers to spell out: (1) an overview of the case study project; (2) research procedures – accessing the participants, etc.; (3) the schedule of questions; and (4) the guide for data analysis and reporting.

2. **Sources of bias and reliability:** As noted above, the autobiographical account provided by the participant is considered to be fully authentic in life history research. Nevertheless, Cohen, Manion and Morrison (2007) suggest several possible sources of 'bias'. They use a famous table in the form of a checklist from Plummer (1983: 103), which we also reproduce:

   Principal sources of bias in life history research

   Source: Informant

   Is misinformation (unintended) given?

   Has there been evasion?

   Is there evidence of direct lying and deception?

Is a 'front' being presented?

What may the informant 'take for granted' and hence not reveal?

How far is the informant 'pleasing you'?

How much has been forgotten?

How much may be self-deception?

Source: Researcher

Attitudes of researcher: age, gender, class, race, religion, politics, etc.

Demeanour of researcher: dress, speech, body language, etc.

Personality of researcher: anxiety, need for approval, hostility, warmth, etc.

Scientific role of researcher: theory held, researcher expectancy.

Source: The interaction

The encounter needs to be examined. Is bias coming from:

The physical setting – 'social space'?

The prior interaction?

Non-verbal communication?

Vocal behaviour?

3. **Improving validity**: Cohen, Manion and Morrison (2007) again précis Plummer (1983) in identifying three ways in which the validity of a life history can be gauged or improved. Please note that we are not convinced that these techniques are used much by life historians. They are: (i) Ask the participant to read and critique the completed life history; (ii) Compare the life history with other life histories (if available); (iii) Compare the interview material with secondary research.

4. **Narrative analysis**: Above we mentioned that the majority of practitioners of life history research are allied with a social realist epistemology, and hence have an interest in proving/improving reliability and validity. However, there is also a strong element within the approach that champions the notion of 'narrative analysis' and more or less rejects positivist (inspired) notions of reliability and validity. Liamputtong and Ezzy (2005: 125) describe this form of analysis as one that 'emphasises the narrative of story-telling, based on the nature of human understanding'. This involves a rejection of forms of 'scientific rationality'. 'In contrast, narrative rationality is formed through telling a good story that is designed to convince through its "life-likedness", and can be tested through ordinary interpersonal checking' (2005: 125). Daniel Bertaux (1981: 415 original italics) famously argued that: 'Empirical sociology has been overloaded and sterilized by the *burden of proof*. Let us simply drop it.'

5. **Saturation of knowledge**: Bertaux also argued that the positivist standards of reliability and validity based on many cases and few variables proved only a surface and facile understanding of social relations (Bertaux, 1981; Bertaux and Bertaux-Wiam, 1981). He argued that case-centric research allowed for an understanding of social relations in depth (and as a corollary supports the tenet of analytical induction that a fairly small number of confirming cases is sufficient to prove a new theory). He describes this as a process of *saturation of knowledge*, in which a limited number of life histories provides a fuller understanding than, for example, a survey (see Chapter 6):

> In our [Bertaux and Bertaux-Wiam, 1981] study of the bakers' trade, we were confronted with a population of about 160,000 people (90,000 bakers and bakers' wives, 70,000 bakery workers). No 'representative sample' was ever drawn. We gathered life stories following what is pompously called 'a snowball strategy'. For instance, we gathered about thirty life stories from bakery workers. The first life story taught us a great deal; so did the second and the third. By the fifteenth we had begun to understand the pattern of sociostructural relations which makes up the life of a bakery worker. By the twenty-fifth, adding the knowledge we had from life stories of bakers, we knew we had it: a clear picture of this structural pattern and of its recent transformations. New life stories only confirmed what we had understood, adding slight variations. We stopped at thirty: there was no point going further. We knew already what we wanted to know.

CONCEPTUAL CONCERNS 3

The 'problem' with life histories is that shared by all case-centric approaches. The low number of cases, including single-case research, means they are not amenable to the sorts of tests of reliability and validity that are associated with forms of predominantly positivist social science. However, the majority of life historians are allied with a social realist epistemology, and hence have an interest in proving/improving reliability and validity.

PUTTING THE APPROACH IN CONTEXT

Life history research is a case-centric and often a single-case approach that is based on parallel or alternating moments of semi-structured interviewing and triangulation in the form of secondary research. Life history research is highly individualistic and very fluid in the way it is undertaken. The life historian has great discretion to explore some aspects of biography in more depth than others, or to focus in greater detail at different moments in the chronology. At the same time, the alternating moments of interviewing and secondary research impose their own 'rhythm' and therefore constraints on the researcher. Once started, the series of interviews must proceed at a fairly regular pace which reflects both the need of the participant for regularity, convenience and respect, and the needs of the researcher to write up the interviews and do secondary research.

CONCEPTUAL CONCERNS 4

Like most case-centric, case-first approaches, life history research enjoys a fluid framing of research. At the same time, the alternating moments of interviewing and secondary research impose their own 'rhythm' and therefore constraints on the researcher.

Life history research has not been much affected by new technologies. Modern digital technologies have impacted the recording, storage, transcription and retrieval of interview data. The flowering of the internet has greatly expanded the possibilities for secondary research (see Chapter 10). But, the core of the approach, a series of in-depth, semi-structured interviews remains more or less unchanged. These interviews are overwhelmingly conducted on a face-to-face basis and there doesn't seem a great likelihood of technology mediating the process in the immediate future. (So brush up your interviewing skills – see Chapter 2, In-Depth Interviewing).

CONCLUSION

Life history research is a form of case-centric research. It can be either a single-case variant (and most normally is) or can combine a limited number of cases. It is somewhat fluid in the way it is undertaken. The life historian has considerable discretion, but is somewhat constrained by the demands of the regular interview, interspersed with secondary research.

Like most case-centric approaches, life history suffers when viewed from a positivistic stance on issues of reliability. Because most practitioners of life history research are allied with a social realist epistemology, there are efforts to prove/improve rigour in terms of the standard measures. The main responses are: case protocols, identifying interviewing bias and, possibly, seeking a participant critique of the finished life history. There is also a weak social constructivist tendency that rejects the positivist demands for 'science'. Most famously, Daniel Bertaux (1981: 41, original italics) asserted that: 'Empirical sociology has been overloaded and sterilized by the *burden of proof*. Let us simply drop it.' This has remained a minority position in the approach but yet the approach remains unstandardised (Sedgwick, 1980).

Rather than standardisation, Blackman (2009: 25) points to commonalities in life history research:

- That the life history emerges through discourse with another.

- That it is a collaboration between the interviewer and the participant.

- That it is a tale told twice – to the interviewer and then by the interviewer to readers.

- That it is shaped by socio-cultural contexts involving participant, interviewer and audience.

- That it makes claims to represent a life, rather than to accurately detail a life.

Blackman expresses the contemporary, anthropological stance. However, the realm of life history is flexible and rich, and as a result we expect the approach to be of enduring interest to social scientists.

FURTHER READINGS

The four-volume set on *Documentary research* edited by John Scott (2006) is a great reference source.
The 'Step-by-step guide to oral history' website by Moyer, J. (1999) contains a wealth of how-to-do advice.

REFERENCES

Becker, H. S. 1993. How I learned what a crock was. *Journal of Contemporary Ethnography*, 22, 28–35.
Becker, H. S. 1998. *Tricks of the trade: How to think about your research while you're doing it*. Chicago: University of Chicago Press.
Becker, H. S. 2009. The life history and scientific mosaic. In: Harrison, B. (ed.), *Life story research*. London: Sage.
Bertaux, D. 1981. From the life-history approach to the transformation of sociological practice. In: Bertaux, D. (ed.), *Biography and society: The life history approach in the social sciences*. London: Sage.
Bertaux, D. & Bertaux-Wiam, I. 1981. Life stories in the bakers' trade. In: Bertaux, D. (ed.), *Biography and society: The life history approach in social sciences*. London: Sage.
Blackman, M. B. 2009. Introduction: The afterlife of the life history. In: Fielding, N. (ed.), *Interviewing II*. London: Sage.
Brown, P. & Levinson, S. 1978. Universals in language usage: Politeness phenomena. In: Goody, E. N. (ed.), *Questions and politeness: Strategies in social interaction*. Cambridge: Cambridge University Press.

Cohen, L., Manion, L. & Morrison, K. 2007. *Research methods in education*. London: Routledge.

Curtis, B. 2007. Doing research. In: Matthewman, S., West-Newman, C. L. & Curtis, B. (eds.), *Being sociological*. London: Palgrave Macmillan.

Dando, C., Wilcox, R. & Milne, R. 2009. The cognitive interview: The efficacy of a modified mental reinstatement of context procedure for frontline police investigators. *Applied Cognitive Psychology*, 23, 138–147.

Harrison, B. (ed.), 2009. *Life story research*. London: Sage.

Leech, B. L. 2002. Asking questions: Techniques for semistructured interviewing. *PSOnline*, December, 665–668.

Lewis, O. 1961. *Children of Sanchez: Autobiography of a Mexican family*. New York: Random House.

Liamputtong, P. & Ezzy, D. 2005. *Qualitative research methods* (2nd edn). Melbourne: Oxford University Press.

Memon, A. & Bull, R. 1991. The cognitive interview: Its origins, empirical support, evaluation and practical implications. *Journal of Community and Applied Social Psychology*, 1(4): 291–307.

Mills, C. W. 1959. *The sociological imagination*. New York: Oxford University Press.

Moyer, J. 1999. Step-by-step guide to oral history. Accessed at://http://dohistory.org/onyour owntoolkit/oralHistory.html [Accessed 10 May].

Plummer, K. 1983. *Documents of life: An introduction to the problems and literature of a humanistic method*. London: Allen & Unwin.

Plummer, K. 2009. Herbert Blumer and the life history tradition. In: Harrison, B. (ed.), *Life story research*. London: Sage.

Ragin, C. 1994. *Constructing social research: The unity and diversity of method*. Thousand Oaks, CA: Pine Forge Press.

Robinson, W. S. 1951. The logical structure of analytical induction. *American Sociological Review*, 16, 812–818.

Rustin, M. 2009. Reflections on the biographical turn in social science. In: Harrison, B. (ed.), *Life story research*. London: Sage.

Scott, J. (ed.) 2006. *Documentary research* (4 vols). London: Sage.

Sedgwick, C. P. 1980. *The life history: A method, with issues, troubles and a future*. Christchurch, NZ: Department of Sociology, University of Canterbury.

Spradley, J. P. 1979. *The ethnographic interview*. New York: Hold, Rinehart and Winston.

Terkel, S. 1974. *Working people talk about what they do all day and how they feel about what they do*. New York: Pantheon Books.

Terkel, S. 1986 [1970]. *Hard times: An oral history of the Great Depression*. New York: Pantheon Books.

Thomas, W. I. & Znaniecki, F. 1918. *The Polish peasant in Europe and America: Monograph of an immigrant group*. Chicago: University of Chicago Press.

Thomson, A. 2006. Four paradigm transformations in oral history. *The Oral History Review*, 34, 49–70.

Yin, R. K. 2003. *Case study research: Design and methods*. London: Sage.

FOUR

ETHNOGRAPHIC RESEARCH – STUDYING GROUPS IN NATURAL SETTINGS

CONTENTS LIST

Key words: ethnography – ethnographic research – cultural groups – communities – natural settings – participant observation – observation

SUMMARY

An outline of the key elements and history of ethnographic research across the social sciences, including: (i) classic examples of ethnographic research; (ii) the practicalities of ethnographic research and how it is shaped by epistemological and methodological issues and resource limitations; (iii) the impact of new technology on ethnographic research; and (iv) some of the key ethical issues relevant to ethnographic research.

In this chapter we discuss ethnographic research – the study of cultural groups or communities in their natural settings. These settings include villages, neighbourhoods, workplaces, and any other venue in which a group of people with some shared characteristic may be found. The primary method used by ethnographers is participant observation – a form of fieldwork. In ethnographic research, such observation is often accompanied by other methods, particularly in-depth interviews (see Chapter 2) and the analysis of existing records (see Chapter 8). Ethnography also has some parallels to life history research (the Chapter 3) and of course is strongly related to autoethnographic research (Chapter 12).

We begin by defining ethnography and elaborating some key elements, before briefly reviewing the history of ethnography across the social sciences. We include some classic examples of ethnographic research within and beyond anthropology (the historical 'home' of ethnography). We then move on to the practicalities of ethnographic research: data collection (comprising entering the field – gaining access to a group – the practice of observation, exiting the field) and data analysis and presentation. We then discuss key epistemological and methodological issues and how these shape practice, as well as the ways in which resource limitations (time, space and costs) impact on the research approach. The impacts of new technologies on ethnography and ethical issues of particular relevance to ethnography are then discussed. We conclude with a review of key points and some thoughts on the future of ethnography.

DOING DATA COLLECTION AND ANALYSIS

Ethnographic research may be defined as the study of a culture. The term comes from the Greek *ethnos,* meaning nation, and *graphia,* meaning writing. It is most commonly associated with anthropology, with Margaret Mead's work perhaps being the best known, along with that of George Bateson and Bronislaw Malinowski. This research generally describes the cultures of specific social groups, often (at least until recent decades) involving First World (western) researchers investigating developing communities (Griffin and Bengry-Howell, 2008). Classic examples include Mead's work focusing on the sexual practices of Pacific Islanders, including Samoans (Mead, 1928), and the Balinese (Bateson and Mead, 1942), while Malinowski conducted ethnographic work among the Trobriand Islanders of Melanesia (Malinowski, 1922).

CONCEPTUAL CONCERN 1

Ethnographic research focuses on a specific group of people, to understand culturally significant behaviour.

Ethnographic research has a history across the social sciences. Classic examples beyond anthropology include sociological ethnographies of working-class communities (Whyte, 1955; Willis, 1977), investigation of the social and psychological impacts of unemployment in an Austrian community (Jahoda et al., 1972), and the admission and discharge practices of mental hospitals (Rosenhan, 1973), which will be discussed in more depth below.

CONCEPTUAL CONCERN 2

Ethnographic research is a case-centric, single-case approach. A group, bounded by time, geographical location and/or cultural practices, is explored through many variables and values.

Key elements of ethnography include:

- An interest in shared cultural activities and their meanings.
- An examination of social phenomena within a specific group in their natural setting.
- A focus on the understandings and interpretations of the people who comprise the case (the insiders' perspective).
- An inductive research process, working primarily with case-centric techniques.
- A multi-method approach (usually), incorporating an extended period of fieldwork (Liamputtong, 2009).

A CLASSIC EXAMPLE: ON BEING SANE IN INSANE PLACES

Rosenhan's work comprised participant observation, later supplemented by hospital records (Rosenhan, 1973). Rosenhan was interested in the question of how sanity and insanity are recognised in psychiatric institutions. Though the processes of treatment have changed markedly in the intervening decades, the subject matter remains relevant, as does the research approach undertaken.

Rosenhan and seven colleagues arranged appointments at psychiatric hospitals, telling the admissions staff that they had been hearing voices (which was not true), and were admitted. Once admitted, the researchers behaved normally and neither exhibited nor reported any particular symptoms of mental illness, though they experienced some initial nervousness. The researchers initially took secret notes of their observations. These included such things as the amount of time staff spent interacting with patients and the quality of those interactions (e.g., making eye contact, stopping to chat as opposed to responding minimally to a question and moving on, and, disturbingly, both verbal and physical abuse). It quickly transpired that no one was interested in reading this material, so extensive notes were taken in public places. Some nursing records subsequently revealed that this note-taking was considered symptomatic of psychiatric disturbance, and the notes taken by the researchers contain many observations of patient behaviours that were misinterpreted by staff. For example, emotional distress was construed as being due to illness, rather than something happening to disturb the patient (social psychologists will recognise this as an example of the fundamental attribution error). Length of hospitalisation varied from seven to 52 days, with 19 days being the average. Each was discharged with the diagnosis of 'schizophrenia in remission', though it is interesting to note that many of the other patients suspected that the researchers were not mentally ill.

Rosenhan's classic 'field stimulation' project (Rosenhan, 1973) is liminal to the experimental method and unobtrusive research (see Chapters 7 and 8 respectively) because of the use of deception, and is unusual in this regard (for ethnographic research).

Origins of the approach

The history and evolution of ethnographic research is well documented. Early work includes *A view of society and manners in America* (Wright, 1821) and *Society in America* (Martineau, 1827) (both cited by Banister et al., 1994). Hays considered Schoolcraft's work regarding native Americans in the 1830s to be the first true ethnography in the sense of living among native peoples, though he does mention the work of Lafiteau in the 1720s (also regarding native Americans), and of German scholars in the mid-nineteenth century (Hays, 1958). As well as Mead, Bronislaw Malinowski is a prominent figure in the development of ethnography, making the point that the goal is to 'Grasp the native's point of view … [to understand] his vision of the world' (Malinowski, 1922: 25).

PRACTICE POINT 1

Ethnographic research may use several methods, but is based on an extended period of participant observation, utilising a process of analytical induction.

True ethnography, then, involves undertaking fieldwork (at least according to Hays (1958), Stocking (1983) and others), and for many years this meant travelling to distant lands to study vastly different cultures, particularly for anthropologists, though considerably less so for other social scientists, especially psychologists. However, by the 1970s few ethnographers, including anthropologists, continued to consider this exotic experience essential (Messerschmidt, 1981); if the subject is culture and social interaction, then 'at home' is as worthy of study as elsewhere.

Blackman (2009) alludes to an anthropological angst about the status of participants/informants, interviewers/anthropologists and audiences in a post-colonial world (see Chapter 4, Life Histories, and Chapter 12, Autoethnographic Research). This reflects the origins of anthropology and its operation as an academic discipline that reported back on exotic others (indigenous peoples) to scholarly and popular audiences in the imperialist powers. As a result, to be a contemporary anthropologist necessitates dealing with a certain disciplinary 'guilt' about this record of (mis)representing indigenous peoples. Geertz (1972) talked eloquently about this problem of translation, and increasingly anthropologists have eschewed the study of the exotic other for the more humdrum focus of sociology and social psychology on industrial societies. We discuss related epistemological and ethical challenges below. At this point we shift focus from *where* ethnography has historically been undertaken to *how* it is done.

Data collection

Data is usually collected using participant observation (as distinct from non-participant observation, discussed in Chapter 8, Unobtrusive Research). This data is often supplemented by other techniques, such as in-depth interviews (see Chapter 2) or analysis of statistical information which may be pre-existing, having been gathered for other purposes, or personal documents such as letters or diaries. Researchers may ask informants (participants) to keep a journal for the duration or a part of the project.

The researcher participates in people's everyday lives for an extended period – usually several months – watching, listening and often discussing what is observed. A crucial element of the success of the research, then, is negotiating extended entry to the field (the setting in which the group of interest is located) and developing relationships that will allow for a productive project.

Entering the field

As noted above, in the past ethnographic research was frequently conducted with people of vastly different cultures from the researcher's own, in distant locales. This meant that particular challenges had to be overcome, such as language barriers, though this was certainly not the only hurdle. The experience of Geertz and his wife (and co-researcher) during their time in Bali in the 1950s as observers observed is an exemplar:

> ... We were intruders, professional ones, and the villagers dealt with us ... as though we were not there. For them, and to a degree for ourselves, we were nonpersons, specters, invisible men.

> ... As we wandered around, uncertain, wistful, eager to please, people seemed to look right through us with a gaze focused several yards behind us on some more actual stone or tree. Almost nobody greeted us; but nobody scowled or said anything unpleasant to us either, which would have been almost as satisfactory. If we ventured to approach someone ... he moved, negligently but definitively, away. ... The villagers were watching every move we made and they had an enormous amount of accurate information about who we were and what we were going to be doing. But they acted as if we simply did not exist... (Geertz, 1972: 1–2)

Fortunately for Geertz, this situation was dramatically and entirely incidentally resolved ten days after their arrival. Geertz and his (unnamed) wife found themselves fleeing from the police along with hundreds of villagers. As a result of this event, Geertz was catapulted from the invisible 'outsider' position to an 'insider'.

Most ethnographers, though, will not experience the instant camaraderie evoked by being 'on the run' from the police alongside the group with which they wish to engage, and must find other means of entering the field and gaining the confidence of the group. However, it is entirely possible to conduct ethnography with a group to which the researcher belongs. This may entail another set of problems, for example, concerns that informants will not behave naturally towards the researcher if she/he is *too* close to them, that informants will not wish to impact an existing friendship, or that they may feel obligated to participate, which would raise ethical issues (see Chapter 1).

A graduate student of our acquaintance conducted research with local 'bogans' (a group that some Britons refer to as 'chavs', and that bears some similarities to so-called 'white trash' in the USA and Canada). Typically, these are people aged in their teens to their thirties, who listen to heavy metal music, are usually in low-paid jobs or unemployed, often wear jeans and black t-shirts with images relating to their favourite bands, and share an interest in cars and/or motorbikes. It is a perfectly appropriate subculture with which to engage. Nonetheless, the student gained a great deal of media attention when it was revealed that he had received a prestigious scholarship, the research sites included pubs, parties and concerts, and he would be interviewing his friends. The obvious assumption was that he was being 'paid to hang out with his friends'. On the other hand, personal experience is considered by some to be necessary, especially when researching sensitive topics (O'Brien, 2010). We'll leave it to you to consider the pros and cons of this situation.

Most ethnographers will find that the groups they are interested in studying fall between these two extremes – neither friends nor completely foreign. This insider/outsider distinction has been the source of some debate. Naples (2004) argues that this apparently clear distinction falls away when we consider the differences that structure our lives, and our research, such as gender, age, class, sexuality, marital status and ethnicity. These multiple identities come with us into the field and may influence our insider/outsider-ness. We would also argue that individuals within the groups we seek to research will also have multiple identities that affect both their group integration and their potential relationship to us. It is clearly an error to assume homogeneity within the group based on the group identity that is salient to the researcher.

Notwithstanding these issues, entry into the field will often have two stages:

- **Gaining permission from a 'gate-keeper':** This permission may be formal, for example, requiring meetings, presentations about the intended research and a formal exchange of documents with a government or other official, or the executive of an organisation. It may be informal, involving a casual chat with a key person such as a club secretary or an influential member of a social group.

- **Gaining the co-operation of the community:** Having permission (as Geertz had in the situation described above) does not guarantee co-operation from the people with which you wish to interact.

PRACTICE POINT 2

In order to successfully undertake fieldwork comprising participant observation, the researcher must carefully consider how they will gain access to – be accepted by – the group/community of interest.

There are several steps which if carefully attended to, will facilitate acceptance of the researcher(s) into the group. These steps are essential for successful participant observation (we also recommend that you read Chapter 3 on life histories regarding building rapport):

What and where is 'the field'? Who are the 'participants'?

In the days in which ethnographical research was conducted in far-flung lands, these questions were easily answered: the field was the village or neighbourhood in which the research was to take place – that is, it was bounded geographically – and the participants (or 'informants') were the people who lived in that place. Contemporary 'fields' may not be so easily defined (Nadai and Maeder, 2005), and therefore the definition of the participant is also contestable. Nadai and Maeder (2005), following

Marcus (1995), argue that the field is a social world constituted by a set of actors with a common concern. These actors are the potential informants. Therefore, the field may in fact be spread over several (geographical) sites, or indeed, may include or consist of virtual sites (see below on the impacts of new technologies and on ethics). As an example, Finley (2010) spent two years attending games, practice sessions, fund-raisers and public appearances in her research on women's roller derby, conducting informal conversations and in-depth interviews with skaters, fans, referees and volunteers, and undertaking unobtrusive observation of 11 leagues across the southern United States. Data also included player and crowd comments and casual discussions. Many of the informants providing this data would not have known they were doing so, though Finley did identify herself as a researcher when engaged in more formal interactions.

Prior to entering the field

The researcher should learn as much as possible about the group or community in advance (obviously this is unnecessary if she/he is an 'insider' – a group member). Points to consider include:

1. Is there a particular person or gate-keeper who should be approached first?

2. What would be the most appropriate way of making the initial approach?

3. Is there an intermediary who could provide an introduction?

4. Or would it be best to simply 'hang around' and develop a relationship with group members?

Presentation of research and self

This may include the presentation of the research – for some groups, such as a workplace or other organisation, it may be appropriate to undertake a power-point presentation or similar, though for others this would be entirely inappropriate. Especially in formal settings it may be important to make explicit how your own subject position, commitments and experiences shape your engagement in the research (O'Brien, 2010) – put simply, why are you interested in it? Do you have any personal experience with the topic of interest, or is it aligned in some way with your own experiences?

Consider how to present *yourself*. What will you wear? Will you speak formally, 'professionally', or in a more relaxed manner? You may find it best to present yourself as a 'researcher', i.e., in a formal manner, as (supposedly) befits an academic when first meeting a gate-keeper, but as a 'participant' when meeting members of the group/community. We are not suggesting that you try to pretend that you are something you are not: this would be unethical, potentially embarrassing and damaging to the research when who you really are is inevitably revealed. However, we all adapt the way we present ourselves according to the situation: compare a job interview with a night out with friends. Decide which one of *your* multiple identities would be most appropriate to emphasise for these encounters.

Materiality

Are there some material objects that could enhance your acceptance into the group? Griffin and Bengry-Howell (2008) discuss fieldwork involving young men who modify their cars, 'cruisers' or 'boy racers'. An important part of gaining entry to this group was the researcher agreeing to go for a rather hair-raising ride with one of them. We assume this 'test' would not have been necessary if he had had his own modified car. Of course, it is unlikely to be practicable or even advisable for a researcher to buy a car specifically in order to 'fit in', but there may be other ways that social distance can be minimised, if this is considered necessary. At the same time, a researcher should not be disingenuous. Again, we suggest you think about what you do have in common with the group, and find ways of making this apparent.

Location

In the days in which ethnography meant travelling to another location, total immersion in the cultural group was common, though it was usual to have separate lodgings to which the researcher could 'retreat'. However, this physical distance could lead to social distancing and reluctance for members of the group to engage, particularly if the living conditions were markedly different (better) from that of the group. Contemporary ethnographers are less likely to live with the group of interest, although the ease of data collection and its richness and completion can generally be expected to be enhanced by spending as much time as possible with the group. Depending on the topic or community of interest, researchers may find themselves spending all their working hours with the group, or the leisure hours of the group (e.g., as with the study of 'car modifiers' mentioned above, Griffin and Bengry-Howell, 2008).

Of course (as discussed above) not only may the researcher engage with the same group in multiple places, but the research could be spread across multiple sites with different groups who share the same characteristics (as in Rosenhan's study (1973), which was sited in twelve psychiatric hospitals; also see the 'Further readings' section below).

Disclosure versus deception

Rosenhan (1973) and his co-researchers clearly used deception to gain entry to psychiatric hospitals, posing as patients. The informants (the staff and other patients) were unaware of the fact that they were being studied. In this way the project was akin to unobtrusive research (see Chapter 8). This was essential to the success of the research. However, the use of deception in ethnographic research is fairly unusual and is somewhat controversial.

A more subtle issue is that of non-disclosure. Generally speaking, it is considered preferable to fully discuss the purpose and process of the research with all concerned, unless this could jeopardise the findings. At times, though, it is simply impractical, as with Finley's research on women's roller derby, mentioned above. Her data included skater and crowd comments at games. See below and Chapter 1 for further discussions of deception in research.

Observation in practice

As discussed elsewhere, participant observation is *the* key research method for ethnographers. Supplementary methods, such as interviews, have been discussed in other chapters. Research involving observation will also be discussed elsewhere (see Chapter 8, Unobtrusive Research). Readers considering including existing documents in their work are also advised to read Chapter 10 on secondary research.

Ethnographic research is a very fluid approach. The researcher is unlikely to know all the variables of interest before she/he begins the research, and variables may be changed and added to as the research progresses. Additional supplementary material may be added, and the sites of the research may also change or be added to.

CONCEPTUAL CONCERN 3

Ethnographic research is a very fluid approach. The variables, supplementary materials, informants and sites may all be easily changed or added to as the research progresses.

Sites for ethnography (and, indeed, all social settings) have several dimensions, all of which provide opportunities for observation. The following list is adapted from Flick (2006: 222):

- Space: the physical place.
- Objects: physical things in the environment.
- Actors: the people involved.
- Acts: actions or behaviours.
- Events: activities, often engaged in by several actors.
- Goals: things actors are trying to accomplish and/or towards which acts are directed.
- Emotions: as expressed by actors.

Detailed research field notes are essential to participant observation. These notes can be taken in a number of ways, including hand-written notes taken openly, or audio- or video-recording. However, in some situations this may be intrusive – informants may feel uncomfortable and knowingly or unknowingly change their behaviour, even if the researcher has obtained their informed consent. It may be more appropriate to record crucial memos discreetly on a mobile phone or digital recorder, to be elaborated on in private as soon as possible.

Field notes can take the form of descriptions of actions and social processes, and will often be in narrative form, describing an incident or observed behaviour. Thorough field notes should answer as many of the following questions as possible (adapted from Flick, 2006: 300):

Who? Which actors are involved/being observed? What roles are they playing?
When? Time and duration of the action or event being observed.
Where? Location.
What? What is happening?
Why? For what apparent purpose?

Field notes may also take a quantitative or numeric form, for example, recording the frequency with which a particular event occurs, how many people are involved, coding verbal responses, etc. The recording of such observations is discussed in detail in Chapter 8.

PRACTICE POINT 3

Ethnography involves immersion in a culture, with the goal of coming to experience events and interactions in the same way as the group/community (Liamputtong, 2009), though the degree to which this is possible is limited and debatable.

Reflexive notes are also very valuable if not essential (Griffin and Bengry-Howell, 2008). These reflexive notes may be of the researchers' thoughts and feelings about what is observed, initial interpretations, and reminders, such as to seek out more information on a particular social behaviour. These reflexive notes are akin to the journaling process discussed with regard to interview transcriptions in Chapter 2. However, reflexivity is primarily concerned with assessing oneself and one's engagement with the research process. Alvesson, Hardy and Harley (2008) take a relativist approach (see below), arguing for consideration of the question: 'What are the different ways in which a phenomenon can be understood?' The motivations and assumptions of the author have to be exposed, explained and their limitations assessed, examining the way in which one interpretation of an observation is favoured over another.

PRACTICE POINT 4

Reflexivity begins with an awareness of your skills and assumptions. It should move on to challenge those assumptions.

We advise researchers to review each day's field notes, to consider items that require further elaboration, to note topics on which further research is required, possible new topics and preliminary coding for analysis.

One final key consideration in participant observation which seems to be surprisingly rarely discussed is personal risk and safety. Of course, all researchers who put themselves in other people's 'personal spaces' put themselves at risk, for example, interviewers conducting a door-to-door survey. Risk can come in many forms; some are easily anticipated, others less so. For example, Bengry-Howell put himself at risk when accepting a ride with a 'car modifier' (Griffin and Bengry-Howell, 2008), Rosenhan and colleagues put themselves at risk of institutional commitment and permanent diagnosis of psychiatric illnesses when they had themselves admitted to psychiatric hospitals (Rosenhan, 1973), Jenness put herself and her colleagues at risk of being offended against when they entered prisons to undertake research (see Jenness, 2010 and Further readings section at the end of the chapter). Though many sites of ethnographic research will not carry particular inherent dangers, it is often wise to take some precautions when spending time in an unknown place with unknown people. This may be as simple as ensuring someone reliable knows where you are going and when you expect to return, and to follow up if you don't return as arranged, as well as having that person's telephone number on speed-dial on your mobile phone. Other practical measures include knowing how to deal with a threatening dog, how to tactfully refuse an invitation into someone's home, always knowing exactly where you are and having enough money for a taxi fare (or at least the ability to get to a safe place if for some reason your anticipated mode of transport isn't available).

Exiting the field

Researchers should consider in advance how they will leave the field. It is likely that close relationships will have been formed. Is it necessary to completely sever these relationships? If so, how will this be done in an ethical manner? Is it appropriate to 'give something back' to the research participants, and if so, what? Are there, or should there be, continuing obligations to the community? Consider providing participants with a copy of your findings, perhaps modified to suit their needs, or giving a presentation. If visual methods (see below) have been used, perhaps a copy can be provided, or an exhibition held. Are there other resources that have been used or developed that may be of value to the informants or their community?

Data analysis and presentation

The processes of data analysis and presentation have been covered in other chapters. Ethnographic research is usually associated with analytical induction. Chapter 2 deals with grounded theory and thematic analysis, processes likely to be useful for analysing field notes, while Chapters 8 and 9 may be useful regarding the analysis of other types of data. Chapter 3 discusses analytical induction in depth. These chapters also discuss the presentation of relevant data, although some particular issues with the presentation of visual data are discussed below. It should be noted, however, that grounded theory is an inductive approach; theory is derived from the interrogation of the data. However, there are alternatives for researchers who wish to take a theory-driven approach to case-centric research, to further develop or modify *existing* theory. One is the extended case method. Thematic analysis can be applied to either, but if applied to a theory-driven approach, the researcher would begin with some key themes they wished to explore and would seek to confirm or disconfirm these through an analysis of the data.

CONCEPTUAL CONCERN 4

As with other case-centric approaches, ethnographic research is primarily associated with analytical induction (the development of new theory).

SOME ISSUES IN RESEARCH

In this section we discuss key epistemological and methodological issues and how these shape practice, as well as the ways in which resource limitations (time, space and costs) impact on the research approach.

Epistemology and claims for validity and reliability

It is generally accepted that researchers engaged in ethnography cannot occupy an objective position (O'Brien, 2010). At the same time, practising ongoing reflexivity can allow for a degree of distance or disengagement that allows the researcher to understand their own subjectivity and therefore peel away some of the issues of concern to positivists and relativists alike, and approach research 'scientifically'. Reliability and validity are essential components of research approaches that aim to be scientific, yet they have been topics of longstanding concern in ethnography (O'Brien, 2010). Reliability measures the extent to which the analysis of data yields results that can be replicated at different times or by different researchers. Validity measures the extent to which the research is accurate and describes the topic it set out to examine and therefore the extent to which claims can be made based on the findings.

A case study protocol can assist reliability in single-case research. Such a protocol provides at least a hypothetical basis for other researchers to repeat the study. The protocol requires researchers to provide an overview of the case study project, field procedures, such as accessing the informants, etc., interview schedules or other guidelines for data collection, and a description of data analysis (Yin, 2003).

A key aspect of validity is the comprehensiveness of the variables used. This comprehensiveness can be enhanced by using multiple sources of evidence. As stated above, participant observation is the primary method used by ethnographers. However, additional data sources can include personal documents (e.g., informant letters, diaries), statutory information, visual material (see below) and other related items. If multiple researchers are involved, they can be invited to review each other's accounts to verify interpretations of events. Chapter 12, Autoethnography, discusses issues of reliability and validity further.

However, concerns with 'science' are mostly associated with a positivist stance. In contrast to positivism, contemporary ethnography draws from the naturalist tradition, which emphasises cultural practices and their meanings within everyday contexts (Griffin and Bengry-Howell, 2008). Many contemporary ethnographers work from a social constructivist approach: researchers are aware of their role in constructing the data and informants' stories are viewed as informed constructions rather than objective truths. Social constructivists have little faith in science as a project that generates anything resembling universal rules, laws or theorems. This means that the positivist notion of the objective scientific observer is rejected.

For social realists doing science is a legitimate goal, but it is understood as a project that is limited by factors that social scientists have great difficulty in controlling for or being objective about. The realist believes that careful observation over time can lead to rich data that accurately represents the social setting and the people who inhabit it. Concepts and theories emerge from the data examined, rather than being imposed upon it from the outset, in accordance with the case-centric approaches predominantly used by ethnographers. This perspective lends itself to thematic analysis and grounded theory, which is discussed in Chapter 2. Social realists emphasise the appreciation of factors like power, meaning and the need for researcher reflexivity. As a result, any search for truth is always clouded by, among other things, the ways in which researchers and institutions impose bias.

The perspectives of the researcher and the researched are necessarily structured by the macro-social factors of class, race and gender, which nonetheless may not be overt or explicit. This can lead to a focus on the micro- (or at best meso-) social factors, i.e., individual relationships (Bronfenbrenner, 1979). The most overt, observable actions are recorded. This can be problematic when researchers' interpretations are presented as reality, but implicit structural factors are overlooked. As Burawoy (1998: 20) notes, 'These social forces are the effects of other social processes that for the most part lie outside the realm of investigation'.

Some ethnographers, principally relativists/postmodernists, argue that the desire of some researchers who wish to 'give voice' to marginalised groups through their work is misplaced (Richardson, 2000). It is inappropriate to speak on behalf of informants, and researchers' conclusions are imbued with their own pre-existing beliefs. Deborah Reed-Danahay (1997) locates the origins of autoethnography (the ethnography of the self – see Chapter 12) in part as a reaction to 'anthropological angst' in which the role of anthropologists in reporting to audiences about exotic peoples and locales became problematic. Autoethnography circumvents these dilemmas.

Resource limitations

Ethnographic research always requires a heavy investment of time, necessitated by fieldwork. However, the perception of this depends to some extent on the status of the researcher as insider or outsider, coupled with the depth of immersion and the location. The perceived experience and thus the drain on resources may be very different for, say, the insider who is spending time with their close associates and returning to their own bed each night, and the outsider interpreting unfamiliar customs far from home with little support, even if both researchers spend the same amount of time engaged in fieldwork.

The required financial resources will vary in a similar way. In the case of the former, very little will be required beyond the standard recording and writing equipment, while for the latter the financial investment may run into the thousands of dollars (or pounds) for travel and accommodation costs alone. However, the situation of many contemporary ethnographers will fall between the two – working fairly close to home, with fairly minimal costs.

PUTTING THE APPROACH IN CONTEXT

Although based on what may seem a fairly standardised approach – participant observation – ethnographic research has developed over time both in terms of practice and conceptually. In this section we discuss the increasing use of new technologies and ethical issues both old and new.

The impacts of new technologies on ethnography

The use of visual methods is increasingly popular, but they have, in fact, been used by ethnographers from the earliest studies. Mead advocated the use of photographs in the 1930s (Mead, 1963; also see Chapter 2). As discussed by Pink (2007), photography, video, art and electronic media are incorporated into the work of ethnographers as documents for analysis, and as forms of social interaction. In contrast to photo-elicitation, as used by interviewers (see Chapter 2), visual methods, particularly photography, used by ethnographers and/or anthropologists has tended to involve the researcher deciding what to photograph, though these images may be used as a topic of conversation with informants (Bunster (1977) provides a very interesting and accessible example, if somewhat dated now).

Internet communities are of interest to some ethnographers, both as sites of social interaction in themselves and as data sources for those interested in groups who happen to make use of internet blogs, forums, etc. (see, for example, Garcia et al., 2009; Paccagnella, 2006; Pink, 2007). The general principles of data collection apply, as discussed elsewhere, though these are additional ethical considerations and these are discussed below.

The ethics of ethnography

Ethics in participant observation, particularly regarding informed consent, has been a topic of much discussion. As we have seen, ethnography is not always conducted with fully informed and consenting informants. Sometimes this is due to practical difficulties in gaining consent from all those present, for example, in public spaces. However, this is not always the case. Rosenhan's research (1973), discussed above, is an example of covert research involving deliberate deception, and there are many more. Such covert research is often rationalised by the 'ends justify the means argument' – if the participants knew the truth about the research, the research itself would be compromised because they would behave differently (Bryman, 2008). This issue has been discussed in depth in Chapter 1 and is also relevant to Chapter 8 (Unobtrusive Research). Another consideration is the intrusive nature of the process of gaining informed consent – discussing what it means, reading information sheets, requesting a signature on a form, and so forth – which may be off-putting to potential informants. The authors of this text have not found this process to be problematic. Informants have appeared grateful for the opportunity to ask questions and pleased that their needs are considered, but it has been a concern for some (Fluehr-Lobban, 1994). A particular issue regarding informed consent in an ethnographic environment involves the possibility of some members of the community giving consent and others refusing, or people joining the group after the consent process has been completed. In addition, obtaining informed consent does not necessarily deal with all possible ethical dilemmas when undertaking ethnography.

Because ethnography requires an extended period of fieldwork particular issues of privacy may arise. It is possible that members of the community or group under observation become so used to the researcher's presence that they allow illegal or immoral activities to be witnessed (or they may believe that assurances of confidentiality apply). In some situations the researcher may be legally obliged to report the matter to the police; in others she/he will need to weigh up the severity of the act and its consequences against the implications for the research (e.g., consideration of whether reporting a traffic infringement is worth jeopardising the continuation of the project). While it is impossible to anticipate all such situations, researchers should consider how they would respond in hypothetical situations as part of their preparation for entering the field.

PRACTICE POINT 5

Although ethnographic researchers usually undertake an informed consent process with interview participants and other informants they directly engage with, it can be impractical to seek consent from all stakeholders and bystanders. In some cases, deliberate deception is used and researchers do not disclose their true purpose.

Another situation to consider is that of partial consent. By this we mean the situation in which some informants have agreed to participate and others have not. Borchard (2010) conducted research with homeless people in Las Vegas. His work included in-depth interviews with 48 homeless people, conducted in public parks and libraries, soup kitchens, bus depots and other places where homeless people are to be found. Each of these people signed an informed consent statement. In addition, he 'hung around' with homeless people. Borchard notes that he did not engage in a formal informed consent process during all aspects of his observations. While simply observing, he chose not to intrude on conversations and events, and presumably service providers and facility (e.g., library) staff were the subjects of some of his observations. Borchard explains that 'to avoid causing any harm to anyone involved in the study, I changed all the names of homeless men and any social service providers I directly studied' (2010: 445). Presumably, as other observations took place in public settings it was not considered necessary to obtain formal consent.

Paccagnella (2006) problematises the notion that internet forums and chat-rooms are public spaces and therefore 'fair game' for covert observation. Collection of data from these settings is likened to eavesdropping on a private conversation in a café or similar semi-public space, yet the usual processes of gaining informed consent may be difficult to complete. This position conflicts with the views of other researchers, as discussed in Chapter 1. In contrast, blogs are written with the express purpose of public dissemination, akin to a speech from a soap-box in Hyde Park, and using them for research purposes is relatively unproblematic.

CONCEPTUAL CONCERN 5

The ethics of using information available from internet sources such as forums and chat-rooms (without requesting permission) continues to be debated. Some liken it to using private conversations overheard in public places, while others consider that as the people who post to these forums know that the postings are publicly available, ethical concerns are unfounded.

Finally, specific ethical issues may arise from the use of visual methods. In particular, the question of ownership of images arises, and the appropriate use of these images by the researcher. Informants might be comfortable with images of themselves being used to supplement conversations and observations, but this does not mean they will be happy for these images to be published or otherwise publicly exhibited. Conversely, informants may have produced images with the expectation that they would be exhibited as a way of disseminating information that is important to the informant. However, the researcher may decide not to use all such images. Anticipating such situations and discussing them at the outset – or at the very least discussing them openly as soon as they arise – is usually the best way of dealing with them.

CONCLUSION

Ethnographic research may be briefly defined as the study of a culture. It is most commonly associated with anthropology, with Mead, Bateson and Malinowski's work being among the best known, although it has a history across the social sciences. The research typically describes the cultures of specific social groups in a case-centric, single-case approach, i.e., a group bounded by time, geographical location and/or cultural practices is explored through many variables and values.

Originally, ethnographic research described the cultures of specific social groups, often involving First World (western) researchers investigating developing communities and attempting to represent them in a scientific manner. However, by the 1970s this view was seen as problematic and few ethnographers now consider this exotic experience as essential. The value of examining groups within our own communities, and ourselves, is now recognised.

Data is usually collected using participant observation, and is often supplemented by other techniques such as interviews or analysis of documents such as statistics, letters or diaries. A crucial element of the success of the research, then, is negotiating extended entry to the field – the setting in which the group of interest is located – and developing relationships that will allow for a productive project.

Detailed research field notes are essential to participant observation and the best means of recording material should be considered before entering the field. Field notes can take the form of descriptions of actions and social processes, and will often be in narrative form, describing an incident or observed behaviour. Field notes may also take a quantitative or numeric form, for example, the frequency with which an activity takes place and the number of people involved. Reflexive notes are also essential. Reflexivity begins with an awareness of the researcher's skills and assumptions; it should move on to interrogating those assumptions and challenging preconceived ideas and interpretations of events that may be influenced by the researcher's own experiences and belief systems.

Contemporary ethnography emphasises cultural practices and their meanings within everyday contexts. Most contemporary ethnographers work from a social constructivist or a social realist (rather than positivist) approach. The social realist believes that careful observation over time can lead to rich data that accurately represents the social setting and the people who inhabit it. Concepts and theories emerge from the data examined, rather than being imposed upon it from the outset, in accordance with the case-centric approaches predominantly used by ethnographers. Social realists emphasise the appreciation of factors like power, meaning and the need for researcher reflexivity. As a result, any search for truth is always clouded by, among other things, the ways in which researchers and institutions impose bias.

Although the use of visual methods is increasingly popular, they have, in fact, been used by ethnographers for decades. Photography, video, art and electronic media are incorporated into the work of ethnographers as forms of social interaction and as documents appropriate for analysis. Internet communities and communications are also potential data sources, again either as a topic in themselves or as means of triangulating data sourced by more traditional means. The continually-evolving visual and computer-mediated approaches promise further enrichment of data collection and we anticipate the continued development of the method.

FURTHER READINGS

As noted, ethnographic research often combines observation with other methods, particularly interviews and the analysis of existing records. It also has some parallels to life history research. We therefore strongly recommend that you read Chapters 2, 3 and 8 for information on these supplementary approaches.

Those interested in the history of ethnography and/or anthropology are encouraged to read the work of George W. Stocking, Jr. Stocking provides an entertaining account of early British anthropologists and ethnographers, including a critique of Malinowski's eminence (Stocking, 1983).

Sociologists interested in the historical development of field research methods in their discipline may enjoy Martin Bulmer's work, although it is limited to the US history, focusing on the Chicago School (Bulmer, 1984).

Carolyn Fluehr-Lobban presents an argument for undertaking an informed consent process 'without the intrusive and necessarily legalistic use of a signed form', and provides a history of the concept in the USA (Fluehr-Lobban, 1994: 1).

Clifford Geertz's 'Deep play: Notes on the Balinese cockfight' (1972) is a classic work that is both entertaining to read and an excellent example of ethnographic work primarily using observation. Similarly, Erving Goffman's *Asylum* (1961) is valuable reading.

More recent examples that we recommend are Nadai and Maeder (2005) and Marcus (1995), who address the possibilities and challenges of conducting multi-sited ethnography, while Val Jenness' work with transgender prisoners (2010) covers many issues:

- Accessing a population that is hard to reach (for multiple reasons).
- Combining planned interviews with observations and informal, serendipitous conversations with various stakeholders.
- Negotiating ideas of reliability and validity.
- Researcher reflexivity and debriefing.

Those interested in undertaking visual ethnography should find Sarah Pink's text useful (Pink, 2007). Pink also has a website: http://www.lboro.ac.uk/departments/ss/visualising_ethnography/. Harper's 'Argument for visual sociology' (1998) is often cited and provides an interesting history of visual methods, although it tends to focus on still photographs.

REFERENCES

Alvesson, M., Hardy, C. & Harley, B. 2008. Reflecting on reflexivity: Reflexive textual practices in organization and management theory. *Journal of Management Studies*, 45, 480–501.

Banister, P., Burman, E., Parker, I., Taylor, M. & Tindall, C. 1994. *Qualitative methods in psychology: A research guide*. Buckingham, UK: Open University Press.

Bateson, G. & Mead, M. 1942. *Balinese character: A photographic analysis*. New York: New York Academy of Sciences.

Blackman, M. B. 2009. Introduction: The afterlife of the life history. In: Fielding, N. (ed.), *Interviewing II*. London: Sage.

Borchard, K. 2010. Between poverty and a lifestyle: The leisure activities of homeless people in Las Vegas. *Journal of Contemporary Ethnography*, 39, 441–466.

Bronfenbrenner, U. 1979. *The ecology of human development*. Cambridge, MA: Harvard University Press.

Bryman, A. 2008. *Social research methods*. Oxford: Oxford University Press.

Bulmer, M. 1984. *The Chicago School of Sociology: Institutionalization diversity and the rise of sociological research*. Chicago: Chicago University Press.

Bunster, X. 1977. Talking pictures: Field method and visual mode. *Signs*, 3, 278–293.

Burawoy, M. 1998. The extended case method. *Sociological Theory*, 16, 4–30.

Finley, N. J. 2010. Skating femininity: Gender maneuvering in women's roller derby. *Journal of Contemporary Ethnography*, 39, 359–387.

Flick, U. 2006. *An introduction to qualitative research*. London: Sage.

Fluehr-Lobban, C. 1994. Informed consent in anthropological research: We are not exempt. *Human Organization*, 53, 1–10.

Garcia, A. C., Standlee, A. I., Bechkoff, J. & Cui, Y. 2009. Ethnographic approaches to the internet and computer-mediated communication. *Journal of Contemporary Ethnography*, 38, 52–84.

Geertz, C. 1972. Deep play: Notes on the Balinese cockfight. *Daedalus*, 101, 1–37.

Goffman, E. 1961. *Asylum: Essays on the social situation of mental patients and other inmates*. New York: Doubleday.

Griffin, C. & Bengry-Howell, A. 2008. Ethnography. In: Willig, C. & Stainton-Rogers, W. (eds.), *The Sage handbook of qualitative research in psychology*. London: Sage.

Harper, D. 1998. An argument for visual sociology. In: Prosser, J. (ed.), *Image-based Research: A source book for qualitative researchers*. London: Falmer Press.

Hays, H. R. 1958. *From ape to angel: An informal history of social anthropology*. London: Methuen.

Jahoda, M., Lazarsfeld, P. F. & Zeisel, H. 1972. *Marienthal: The sociography of an unemployed community*. London: Tavistock.

Jenness, V. 2010. From policy to prisoners to people: A 'soft mixed methods' approach to studying transgender prisoners. *Journal of Contemporary Ethnography*, 39, 517–533.

Liamputtong, P. 2009. *Qualitative research methods*. Melbourne: Oxford University Press.

Malinowski, B. 1922. *Argonauts of the western Pacific*. London: Routledge.

Marcus, G. 1995. Ethnography in/of the world system: The emergence of multi-sited ethnography. *Annual Review of Anthropology*, 24, 95–117.

Martineau, H. 1827. *Society in America*. London: Saunders and Otley.

Mead, M. 1928. *Coming of age in Samoa*. New York: Morrow.

Mead, M. 1963. Anthropology and the camera. In: Morgan, W. D. (ed.), *The encyclopedia of photography*. New York: Greystone Press.

Messerschmidt, D. A. 1981. *Anthropologists at home in North America: Method and issues in the study of one's own society*. Pullman, WA: Washington State University.

Nadai, E. & Maeder, C. 2005. Fuzzy fields: Multi-sited ethnography in sociological research. *Forum: Qualitative Social Research*, 6, Art. 28 [online].

Naples, N. A. 2004. The outsider phenomenon. In: Hesse-Beiber, S. & Yaiser, M. L. (eds.), *Feminist perspectives on social research*. New York: Oxford University Press.

O'Brien, J. 2010. Seldom told tales from the field: Guest editor's introduction to the special issue. *Journal of Contemporary Ethnography*, 39, 471–482.

Paccagnella, L. 2006. Getting the seat of your pants dirty: Strategies for ethnographic research on virtual communities. *Journal of Computer-Mediated Communication*, 3, online.

Pink, S. 2007. *Doing visual ethnography: Images, media and representation in research*. London: Sage.

Reed-Danahay, D. E. 1997. *Auto/Ethnography: Rewriting the self and the social*. Oxford: Berg.

Richardson, L. 2000. Evaluating ethnography. *Qualitative Inquiry*, 6, 253–254.

Rosenhan, D. L. 1973. On being sane in insane places. *Science*, 179, 350–358.

Stocking, G. W. J. 1983. *Observers observed: Essays on ethnographic fieldwork*. Madison, WI: University of Wisconsin Press.

Whyte, W. F. 1955. *Street corner society*. Chicago: University of Chicago Press.

Willis, P. 1977. *Learning to labour: How working class kids get working class jobs*. Farnborough: Saxon House.

Wright, F. 1821. *A view of society and manners in America*. New York: E. Bliss & E. White.

Yin, R. K. 2003. *Case study research: Design and methods*. London: Sage.

FIVE

FOCUS GROUPS – STUDYING ARTIFICIAL GROUPS

CONTENTS LIST

Key words: focus groups – artificial groups – qualitative – one-to-many – market research – moderation – group research

SUMMARY

An outline of the case-centric approach of using focus groups, including: (i) the history of focus groups; (ii) the practicalities of conducting focus groups; (iii) the impact of new technologies on this method; and (iv) epistemological issues relevant to focus groups.

The previous chapter discussed ethnographic research – studying naturally-occurring groups. In this chapter we discuss a very different process of conducting research, this time with a contrived group – a group of people who come together for the express purpose of the research.

We begin by defining the term 'focus group' and providing some history to introduce you to the development and processes of this method. Though the conduct of a focus group has some similarities to an interview – they are both case-centric approaches, for example, led by the researcher in a semi-conversational format – the differences are significant. We discuss the practicalities of conducting focus groups in detail, including the use of new technologies such as the internet. We also consider epistemological issues.

DOING DATA COLLECTION AND ANALYSIS

Travers (2006) notes that the term 'focus group' provides a pretty good indication of what the approach involves: 'focus' suggests that the approach has a limited (focused) area of interest; and 'group' points to a number of participants occupied in the interview and even suggests that they may have some things in common. However, a focus group is not merely (or necessarily) a way of quickly gathering data from several participants. Although the approach incorporates the strengths of qualitative research in terms of gathering rich, contextualised material (thick data, according to Geertz, 1973), the aim is also to generate additional opinions and insights through the interactions of the group participants. The idea behind this is that group involvement assists people to reflect on and to clarify their perspectives as a collective (Liamputtong and Ezzy, 2005).

The focus group approach uses the interactive techniques of interviewing we discussed in Chapter 2 (In-Depth Interviewing). The novelty of focus groups is that rather than a series of one-to-one interviews (which is one way of obtaining multiple responses) the focus group uses a one-to-many approach. The core of the focus group is that a single researcher – the moderator (also referred to as the facilitator) – poses questions to a group of participants.

The core premise of the focus group is that a single researcher – the moderator – poses questions to a group of participants, who respond as a collective.

Exceptional focus groups

Focus groups are an example of a case-centric or case-first research approach. By this we mean that there are few cases and many variables associated with the research. The number of cases is either singular, if we wish to count the group as a collective (as in, one focus group) or several, if we wish to count the number of participants in the group (that is, typically six to nine people). At the same time, the 'focus' of focus groups is interaction between its participants and moderator(s) and this raises the possibility for a very great number of variables and values (e.g., questions to be posed and answered in a variety of ways).

CONCEPTUAL CONCERN 1

The focus group is a case-centric approach to research. There are one or few cases – in this instance, the case is the group of participants. There are multiple variables and values, which arise from the interaction between participants and moderator.

Hopefully, the designation of a focus group as case-centric is fairly obvious. If we accept the group as a collective, it would count as a single case approach. However, focus group research is only *weakly* case-centric. It only just fits this designation and has a number of variable-centric aspects. The most obvious of these is that the approach uses a deductive, top-down or even outright hypothesis-testing logic. For example, the moderator or facilitator of a focus group often begins with a thoroughly detailed schedule of topics and questions. There is limited scope for analytical induction. This is very unusual for case-centric approaches (see Chapter 1). It can be explained by the considerable pressure of space and time constraints.

The clearest example of the link between case-centric research and analytical induction is ethnography (see Chapter 4). In a traditional ethnography, the researcher would spend a sustained period of time in the field studying groups in their natural settings. But, focus group research does not take place in a community, a village, a factory, a nudist beach, etc.; it is undertaken in a rented room. Rather than taking weeks, months or years (like an ethnography), a focus group lasts only one or two hours. These space and time restrictions stymie most of the possibilities for inductive research. As a result, focus group research is hypothesis-testing and deductive in its character.

CONCEPTUAL CONCERN 2

Unlike most case-centric, case-first approaches, the focus group deploys a hypothesis-testing or deductive logic of research. This is largely the result of the pressures of time, which limit the inductive elements of research most commonly associated with case-centric approaches. By necessity, the research questions used in focus groups are developed in advance of the meeting and are applied in a 'top-down' manner by the moderator.

For the same reason, pressures of time mainly, focus groups are more fixed than fluid in their framing of research. Fluidity requires time to collect data and to analysis and to reflect. Ample time is not a feature of focus group research. We note below that the moderator of a focus group has to 'hit the ground running'. This means the designer of the research has to have fully prepared the moderator (designed questions, etc.) well in advance. There is very little opportunity for a fluid framing in focus groups research. This fixed analytical framing is also unusual for case-centric research (see Chapter 1).

CONCEPTUAL CONCERN 3

Focus groups usually involve a fixed framing. This is especially so when the purpose is to evaluate a questionnaire prior to a survey or supplement some other research, or when the research is a preliminary to a marketing campaign. In these situations, the variables and questions are likely to be predetermined, though there will sometimes be opportunities to add further material.

More generally, focus groups are located across a number of methodological boundaries or oppositions that we discuss in this textbook. For example: between structured and unstructured questions (see Chapter 2 on in-depth interviewing); between naturalistic settings (see Chapter 4 on ethnographic research) and laboratories and experimental research (see Chapter 7 on experimental research); and between individuals or collectives as the basic units of analysis or as measures of what constitutes a case. It is the latter, the participation of multiple respondents, a collective, at the point of data collection that most distinguishes the focus group as a very useful approach.

Origins of the approach

Focus groups are a popular way of collecting data. The ubiquity of the focus group is in part explained by its long and mixed history. It is one of the oldest laboratory-based research approaches used by contemporary social scientists, especially by social psychologists and sociologists (we use the term 'laboratory' in a broad sense here, to refer to an artificial environment in which research is conducted). These foundational developments in psychological and sociological research took place in the 1910s, 1920s and 1930s. Indeed, the development of a coherent approach or methodology around the focus group was undertaken by some of the original university-based practitioners of sociology and psychology/social psychology, but without, it should be noted, much input from the practitioners of the discipline of anthropology, who tended to eschew laboratories for the field.[1]

Social scientists were joined in this methodological undertaking by non-academics who were also interested in focus group research, not for scholarly reasons however, but to inform marketing and advertising campaigns. As a result, the history of the focus group includes work at the intersection of the social sciences and what we would now call private and public marketing. For example, Edward K. Strong, Jr (1884–1963), one of the founders of American psychology, wrote an article called 'Psychological methods as applied to advertising' (Strong, 1913). He used a focus group approach (although he did not use that term) to assess the effectiveness of five newspaper adverts for tungsten lamps (which were an exciting new consumer product at the time, and alternatively called the electric light bulb). Such early work was published in mainstream psychology (Poffenberger, 1925) and sociology journals (Bogardus, 1926) in the decades prior to the Second World War (Morgan, 1996).

The Second World War (1939–45) provided an important fillip for focus groups as the British and United States governments, among others, used the approach to assess their domestic propaganda campaigns around the war effort (Merton, 1987; Moran, 2008; Morgan, 1996). Moran (2008: 827) notes that:

> [T]he focus group can be traced back to a much larger series of connections between market research, a growth industry in Britain since the mid-1930s, and political culture. The roots of this crossover between market and political research lie in the work of the eclectic social research organization Mass-Observation, founded in 1937, and rival organizations emerging around the same time.

---

[1]Anthropologists were not initially interested in focus groups, largely because their focus in the early part of the twentieth century was still bound up with ethnographic, naturalistic, fieldwork among isolated 'traditional' peoples. At this time the discipline of anthropology was focused on studying 'them' (the cultures of traditional societies) rather than 'us' – in other words, the cultures from where anthropologists originated (see Darnell, 2001).

In the USA, Robert K. Merton (1910–2003), one of the most influential sociologists of the twentieth century, played a leading role in the standardisation of the approach (Merton et al., 1956; Merton and Kendall, 1946). Merton was the great 'methodologizer' of the social sciences. Indeed, Crothers argues more broadly that:

> [S]ome of the praise for the successful development of American sociology in the post-war period can be given to Merton's methodological writings, together for some of the blame for the deficiencies of the empiricism (the doctrine that theory unproblematically flows from social facts) that it unintentionally seemed to support. (Crothers, 1987: 52)

Interestingly, in a late career review of his contribution to focus groups, Merton (1987) admits that he didn't pay much attention to the approach following his initial work in the 1940s and 1950s, and was later surprised to find it so popular among marketers. Regardless, his initial discussion is instructive primarily because it locates focus groups within a positivist (in Crothers' terminology, empiricist) epistemology. It is also instructive because it urges caution in data collection and analysis, especially the need for reliability and validity, which contemporary researchers and especially emergent researchers should consider, even though the dominance of positivists like Merton is long-gone.

DATA COLLECTION

There are multiple examples of data collection that can be categorised as a focus group. As noted, focus groups are interactive, involve multiple respondents and a moderator. We suggest that the main reason for doing social research through focus groups is for in-depth interviewing of a collectivity, or for finding out about collectively held beliefs and attitudes.

CONCEPTUAL CONCERN 4

Focus groups are most useful for finding out about collectively held beliefs and attitudes.

In this section we identify three areas of importance in organising a focus group. These are:

1. Determine the purpose of the focus group.

2. Determine the role of the moderator.

3. Determine the composition of the group.

The areas are broadly sequential, in that it is important to decide on what you want to research before recruiting participants, for example. Nevertheless, the areas are also interactive – decisions made in one area will affect those in others. Like all social research, the process of organising a focus group is in practice far more messy than suggested by the lists of things to do that many textbook authors come up with.

Determine the purpose of the focus group

Before organising a focus group it is imperative that the purpose of the focus group is thought through, as well as determining the specific questions that are intended to illuminate the various research variables. The focus group approach attempts to understand and contextualise a case that is both somewhat experimental and transitory. A group of people (often, but not always, strangers) are brought together in an unfamiliar place and subjected to a process of which they have little knowledge and over which they have little control, and for only a short time. Time constraints alone mean that a moderator and the focus group must 'hit the ground running'. Some of the key issues facing focus group researchers include:

- **Testing individual or collectively held beliefs**: Focus groups are very useful for finding out about collectively held beliefs and attitudes. The responses to questions posed by the moderator are both singular – they are made by individuals – and, at the same time, collective – they are typically the result of by-play and discussion between participants. For this reason, focus groups can be thought of as a way of interviewing a collectivity of participants or of gauging attitudes and beliefs that are held as a group.

- **Stand-alone, preliminary or follow-up research**: Focus groups can take one of these three forms. They are used in small-scale research as a form of stand-alone data collection. Commonly, they figure in either the preliminary or follow-up phases of large-scale research projects:

  1. Focus groups are very fast and cost-effective ways of generating data. They have considerable appeal to the sole researcher for this reason. They are also viewed favourably by government agencies and other potential sponsors seeking data in a restricted time frame.

  2. Almost every large-scale survey or census will have 'focus grouped' its questions to ensure that the questions used are valid and reliable. They are particularly useful in the context of questionnaire design, showing where there is or isn't a consensus of opinion about terms and concepts. When social scientists want to ensure that the terms they use in a survey (such as 'household' or 'marriage', etc.) that is sent to multiple recipients (perhaps millions of recipients, as is the case with national censuses) are reliable and valid, they will often use focus groups to check and refine their wording. This capacity of focus groups to show the presence or lack of a consensus is also what makes them attractive to political pollsters and marketers. (Indeed, when the authors of this textbook were starving graduate students, they got a free meal and NZ $50 each as participants in a focus

group that was trying to decide if blue was a more upmarket colour than red. The consensus was for blue, although Bruce still liked red.)

3. Focus groups can also feature in the follow-up phases of research, to elaborate, provide feedback or check on research findings. This almost always is subsequent to a survey. The researchers may wish to gain more information on the responses to a specific question, to gain richer data or to contextualise the findings. This can be done either with a subset of the survey respondents (in which case respondents will have been asked if they would be willing to take part in a focus group at the end of the survey), or with different participants. They may wish to gain feedback from respondents on the survey, such as whether, in the opinion of the respondents, all the relevant areas were covered. Finally, they may wish to confirm or seek further explanation from survey respondents about their answers to questions (e.g., if they seem to be contradictory).

- **The quantification of research**: Focus groups may play an important part in the broad trend towards the 'quantification of research' (alongside content research – see Chapter 9 – and survey research – see Chapter 6). The quantification of research is a trend in which the social world is increasingly represented through numbers and statistics (for an interesting discussion of this, see Best, 1995). With case-centric research this means that (often undue) weight is given to the frequency with which responses occur, rather than to the deeper meaning of the responses. Bertaux (1981) discusses the validity and reliability of meaning, rather than frequency of response in terms of the 'saturation of knowledge'. He argues that a few meaningful responses are more significant than counts or frequencies (see Chapter 12, Autoethnographic Research).

PRACTICE POINT 2

It is crucial for the researcher/moderator to have a clear sense of the research goal and to have ready all the questions or prompts required for the group.

Determine the role of the moderator

The role of the moderator is central to a successful focus group. Here are some key issues to consider:

- **Avoiding a false consensus**: A key concern is avoiding a false consensus. Exploring consensus or its opposite is a research activity requiring sensitivity and skill on the part of the moderator. Of particular concern is ensuring that the moderator or a dominant participant does not influence the discussion, resulting in participants giving the responses they think are desired, rather than what they actually think. For this reason, focus groups are often structured around a series of projective techniques that are common to psychological research, rather than direct questions, such as 'Do you think blue is a more upmarket colour than red?'[2]

- **Projective techniques**: Projective techniques (see Murstein, 1965) operate by exploring participants' reactions to somewhat ambiguous images or situations. The most famous such test is the Rorschach inkblot test, where people (often psychiatric patients) are shown a symmetrical inkblot and asked to tell the interviewer what it reminds them of. Supposedly, differing answers, such as 'I see a beautiful butterfly' or 'I see a decapitated baby', illuminate the psychological state of the patient and aid diagnosis. In a focus group the aim is to gather collectively-generated data. Group participants may be shown a video of something related to the research (e.g., an advertisement to be used in a health campaign) and asked to comment on it. At the very least, social researchers (especially psychologists) are concerned to avoid 'leading' participants, so will formulate neutral questions as often as possible: 'What does this inkblot remind you of?', not 'What kind of violent image do you see in this inkblot?'

- **Save direct questions to the end**: Focus groups are highly deductive forms of hypothesis-testing, in the sense that, like the questionnaire in a survey, there is often a clear and consistent research agenda. A moderator may work from a predetermined sequence of questions and/or prompts. However, because of the collective nature of the approach, and the importance of not over-directing the group, the direct questioning of research participants will in all likelihood occur only at the final stages of the session, for the purposes of clarification, for example. The initial discussions are far more likely to focus on a range of projective techniques.

- **Forms of moderation**: Flick (2006) also offers three forms of moderation that might shape your thoughts on this:

  1. Formal direction, in which moderation is limited to directing the beginning and end of the discussion and ensuring key topics are discussed.

  2. Topical steering additionally incorporates steering the discussion towards more detailed, deeper understandings, including asking additional (new) questions when appropriate.

  3. Steering the dynamics may include asking provocative questions to stimulate further discussion, playing 'devil's advocate', that is, taking an opposing or polarising viewpoint to encourage argument and reflection and directly addressing issues of group dynamics.

---

[2]By 'projective techniques' we are referring to methods of stimulating responses that keep to the topic of interest and at the same time encourage a free flow of information. One common example is the open-ended question.

PRACTICE POINT 3

The role of the moderator is crucial to the success of any focus group. They must help create a naturalistic or life-like experience.

Overall, the ability to manage or balance focus group dynamics is a key requirement for successful moderators. On the one hand, in order for the discussion to feel 'natural' and thereby allow for participants to discuss the topics of interest in an everyday, relaxed way, it is argued that the moderator's interruption should be kept to a minimum; her/his role is to create a space in which the discussion unfolds through an unfettered exchange, rather than disturbing the group's processes. On the other hand, group dynamics can become destructive. For example, one participant may be more forceful in stating his or her views than others in the group, with the result that others agree with the dominant personality, or become reluctant to say anything at all. Arguably, this may be more likely to happen in an already established group, for example, a group of friends or workmates.

PRACTICE POINT 4

A key aspect of the focus group is the ability for group interaction to generate data as participants are encouraged to think about the topics in new ways (Brannen and Pattman, 2005). For this reason close attention must be paid to group dynamics as well as broader issues of power differences between and within group members and between researchers and participants (Farnsworth and Boon, 2010; Willis et al., 2005).

- **Dealing with problems:** Focus groups are often used to deal with emotive or sensitive topics. If moderated well, they can be of benefit not only to the researcher, but also to the participants, if they get an opportunity to speak honestly about the topic and have their opinion validated. A strong sense of group camaraderie can develop in this situation. However, there is also the potential for distress to occur. As with managing groups more generally, the best way to avoid this is by being clear about the ground rules from the start, for example with statements like: 'This is potentially a sensitive topic, so we need to make a commitment to treat each other with respect' or 'If you feel you don't want to contribute for a while, or to leave the room, that's fine'. While the moderator should stress the importance of the topic, he or she may be able to lighten the mood by telling a humorous anecdote about his or her own experience. Sometimes despite our best efforts, though, participants may become uncomfortable. If you think this is about to occur (or already has occurred – it can happen quickly!), possible ways of dealing with it include statements like: 'This is a pretty difficult topic, so let's take a breather for a few minutes' or 'It seems that some people's opinion is quite at odds with others. To avoid that becoming an issue, let's talk about x for a while. We can come back to this topic later (or in an individual discussion)'.

Determine the composition of the group

The composition of focus groups can also take various forms. Sometimes the heterogeneity of the group is preferred, sometimes the possibilities for affinity are stressed.

- **Heterogeneous groups**: These groups tend to maximise the differences between members/participants. They are favoured when: (1) only a few focus groups are being run, (2) there is a broad topic of discussion, (3) the topic is relatively 'safe' (not covering sensitive topics, such as sexuality, abuse or traumatic events). Also, heterogeneous groups require the most capable moderators. This requirement is somewhat offset by the relative ease of recruitment of participants. Selection criteria can be relatively loose and random.

- **Affinity groups**: As discussed above, interaction between participants is a key feature and advantage of focus groups. This interaction can be affected by the degree to which the participants feel comfortable with each other. Affinity group participants are recruited in order to increase the likelihood of good group dynamics (for example, participants may know each other or share characteristics such as gender or age), or to ensure that specific sectors of society are included in the research. Affinity groups may ease the process of relationship building which occurs at the beginning of a focus group meeting, encouraging frank and open discussion and limiting the power differential between the moderator and the participants (Barbour, 2005). Affinity groups are favoured when: (1) multiple focus groups are being run, (2) there is a narrow, specialised topic of discussion, (3) the topic is highly sensitive. Affinity groups are typically recruited using purposive sampling.

An example of affinity groups

To cover all the necessary demographic groups may require a number of affinity groups. For example, if the topic is perceptions of drinking alcohol during pregnancy, it may be decided that it is important to include women of child-bearing age and their partners (because their partners may influence drinking), but not men in general or older women because they may have both less interest in the topic and not have spent much time considering the issue. It may also be decided to split the groups according to motherhood status (i.e., have had or have not had children), age and socio-economic status (SES), or ethnicity, or geographical location. So a matrix of the necessary groups might look like that shown in Table 5.1.

TABLE 5.1 Example focus group demographic matrix

Women aged 16–25	Women aged 26–35	Women aged 36–45
Low SES	Low SES	Low SES
Middle SES	Middle SES	Middle SES
High SES	High SES	High SES
Mothers (any SES)	Mothers (any SES)	Mothers (any SES)
No children (any SES)	No children (any SES)	No children (any SES)

That gives a total of 15 groups: three age groups times five categories within each age group. Further consideration might also need to be given to how partners would be involved. If they are included with the women, they may influence each other's input (but having separate groups for partners would double the number of focus groups). Would it matter if participants included same-sex partners? How would female partners be dealt with? Would a separate group be appropriate?

The ways of recruiting focus group participants are fairly well established:

- **Random telephone selection** – selecting participants from the telephone directory. This method would generally only be suitable for a topic of broad interest, and even then, it is likely that screening processes would be used. Care must be taken when approaching people directly. Usually an information sheet or letter would be sent asking for interested people to contact the researcher. If no contact is received, no follow-up is undertaken.

- **Snowball** – participants are invited to bring a friend.

- **Piggyback** – participants suggest another person who may be suitable (as with random telephone selection, for ethical reasons, it is unusual for the researcher to directly approach people without the person's interest first being confirmed).

- **Existing groups** – such as clubs, workplaces or service users. In this case a letter, flyers, posters or other advertising material would generally be sent to the organisation inviting interested people to contact the researcher.

- **Revisiting respondents** from earlier phases of research.

PRACTICE POINT 5

Participants in focus groups may be recruited by purposive sampling across significant factors (e.g., age, gender, sexual orientation and life experience), thus creating an affinity group. This sense of affinity, or similarity, can aid the development of a relaxed discussion.

SOME ISSUES IN RESEARCH

In this section we discuss epistemology, reliability and validity, and some benefits of focus group research.

Epistemology

We have tried to capture the complexities of epistemology through three positions: positivist, social realist, social constructivist (see Chapter 1). To recap: Positivists accept as true a social reality that exists independently of our perceptions of it. They emphasise the techniques of observation and measurement and the potential for scientists to form objective understandings (truth-claims). This assurance informs their practice and is the justification for doing science and for excluding all other forms. Social realists also accept an external and measurable social reality, but one that exists through the mediation of our perceptions and actions. Where positivists strive for objectivity, social realists insist on forms of subjectivity and the appreciation of factors like power, meaning and researcher reflexivity. For social realists, the scientific endeavour is still a legitimate goal but it is understood as a limited and somewhat contextual project. Social realists are, as a result, more inclusive of methodological approaches than their positivist counterparts and now occupy the mainstream position within the social sciences. Social constructivists continue the critique of positivism and have little faith in science as a project that generates anything resembling universal rules, laws or theorems. According to this epistemology, it is impossible to differentiate truth-claims based in science, or folklore, or commonsense, or metaphysics, because individuals or actors actively create the social world and all potential measures of that social world.

Since the end of the second World War the social sciences have been transformed by the decline of positivism as a (the) dominant way of conducting research. We have discussed elsewhere in the textbook how the decline of positivist fascinations with (many would say self-serving) definitions of validity, reliability, science and objectivity opened up new spaces for other approaches. Thus, the rise of post-structural semiotics (see Chapter 11), the use of autoethnography (see Chapter 12), and even Stanley Milgram's (now) ethically ambiguous use of experimental research (see Chapter 7). At the same time, positivism didn't simply go into decline. Rather it was the long-run loser in what are now called the 'science wars' of the 1960s and 1970s. For example, Anne Oakley, a pivotal figure in the struggles in which positivistic formulations were challenged and dismantled by researchers using different paradigms, provides a wonderful retrospective on the role of feminists in opening up the social sciences (Oakley, 1998).

This is not to say that positivism no longer exists and, more significantly, that positivist social scientists no longer hold important positions as teachers, funders, editors and researchers. The decline of positivism has been an uneven process in the social sciences. Sociology and anthropology have been transformed by it. Psychology has more or less splintered into positivist versus non-positivist camps. In psychology, in particular, the focus group approach has suffered until fairly recently from the dominance of positivistic experimental and quantitative methods, and some psychology academics still have limited understandings – and major misunderstandings – of the approach. Here, positivist criticisms of focus groups reflect psychology's ongoing angst to be taken seriously as a 'hard science' with the attendant adoption of forms of the experimentation and quantification that echo what hard scientists purportedly do. The social realist and social constructivist concerns with power, meaning and reflexivity as unavoidable components of research are still given little credence by mainstream, clinical psychologists (much to the detriment of their work, we believe). While the crisis in social psychology which occurred in the 1970s resulted in a broadening of approaches and the incorporation of methods used elsewhere in the social sciences, particularly in Europe, the same cannot be said of psychology more broadly. It is still common for undergraduate psychology research courses to focus on experimental and quantitative methods, and many social psychology textbooks barely mention other methods, such as focus groups.

While focus groups began as part of the positivist movement that helped establish the social sciences in the early twentieth century, the approach now sits squarely within the social realist camp. Similarly, we have noted how psychology came late to focus groups, mainly because it wasn't positivist enough, while sociology and anthropology found its traditional variants too positivistic. Nevertheless, the decline of positivism has led to a flowering of focus group techniques (as with other approaches), especially when coupled with the use of new technologies (see below). However, this flowering, an integration of the approach with social realist and social constructivist concerns, does constitute a relaxation of the issues that positivist scholars like Merton had with ensuring validity and reliability.

CONCEPTUAL CONCERN 5

The decline of positivism as a dominant way of conducting social research has resulted in the flowering of new forms of research. While focus groups began as part of the positivist movement that helped establish the social sciences, the approach now sits squarely within the social realist camp.

Reliability and validity

There are lingering concerns about the reliability and validity of focus groups research. In this respect, the 'problem' with focus groups is that shared by all case-centric approaches. The low number of cases, including single-case research (see Becker, 2009), means they are not amenable to the sorts of tests of reliability and validity that are associated with survey research (Chapter 6) and other forms of predominantly positivist social science. We discuss this issue in some depth, and offer some solutions, in Chapter 3 (Life Histories) and Chapter 12 (Autoethnographic Research). Our focus here is on the unique issues of focus groups. These centre on the moderator.

It is perhaps bizarre that given the challenges of moderation, emergent researchers are nevertheless likely to find themselves being asked to take on the role in large research projects. While Liamputtong and Ezzy (2005) and others may rather glibly list the skills needed by a successful moderator, we feel it is important that emergent researchers aren't put off by this list:

- Sensitivity to participant needs and emotional states.
- Respectfulness and open-mindedness.
- Leadership skills.
- Listening skills.
- Observation skills.
- Patience.
- Flexibility.
- Self-confidence.

Obviously, the moderator plays an extremely important role in the success of the focus group and spending time thinking about how she/he might deal with a range of possible scenarios is essential. A well-run focus group may look to the untrained eye like a free-flowing conversation involving six to ten people. The atmosphere is relaxed and informal, while at the same time all the participants are engaged and contribute to the discussion. The participants in the discussion are likely to be sitting around a table with tea/coffee and light refreshments and taking turns to talk and to listen. But it is crucial to remember that the naturalness in the presentation of a focus group is an artifice. The setting is a laboratory and the conversation is in fact the result of considerable planning on the part of the researcher, and involves any number of assistants, possibly observers viewing from behind a one-way mirror and – most significantly for many emergent researchers – a competent moderator.

To recap: A key concern about focus group research is the rigour of its findings or results. This concern is precisely about validity and reliability (see Chapter 1). The concern is that it is possible that on another day with another moderator and other participants the discussion may turn out very differently. Nonetheless, we think these concerns are overstated. There is now a considerable body of evidence that shows that well designed and moderated focus groups are rigorous. While the details of discussion may differ between groups or over time, the overarching themes and responses are very similar and consistent.

Less defensively, it has been argued that the focus group research is preferable to many other approaches (particularly the in-depth interview and the questionnaire) because the data is collected in a more 'life-like' way. Rather than participants responding to a series of questions, data is gathered in context, as a conversation with participants feeling they have a significant degree of control in the discussion. Flick (2006) suggests that focus groups come closer to simulating everyday life, and therefore to verisimilitude, than other research approaches.

PRACTICE POINT 6

Exploring the presence or absence of a consensus of opinion is an important capacity of focus groups. It is crucial to manage focus groups so as to not develop a false consensus.

PUTTING THE APPROACH IN CONTEXT

We have noted that because of time and space constraints, focus groups are somewhat deductive in their orientation. What flows from this is that focus groups also operationalise a fixed framing of research. This means that the stages or elements in undertaking research are very sequential. On the one hand, the schedule of questions may need to be finalised before the focus group begins. On the other, the moderation of a focus group requires the careful balancing of a predetermined agenda with the need for spontaneity and developing a collective response. However, new technologies, especially those relating to the internet, open up new possibilities for research using focus groups. Stewart and Williams (2005) note that over the last decade the traditional methods of research have been applied to online environments with varying degrees of success, and that these processes continue to evolve. While other forms of new technology, such as audio- and video-conferencing, have been employed to conduct research, the following discussion focuses on online facilities, due to both the greater challenges and the opportunities they afford. In this respect, the use of virtual focus groups via the internet, and also including video- or audio-conferencing, offers both advantages and disadvantages in research (Stewart et al., 2007).

On the plus side, there may be greater potential to preserve anonymity and participants don't need to gather in one place. This may be particularly useful for a hard-to-access group, such as those whose experiences are rare (e.g., research to be conducted with people who have experienced an unusual disease) or for participants who are disabled. It is also easier to encourage less extroverted participants to take part (and they may be more extroverted in a virtual setting). The research may not need to be conducted at a particular time. For example, a website may be open for postings for several hours or even days, although this may raise facilitation challenges. This is known as an asynchronous focus group – it is not conducted in real time (Stewart and Williams, 2005). In the case of written postings to a website or similar, transcribing (surely every researcher's most hated task!) won't be necessary.

On the negative side, there is a risk that participants may not be who they say they are, which might lead to sampling problems and invalidate the results (e.g., if the focus group is about attitudes to abortion and is intended to be composed of young women, but one of the participants is actually an older man with markedly different and strongly-held views). Some of the advantages of the traditional focus group method may be lost, such as the contextualisation of responses. There may be a reduced sense of intimacy compared to face-to-face focus groups, although this may be balanced by greater anonymity, so openness will not necessarily be reduced. Non-verbal communication may be reduced, especially in focus groups conducted via chat-rooms, blogs or message boards, although this can be moderated through the use of webcams, and to a lesser extent, emoticons (☺ ☹). Further, the online discussion may be harder to moderate, especially in regards to dominant participants. Some forms of technologically-mediated conversation, such as conference telephone calls, can be very socially awkward, with people being unsure when one group member has finished, causing 'dead air' or people talking over each other. Finally, there is the potential for technical issues to delay or disrupt proceedings.

PRACTICE POINT 7

New developments, especially in information and communication technologies, have allowed for a relaxing of time and space constraints on focus groups. This relaxation comes with both benefits (greater flexibility, etc.) and potential pitfalls (loss of intimacy, focus and control). The use of technologically-mediated meetings and various software packages has the potential to automate and ease the process of data analysis, but at the risk of oversimplifying the results.

The decline of positivism has resulted in what the champions of social realism and social constructivism would call the diversification of focus groups. However, from the perspective of positivists, this flowering of forms raises many concerns about issues of reliability and validity of social research. This differentiation of focus groups has been accelerated by the rise of the internet and other information and communication technologies. Indeed, many of the cutting-edge ways of doing a focus group would be unrecognisable to the founders of positivistic psychology and sociology at the turn of last century. Yet, the ghost of positivism still haunts the approach in its inherent deductivism and fixed, sequential framing of research. Further, whereas positivist concerns with being objective, and hence scientific, were previously to the forefront of the approach, and were made explicit, the new elements appear as mere technical or procedural demands on the part of the researcher/moderator. We suggest that this relegation of epistemological issues to procedural ones is a worrying development.

At the same time that positivism has declined as an unrivalled research paradigm, there has been a massive increase in demand for research that looks a lot like objectivist, valid and reliable 'science'. This demand isn't simply the result of a proliferation of academic journals in recent decades but, more importantly, comes from the end-users of research: policymakers, politicians, pollsters, lobbyists, activists and marketers. These people constitute a category that Joel Best (1995) calls claims-makers. By claims-makers we mean the public process by which individuals, groups and institutions make demands for change and set about justifying and legitimating those claims. Best, and other writers such as Darrell Huff, whose classic *How to lie with statistics* (1954) remains a must-read, have shown that statistics or quantitative research is highly attractive to all sorts of claims-makers. In short, statistics, numbers and the gloss of science provide compelling material for making a convincing public argument (for example, for more public transport, for longer prison sentences for paedophiles, for taxpayer bailouts of banks, etc.). As we have noted earlier, there is now considerable incentive for 'making qualitative into quantitative research' and new technologies and packages such as NVivo and NUDIST do just that (see Chapter 2 on in-depth interviewing for our discussion on how such software packages tend to quantify the results of qualitative research). They turn conversational analysis into forms of counting and reporting.

Focus groups are a prime location for using these packages – for analysing conversations – and so are an important element of the trend for making qualitative into quantitative research. We consider this regrettable in so far as considered scholarship is undermined by a 'quick and dirty' approach to the social sciences – by this we mean research that is driven more by the demands of the end-user as contractor rather than end-user as enquiring mind. The realities of social research are such that all emergent researchers must come to some sort of accommodation with the demands of earning a living while being ethical. We think it is important to note that we consider a lot of contemporary focus group research to be more or less quick and dirty; it is social research that looks like 'science' but lacks the rigour to truly be so. At the same time, this non-academic component has been part of the approach since its inception (see above).

Commenting on how a commercial for car tyres or a party political campaign made you feel about yourself, the product and the sponsors of the product (campaign) is clearly grist to the mill of political pollsters and marketers using focus groups. From this sort of inquiry we have 'discovered' that men with beards are less trustworthy spokesmen than those without, and that fat people are considered unreliable. It is easy to dismiss this type of research as quick and dirty, which discredits genuine scholarly research. But it is also important to recognise the legitimacy of focus groups and their capacity to illuminate collective responses to very sensitive social issues. Hence, the use of focus groups in the social sciences was developed as a feminist research approach (Wilkinson, 2004), precisely because it could illuminate very difficult issues. For example, through bringing together (in a comfortable yet neutral setting) a group of women who have undergone a similar difficult experience, spending time allowing them to get to know each other, and allowing the group a high degree of control over what and how information is disclosed, a sense of support and camaraderie often develops among participants, such that they will talk more openly and honestly about their experiences than they would do in many other settings.

A real-life example: when focus groups go wrong

Let's conclude this section with an example of how a focus group has been – and (in some respects) should not be – done. The broad topic of a piece of research one of your authors (not the gloriously red-bearded one!) was involved in was users' perceptions of a mental health service in a provincial town. Prepared questions included 'What are the areas of this service that could be improved?' (Note that participants were also asked about the strengths of the service, so as to minimise the risk of eliciting biased data.) Participants spoke passionately and in detail about their experiences, including many specific aspects of the service, such as the availability of respite care, crisis services, residential facilities, community outreach programmes, liaison with general practitioners, community support workers, the personalities and approaches of various staff members and much more. It would have been very difficult, if not impossible, to anticipate the many variables that would arise from the first focus group discussion, and this first pool of data informed the development of subsequent discussion guides. However, for some time each discussion raised new issues, or new aspects of previously discussed issues, due to the different experiences of the group. So far, so good. Yet involvement in this series of focus groups was one of the most stressful and distressing times in the author's career. Why?

Within minutes of the first focus group beginning, two participants were in tears, another was shouting and another was demanding 'Who's in charge of this meeting?'! How did this happen, you may be wondering? The answer is the mishandling of a series of surprisingly simple processes.

The private research company that employed the author at the time of this research was based in another country and lacked an appreciation of local New Zealand culture, particularly in regards to Maori, the indigenous people. However, Maori are disproportionately over-represented as mental health service users and thus comprised the majority of research participants. Normally, appropriate cultural protocols would be undertaken before the commencement of the focus group discussion, such as the opportunity for a formal welcome and prayer. This would be particularly important given the sensitive nature of the topic. In addition, as we've mentioned above, to get the best out of a focus group discussion it is advantageous to spend some time allowing participants to get to know and become comfortable with each other and the moderator. However, in this case there was not even a simple round of introductions.

Instead, as soon as everyone was seated the moderator (NOT the author, who as a new employee was assigned a lowly assistant role) said: 'Right, please sign the consent form and we'll get started. How do you feel about this service?' Note that the normal process of reviewing the purpose of the research and participants' rights in regards to informed consent was not undertaken. The moderator – one of the directors of the company – had an undergraduate degree in economics but no training in social science research methods, or any other research methods for that matter, beyond economic data manipulation. (In addition, as he had spent the night before getting very drunk with his 19-year-old personal assistant, he was perhaps lacking the clear-headedness normally required to conduct a successful focus group.) Nevertheless, the company had a solid reputation in financial research and had diversified into other areas, apparently blissfully unaware of a serious deficit in competence – up until this point. A degree of calm was eventually restored, some ground rules for the process were established by the author, and the rather shaken moderator was given a crash course in focus group and cultural protocols. However, this was a very hierarchical company and your author lost many hours of sleep over the ensuing few weeks while trying to strike a balance between ensuring appropriate and ethical processes were undertaken and the need to pay the mortgage (the author resigned from her position shortly after this experience). *We invite you to consider the reasons why things went wrong, how they could have been avoided, and what YOU would do in this situation.*

CONCLUSION

Focus groups have a long, and somewhat mixed, history in the social sciences. Nevertheless, they have much to offer both the emerging and experienced researcher. The approach is one of the oldest used by contemporary social scientists; initial developments took place in the 1910s though it fell out of favour for several decades within some social science disciplines, while being embraced elsewhere. We suggest that the main reason for doing social research using focus groups is for in-depth interviewing of a collectivity, incorporating the strengths of qualitative research in terms of gathering rich, contextualised material. However, a focus group is not merely a way of quickly gathering data from several participants. The aim is also to generate additional insights through group interactions.

Focus groups are classified as an example of a case-centric or case-first approach – there are few cases and many variables associated with the research. It would be unusual for there to be more than ten or twenty focus groups in a single research project. As the 'focus' of focus groups is the interaction of participants, the possibility is raised of a large number of variables, some or many of which may not have been anticipated.

So, as a final plug for the approach and to ensure that your focus group experiences are positive:

- Consider the participant group demographics: are they likely to be different from you in some significant way, such as ethnicity, gender, age or class? If the answer is yes, consider enlisting the aid of a moderator who is a better match or a consultant who can advise on cultural requirements, for example.

- Is the topic likely to evoke strong emotion? Consider ways you can minimise and/or manage this.

- Ensure that participants are familiar with the purpose of the research, what will happen during the focus group and appropriate behaviour, such as giving everyone an opportunity to voice their opinion in a non-judgemental way.

- Read through the consent form (aloud) before beginning the focus group and ask people if they have any questions. If possible, arrange this so that participants have some privacy to ask questions, or go through this process in a relaxed way, perhaps over refreshments.

- Be alert to signs of distress and tension during the discussion and be ready to intervene.

PRACTICE POINT 8

There are many elements that contribute to a successful focus group, the most important of which is the role of the moderator. Emergent researchers acting as moderators will benefit greatly from familiarising themselves with all aspects of the approach and even contemplating how they might react if things go wrong in the group.

FURTHER READINGS

There are a great number of textbooks on focus groups. A simple search at your library or via Google will throw up dozens. Krueger and Casey's *Focus groups: A practical guide for applied research* is now in its fourth edition (2009) and is very comprehensive, if you can get past the 'down with the kids' use of text icons and related ephemera.

David Morgan (1996) provides an excellent history of the focus group and especially of the centrality of the moderator.

REFERENCES

Barbour, R. S. 2005. Making sense of focus groups. *Medical Education*, 39, 742–750.
Becker, H. S. 2009. The life history and scientific mosaic. In: Harrison, B. (ed.), *Life story research*. London: Sage.
Bertaux, D. 1981. From the life-history approach to the transformation of sociological practice. In: Bertaux, D. (ed.), *Biography and society: The life history approach in the Social Sciences*. London: Sage.
Best, J. 1995. *Images of issues: Typifying contemporary social problems*. New York: De Gruyter.
Bogardus, E. S. 1926. The group interview. *Journal of Applied Sociology*, 10, 372–382.

Brannen, J. & Pattman, R. 2005. Work–family matters in the workplace: The use of focus groups in a study of a UK social services department. *Qualitative Research*, 5, 523–542.

Crothers, C. 1987. *Robert K. Merton*. London: Tavistock.

Darnell, R. 2001. *Invisible genealogies: A history of Americanist anthropology*. Lincoln, NB: University of Nebraska Press.

Farnsworth, J. & Boon, B. 2010. Analysing group dynamics within the focus group. *Qualitative Research*, 10, 605–624.

Flick, U. 2006. *An introduction to qualitative research*. London: Sage.

Geertz, C. 1973. *The interpretation of cultures*. New York: Basic Books.

Huff, D. 1954. *How to lie with statistics*. New York: W. W. Norton.

Krueger, R. A. & Casey, M. A. 2009. *Focus groups: A practical guide for applied research* (4th edn). Los Angeles, CA: Sage.

Liamputtong, P. & Ezzy, D. 2005. *Qualitative research methods* (2nd edn). Melbourne: Oxford University Press.

Merton, R. K. 1987. The focussed interview and focus groups: Continuities and discontinuities. *Public Opinion Quarterly*, 51, 550–566.

Merton, R. K., Fiske, M. & Kendall, P. L. 1956. *The focused interview*. New York: The Free Press.

Merton, R. K. & Kendall, P. L. 1946. The focussed interview. *American Journal of Sociology*, 51, 541–557.

Moran, J. 2008. Mass observation, market research, and the birth of the focus group, 1937–1997. *Journal of British Studies*, 47, 827–851.

Morgan, D. L. 1996. Focus groups. *Annual Review of Sociology*, 22, 129–152.

Murstein, B. 1965. *Handbook of projective techniques*. New York: Basic Books.

Oakley, A. 1998. Gender, methodology and people's ways of knowing: Some problems with feminism and the paradigm debate in social science. *Sociology*, 32, 707–731.

Poffenberger, A. T. 1925. *Psychology in advertising*. Chicago: A. W. Shaw.

Stewart, D. W., Shamdasani, P. N. & Rook, D. W. 2007. *Focus groups: Theory and practice*. London: Sage.

Stewart, K. & Williams, M. 2005. Researching online populations: The use of online focus groups for social research. *Qualitative Research*, 5, 395–416.

Strong, E. K. 1913. Psychological methods as applied to advertising. *Journal of Educational Psychology*, 4, 393–395.

Travers, M. 2006. Qualitative interviewing methods. In: Walter, M. (ed.), *Social research methods: An Australian perspective*. Melbourne: Oxford University Press.

Wilkinson, S. 2004. Focus groups: A feminist method. In: Hesse-biber, S. N. & Yaiser, M. L. (eds.), *Feminist perspectives on social research*. New York: Oxford University Press.

Willis, E., Pearce, M. & Jenkin, T. 2005. Adapting focus group methods to fit Aboriginal community-based research. *Qualitative Research Journal*, 5, 112–123.

SIX

SURVEY RESEARCH – STUDYING MANY CASES

CONTENTS LIST

Key words: survey research – variable-centric – probability – random sampling – margin of error – scales of measurement – survey fatigue – over-sampling – inferential statistics – hypothesis-testing – sampling frame

SUMMARY

An overview of survey research as a variable-centric research approach, including: (i) a brief history of survey research; (ii) the key terms and process, such as probability and random sampling; (iii) the issues and limitations of survey research in the social sciences; and (iv) the impact of recent developments such as internet-based surveys.

The previous chapters have dealt with case-centric research approaches: a key starting point is deciding who or what the case(s) will be, and how to access them. Case-centric research has a small number of cases and a large number of variables, not all of which may be known before the research is begun. Case-centric research is typically inductive. Survey research is the first variable-centric approach we will discuss; it consists of the opposite characteristics.

As with every chapter of this book, we begin by discussing the way(s) in which data collection and analysis are typically worked through, including a brief history of the approach. We explain the key terms and processes, such as probability and random sampling, margin of error and scales of measurement, and discuss the operationalisation of a hypothesis. We provide an overview of some of the issues associated with survey research in the social sciences – the limitations of the positivist framing, survey fatigue and over-sampling, and conclude with recent developments, such as internet-based surveys, which have the potential to help overcome some of these issues.

DOING DATA COLLECTION AND ANALYSIS

Survey research is an approach that collects data through sampling from the population and uses statistical analysis to make inferences about the population. As De Vaus (1986: 3) notes: 'The distinguishing features of surveys are the form of data collection and the method of analysis.'

PRACTICE POINT 1

Survey research is an approach that collects data through sampling from the population and uses statistical analysis.

The combination of sampling and inferential statistics in survey research means that it has enduring strengths as an effective way of identifying and examining general patterns in society without having to talk with all, most or even a large percentage of the population. Because of this, survey research is one of the most important approaches in the social sciences. It remains the bedrock of positivistic social science. At the same time, survey research allows for hypothesis-testing through the use of tried and true (if not universally accepted) statistical methods – most notably techniques used to prove/disprove the 'null hypothesis' (see below).

CONCEPTUAL CONCERN 1

Survey research depends on: (1) probability or random sampling and (2) inferential statistics. This combination allows the researcher to infer general patterns in the population on the basis of the sample.

Origins of the approach

Catherine Marsh (2007 [1982]) provides an overview of the history of the survey. She points to the diversity of forms dating from the nineteenth century. The key elements of the approach took decades to come together, in part because the statistical laws at the core of survey sampling and analysis were also under development. Ian Hacking (1990) provides a fantastic account of the rise of statistics from the nineteenth century. Only when this statistical assemblage was in place did it become possible for the modern survey to come together. Marsh argues that the Second World War provided a stimulus in that both the USA and the UK governments used surveys to assess wartime morale among their citizens.

For several decades, the postal survey was the preferred means of delivery (or administration), with face-to-face administration – either by door-knocking or approaching people in public spaces – being the only alternative. As discussed elsewhere, survey fatigue has largely put paid to these methods. In the latter half of the twentieth century telephone interviewing became the most popular means of survey administration, later supplemented by computer programs, in which the interviewer enters responses into a computer program in real time, thus eliminating the need for subsequent data entry. Such software includes options for randomisation of existing electronic sampling frames, and/or automated random telephone dialling. The last two decades have seen the rapid rise of computer-based surveys in a variety of formats, including face-to-face interviews, in which data is entered using a lap-top or PDA, or self-administered surveys, in which the respondent enters data into the computer system, for example by clicking on a link to a website hosting the survey.

As noted by Dillman (1978, 2007), surveys may be administered by interviewers or be self-administered. However, the primary role of interviewers in surveys is recruitment and ensuring completion of the questionnaire. Only limited (if any) interviewing skills are required beyond this. A well-constructed questionnaire is self-explanatory and does not require assistance for completion (see Chapter 2, In-Depth Interviewing).

Hypothesis-testing: from insights to posing questions

Survey research is a variable-centric approach. The researcher begins at a conceptual level with an intuition or problem that can be posed as a relationship between at least two variables. For example, the question 'What is the relationship between Education (a variable) and Income (another variable)?' The researcher might believe that there is a positive relationship between the variables Education and Income: as Education goes up (measured in some way) so does Income (measured in some way). From this start point the researcher has to transform an insight into a hypothesis and then find ways to test it.

CONCEPTUAL CONCERN 2

A hypothesis takes the form that there is a relationship between variables. Changes in the values of a hypothesised independent variable will result in changes in the values of a hypothesised dependent variable. This relationship is called covariance or correlation, depending on the statistical measure.

This process is often called the operationalisation of a hypothesis.

- **Insights have multiple sources**: A researcher begins with an insight about some aspect of the social world. The insight might be an original idea or someone's theory that the researcher wants to test empirically through scientific means. The insight can come from many sources: a response to a social problem, personal experience, or from secondary research – a literature review may have thrown up a theory that deserves further attention (see Chapter 10 on secondary research). Ragin argues that survey research (and other forms of quantitative research) is particularly good at identifying broad patterns in the social world, at making predictions about social change and at testing theory (Ragin, 1994: 32, 33; see also Curtis, 2007). Survey research is typically used to test theories and therefore plays an important but limited role in building theoretical knowledge.

- **Converting an idea into a series of propositions**: The researcher will probably generate more than one hypothesis from an initial idea. Hypotheses take the form of propositions. For example: (1) That higher Levels of Education are associated with higher Levels of Income; (2) That lower Prices of Petrol are associated with greater Usage of Private Transport; (3) That higher levels of Internet Usage are associated with increased Feelings of Isolation. Of course hypotheses can be more complex and can involve additional variables, but the bare bones of any hypothesis is that some changes in one variable will stimulate changes in another (for a further discussion, see Chapter 7 on experimental research).

- **The different roles of variables**: There are three types of variables used in every piece of research (not just survey research): independent, dependent and intervening variables. Independent and dependent variables relate to cause and effect. Every hypothesis must have them. The independent variable is the cause of change. The dependent variable is where changes are observed. For example, a change in the independent variable Levels of Education is hypothesised to cause changes in the dependent variable Levels of Income. But there may well be intervening variables, sometimes called third variables, that mediate between this cause and effect. For example, an intervening variable between Levels of Education and Levels of Income might be Type of Occupation or Gender. Intervening variables can have no effect, or a strengthening effect or a weakening effect on the hypothesised relationship.

- **Developing mutually exclusive and collectively exhaustive values**: The most important guiding principle of this research design is that of being *mutually exclusive and collectively exhaustive* (MECE). The principle is a way of thinking about how data or data sources are organised so as to avoid any gaps and/ or overlaps that will skew the subsequent analysis. The set of values assigned to a variable are mutually exclusive when only one value can be allotted to any aspect of that variable. The set of values are collectively exhaustive when they describe all the pertinent aspects of the variable. For example, for many decades the variable Gender had two values that were mutually exclusive and collectively exhaustive: Man and Woman. Researchers and the academic community in general were satisfied that the use of these two values captured all the possible responses without gaps or overlaps. However, even such fundamental assumptions change and today Gender would need three values (at least) to be considered truly MECE: Man, Woman, Transgendered.

- **Evaluating the variables**: Ensuring that the variables and values are appropriate is crucial. Imagine that you have just obtained the data arising from your survey of 2,000 people and found that the wording of a key question was incorrect. For example, you intended to ask respondents how strongly they agreed with the statements 'Physical discipline is an important part of parenting' and 'Physical discipline should be illegal', but somehow the questions were run together as 'Parenting should be illegal'. For this reason, questionnaires are often discussed in a focus group comprised of people similar to your intended sample (e.g., parents of small children), to tease out potential problems such as what 'physical discipline' actually means – do the participants have the same understanding as you, or should you rephrase it or include a definition? Pilot surveys are very common, for similar reasons. They provide an opportunity to pick up errors such as poorly worded questions, missing questions and values that are not mutually exclusive and collectively exhaustive.

CONCEPTUAL CONCERN 3

Survey research is a variable-centric approach. There are few variables and many cases. The researcher begins with a problem or an intuition or some secondary research that focuses on some variables or sets of variables. Like most variable-centric approaches, survey research engages in hypothesis-testing.

Attributes, attitudes and behaviour

These are the three main types of surveys:

- **Attributes** describe elements of cases that are considered most important by the researcher. For example, most surveys collect attributional data about age, ethnicity and gender. Other attributional data includes: income, occupation, marital status, location, health status and educational attainment. These attributes are collected and then analysed as potential intervening variables. For example, in the hypothesis above, an intervening variable between Levels of Education and Levels of Income might be Type of Occupation or Gender.

- **Attitudes** are based on perceptions of respondents. Attitudinal surveys are probably the most common variant of the survey approach, especially if we include surveys commissioned by governmental agencies and business. They are the bread and butter of market research. Attitudes are considered important for two reasons. First, because they are seen as shaping, prefiguring or anticipating behaviour. Today's attitudes are commonly regarded as tomorrow's behaviour. For example, the surveys that purport to show how voters will vote on election day are attitudinal surveys. Second, attitudes are important to researchers and persons who commission surveys because attitudes are regarded as changeable. Much of attitudinal surveying is about testing the impact of government programmes, education, social and commercial marketing campaigns.

- **Behaviour** is the measure of what respondents do. Measuring behaviour through a questionnaire has two possible shortcomings. First, respondents assess their behaviour either through recall of previous events or extrapolation into future endeavours. Clearly, neither recall nor speculation are necessarily accurate. Second, Webb and colleagues (1966) suggest that interactive research, including survey research, introduces a 'foreign' or extraneous element into social relations (see Chapter 8 on unobtrusive research). Webb et al. stressed that what respondents say that they do may differ greatly to what they actually do!

Sample size and margin of error

Most survey research focuses on individuals as cases. It is worth noting that survey research can have cases other than individual respondents. For example, research about the provision of healthcare for the elderly could be organised around the comparison of healthcare facilities or perhaps the businesses that own and operate them. This means that a questionnaire might be completed for each case (healthcare facility or business) from the responses of many individuals – perhaps including managers, employees and residents.

Survey research is based on drawing (or selecting) a sample from a population. The population is made up of all the possible cases that could be covered in the survey. It is very rare for populations to be surveyed in their entirety, mainly because of the practical constraints involved in getting full coverage. The only entire surveys of general populations are the censuses that most stable governments conduct on a regular basis. These are extremely expensive to run, are typically made mandatory, with potential prison terms for non-compliance, and even then don't get 100% coverage. There seems to be increasing resistance on the part of some people in English-speaking countries in completing censuses and in subverting the process. For example, up to 1.5% of respondents in recent British, Australian and New Zealand censuses indicated that their religion was that of 'Jedi knight'. This sort of joking and subversion is probably part of a broader dislike of surveys which is increasingly affecting the approaches of academics, governments and market researchers. Dillman (1999) optimistically focuses on the rise of 'self-administered' surveys as the way forward for the approach, when increasing numbers of potential respondents don't have time to talk to an interviewer face-to-face or over the phone. We will return to the issue of survey fatigue below.

Sampling from a population comes in two main forms: a non-probability sample (cluster, quota or convenience sampling) or a probability sample (simple random sampling, systematic sampling, stratified sampling). The key difference between a non-probability and probability sample is that in the latter all potential participating cases have an equal chance of being selected. The randomness of probability sampling makes it the better option because it allows the use of more powerful statistical analysis, called inferential statistics. Inferential statistics let a researcher infer (or deduce) about the population from analysis of the sample. In contrast, a non-probability sample (where the individuals/cases are not picked at random) is a far weaker data set. A non-probability sample can only be analysed using descriptive statistics, which describe the features and patterns of the sample only. In other words, a non-probability sample does not allow the researcher to talk about the population, or at least not with much rigour. When researchers use non-probability samples to discuss populations they have to use moderating, limiting statements like 'indicative' or 'suggestive', etc.

PRACTICE POINT 2

Descriptive statistics are used to describe the features of the data in a sample. But descriptive statistics cannot move beyond describing the sample. They do not allow inferences about the population. *Inferential statistics* transcend descriptive statistics. These statistics allow analysis of sample data that can infer measures and patterns in the population. The underlying rationale of survey research is to conduct inferential statistics.

A reasonable-sized random sample will closely resemble the population and this provides the basis of inference or deduction. Researchers and statisticians are interested in the relationship between sample size and sampling error. Statisticians have proven a positive correlation between larger sample size and greater sampling accuracy (less sampling error). This seems pretty logical: the bigger the random sample, the more likely it is to reflect the population. The relationship between sample size and sampling error is a standardised model and is near universally accepted by researchers (and funders and peer reviewers). Statisticians regard the calculation of sample size and sampling error as straightforward; many social scientists might find it a bit more challenging and we'll just review the main concepts and leave out the formulae. Like all statistical operations it makes a series of simplifying assumptions about social reality. The main points are:

1. Calculating the relationship between sample size and sampling error involves decisions about margin of error, confidence level, the binary nature of variables, and expectations about responses in the population.

2. The relationship between sample size and sampling error is measured in terms of margin of error. The margin of error is a percentage plus or minus around the results from a sample. For example, if 76% of 500 respondents answer 'the Democratic Party' to the survey question 'What Political Party are you voting for in the Election?', this will have a margin of error of (+/−) 4%. This means that the percentage of the population that would do the same range from 72% (76% − 4%) to 80% (76% + 4%). The larger the sample, the lower the margin of error (the greater the accuracy).

3. Margins of error are always calculated in terms of confidence levels. A 95% confidence level means that we have that level of confidence the margin of error will capture what we infer from the sample to the population. For example,

we are 95% confident that 72%–80% of the population will vote for the Democratic Party. Most surveys operate at a 95% confidence level. Sometimes a 99% confidence level is required. The higher the required confidence level, the greater is the sample size for any given margin of error.

4. Margins of error are calculated for questions/variables that are assumed to have binary values (there are only two possible responses). For example, the data for the variable 'Voting Preference' might be collected by asking the question 'What Political Party are you voting for in the Election?' Binary values for this variable might be (1) Democratic Party, (2) Republican Party.

5. Expectations about responses in the population also feature in the calculation of margin of error. This is relatively straightforward in that when we calculate margins of error we need larger samples the more the answers to questions are split 50%/50%. Where there is a clear preference, the sample size can be smaller. So a question where 95% of the respondents say they will vote for the Democratic Party needs a sample size of 1,900 for a 1% margin of error (at the 95% confidence level). If the response was 50% we would need a sample size of 10,000. The norm is for margins of errors to be calculated with an expected response rate of 50%/50%.

Table 6.1 shows the relationship between survey sample size and the margin of error. It assumes a 95% level of confidence and that the expected responses are split 50%/50%.

Sampling frames

Probability sampling is better than non-probability sampling but is usually more expensive and more difficult to do. The first hurdle is that probability sampling

TABLE 6.1   The relationship between sample size and margin of error

Survey sample size	Margin of error (plus or minus percent)
2,000	(+/–) 2%
1,500	(+/–) 3%
1,000	(+/–) 3%
900	(+/–) 3%
800	(+/–) 3%
700	(+/–) 4%
600	(+/–) 4%
500	(+/–) 4%
400	(+/–) 5%
300	(+/–) 6%
200	(+/–) 7%
100	(+/–) 10%
50	(+/–) 14%

requires a sampling frame. Probability sampling (random sampling) is only possible when the researcher has access to a sampling frame.

A sampling frame is a list of all the cases in a population. The two most used sampling frames are the telephone white-pages and electoral rolls. These documents have for at least fifty years been the first port of call for researchers contemplating a survey of the general population (e.g., the entire adult population). However, both are becoming less useful as they become less comprehensive because: (1) fewer people in the developed countries have landline telephones (instead opting for mobile phones, for which there are no directories) and (2) fewer people enrol to vote).

Sampling frames are a prerequisite for all efforts at probability sampling, not just for samples of the general population. Often the most difficult task in implementing a probability survey is finding or creating the sampling frame (a list of all possible cases/respondents). Certainly, creating a sampling frame can raise ethical issues and confidentiality issues. Most countries have strict rules covering the dissemination of personal data, and organisations may not give information to a third party. This means that researchers looking to construct a sampling frame for mental health patients will in all likelihood be out of luck if they write to their local hospital and ask for a list. Researchers interested in psychology students or speeding motorists will be similarly rebuffed by the student records at their local university or the criminal court. Often government-sponsored research will have access to databases and sampling frames that independent researchers simply cannot access.

Survey research is absolutely defined by this reliance on a sampling frame, although readers of survey textbooks get very little advice on the subject. The two leading textbook authors and editors we refer to most in this chapter say little more than 'Obtain a complete sampling frame' (De Vaus, 1986: 53) and provide a definition (Dillman, 2007: 196). However, Leslie Kish (1910–2000), one of the earliest textbook writers on survey methodology, notes:

> The [sampling] frame is perfect if every element [case] appears on the list separately, once, only once, and nothing else appears on the list. … But perfect frames are rare, and we must often use frames with serious deficiencies that must be detected and remedied. Before undertaking a selection, the sampler must probe thoroughly for possible faults in the frame. He can discover some faults by skilful questioning of persons with specialized knowledge of the lists. Other faults may have to be found by empirical investigations. Recognizing the faults may permit dealing with them adequately, economically, and practically. (Kish, 1965: 53, 54)

Kish (1965: 384–439) goes on to dedicate a chapter to 'Sampling from imperfect frames'. This is a rigorous account of the statistical steps required in the combination of different sampling frames. It provides an extremely challenging read for emergent researchers in the social sciences. Kish also identifies likely problems with sampling frames in a non-statistical manner. He applies the principle of being *mutually exclusive and collectively exhaustive,* which we discussed above in terms of assigning values to variables. Kish (1965: 54) noted that there are four types of errors that make sampling frames imperfect:

1. **Missing cases**: Some of the cases in the population are not in the frame.

2. **Duplicate cases**: Some of the cases in the population are repeated in the frame.

3. **Clustered cases**: Some of the cases in the population appear in the frame as clusters or groups.

4. **Foreign cases**: Some of the cases in the frame are not from the population.

Response rates

In the scholarly use of survey research the response rate is the number of respondents (either people who were interviewed or who completed self-administered questionnaires) divided by the number of people in the sample. If the sample was a random selection of 1,000 households in a neighbourhood, using face-to-face interviewing and a lot of door knocking, and the result was 100 completed questionnaires, then the response rate is 100/1,000 = 10%. Response rates are considered important because it is assumed (but not proven) that higher response rates are indicative of better, less biased surveys.

Most organisations that commission survey research will set minimum acceptable response rates. This is a problematic measure of quality and encourages a lot of fudging. For example, commercial researchers often inflate their response rates by calculating it as the number of completed questionnaires divided by the number of requests. In our door-knocking example above, all those households where no one was home would be excluded from the calculation. The result is a higher 'response rate'. For example, say 500 people were not at home or did not open the door to our researcher(s). The response rate would be 100/(1,000–500) = 20%. This sort of fudging is bad social science.

The actual margin of error has to be calculated on the actual number of people who completed a questionnaire and not on the number of responses a researcher hoped to get in sampling. At the same time, response rates are a very poor measure of quality because they do not take into account the difficultly of accessing respondents. Of course sometimes a researcher is engaged in a survey that is likely to gain low response rates. This needs to be recognised when designing the research, especially when allocating time and other resources to meeting the desired sample sizes. We will return to this issue later in our discussion of survey fatigue and the dilemmas of over-sampling. More specifically, Dillman (2007: 9–31) talks about ways in which surveys and questionnaires can be designed and delivered to improve response rates. This doesn't address the issues of accessing respondents but shows that a sensitivity to establishing trust, increasing the social and psychological rewards of completing a survey and reducing the costs of doing so will improve response rates. The most important aspects of his discussion are shown in Table 6.2.

TABLE 6.2   Techniques to improve response rates

Establishing trust in the survey	Increasing social and psychological rewards of completing survey	Reducing social and psychological costs of completing survey
Secure a credible, institutional sponsor for the research	Say thank you	Minimise authoritarian language
Provide tokens of appreciation (gifts)	Seek advice in improving the survey	Minimise embarrassing and personal questions
Emphasise the importance or public good of the survey	Make the questionnaire a reasonable length (not too long or too short)	Minimise the length of the questionnaire
Link the survey with popular institutions/ initiatives	Make the questionnaire attractive and vary the format of the questions	Emphasise the similarity to other requests

Sampling strategies

Deciding what sort of sample should be used is called the sampling strategy. We start with probability sampling:

- **Simple random sampling (SRS)** is the most straightforward approach. It entails the random selection of a sample from a complete sampling frame. Drawing names or numbers from a hat can work, but when the population or sample is large it is more convenient to use some sort of random number generator and to reorder the sampling frame as a numeric list. Today, an online random number generator is only a few keystrokes away. The key is that this sampling strategy must give every case an equal chance of selection. This is the overriding criteria for all probability sampling. SRS works best when the researcher has full confidence that the sampling frame is complete. This approach can be disastrous if there are gaps or overlaps in the sampling frame. It also begs the question about calling something a probability sample when it is suspected that the sample frame is incomplete, as in the approaches below.

- **Systematic sampling** is often used instead of SRS. SRS uses random numbers to pick a sample from the frame or list. Systematic sampling adopts the opposite approach. The sample size is divided by the population size and this sample fraction produces an *n*th number for selection. For example, if the desired sample is 1,000 and the population size is 10,000 then every tenth case in the sample frame will be selected. SRS runs the risk of double sampling or missing respondents where there are gaps or overlaps in the sampling frame precisely because of the randomness of selection. Systematic sampling doesn't face this problem because it selects every nth case from the frame. However, systematic sampling does face the problem of periodicity. This occurs if there is a pattern in the sampling frame. For example, a list of mortgage holders with a bank will have many married couples and it is the cultural norm in English-speaking societies to enter the man's name first. This means that any odd numbered sample fraction/nth case selection is likely to pick up more men than women and the opposite holds for even ones. So while systematic sampling may be preferred if there are some doubts about the completeness of the sampling frame, it is essential when using this strategy that the frame itself has been fully randomised (mixed up).

- **Stratified sampling** is based in further modifications to the sampling frame. Stratified sampling is used to help ensure that the sample matches the population if there is some concern about the completeness of the sampling frame. These strata have to represent the real divisions in the population. For example, in the case of mortgage holders, the sampling frame would be stratified/divided into two: a list of male mortgage holders and a list of female ones. The sample would then be drawn separately from each strata in proportion to the gender balance in the population. This means that if 60% of all mortgage holders were male, then 60% of the sample would be drawn from this strata, this subdivision of the frame. When drawing a sample from a stratified frame, researchers can use either SRS or systematic sampling depending on their assessment of completeness.

To recap: (1) SRS relies on random numbers for probability sampling where the frame is left untouched; (2) systematic sampling requires the randomisation of the sampling frame; and (3) stratified sampling requires the subdivision of the sampling frame into strata.

PRACTICE POINT 3

If you have a complete sampling frame or something near enough to it to be plausible, then do probability sampling. Only this method allows inferential statistics.

Non-probability sampling two main forms:

- **Quota sampling** is a strategy that can be used when the researcher has a good description of a population but no actual sampling frame. Quota sampling tries to capture the benefits of stratified sampling in getting a reasonable spread or representation in the sample. For example, a researcher might have a lot of information about the attributes of students doing Social Sciences 101 at their university but not at the level that would allow probability sampling. The researcher might know that there are 100 students enrolled and that 60% of them are female. Quota sampling would therefore aim for 60% female respondents. This would mean that across one important dimension at least the non-probability sample would be indicative of the population. If the researcher had more information about the percentages of students that were new or returning, or their ethnicity, or in fact any dimension/attribute, then this could be factored in to make the quotas more fine-grained and more likely to be representative of the population. Despite its sophistication, quota sampling doesn't constitute probability sampling and the research can only use descriptive statistics that are indicative or suggestive. This is because without a sampling frame all potential participating cases cannot have an equal chance of being selected in the sample.

- **Convenience sampling** is the worst sampling strategy. Whereas quota sampling attempts to get some representativeness in its sampling, convenience sampling does not. Sometimes it is called accidental or availability sampling. Interviewing the first 10 compliant people you meet is a form of convenience sampling. So are most forms of self-complete surveys. De Vaus (1986: 69) notes these are 'common but must be used with caution and only for specific purposes, and are the least likely of any technique to produce representative samples. Using this approach anyone who will respond will do.' He goes on to note that convenience sampling is often used for pilot surveys, which are preliminary surveys undertaken to test whether a survey questionnaire has been properly designed.

Scales of measurement

In 1946, Stanley Smith Stevens (1906–73) puplished 'On the theory of scales of measurement' (Stevens, 1946). The article argued that data can be judged against four different scales in terms of their accuracy in representing the world (both physical and social) and, in particular, how useful they are for statistical analysis. The scales of measurement are nominal, ordinal, interval and ratio. The first three scales are relevant for the social sciences. The ratio scale requires precise and certain data and it is not feasible to collect such data in the social sciences.

The strength of data – nominal, ordinal, interval and ratio – refers to the relationship between variables and values. Variables are conceptualised as ways of capturing what is interesting about cases. Variables are made measurable by the assignment of values. The scales of measurement refer to how variables and values can be assessed for statistical purposes. The key assessments are:

1. Are there differences between variables?

2. Can the values associated with the variable be ranked?

TABLE 6.3   Scales of measurement

	Nominal	Ordinal	Interval	Ratio
Are there differences between variables?	Yes	Yes	Yes	Yes
Can the values associated with the variable be ranked?	No	Yes	Yes	Yes
Can the intervals between ranked values be determined?	No	No	Yes	Yes
Does the scale have a true zero point?	No	No	No	Yes

3. Can the differences or intervals between such ranked values be determined?

4. Does the scale along which values are ranked have a true zero point? (see Table 6.3).

Nominal data is the weakest type because the values assigned to variables cannot be ranked or ordered or scored. Stevens (1946: 678) noted: 'The nominal scale represents the most unrestricted assignment of numerals. The numerals are used only as labels or type numbers, and words or letters would serve as well.' Stevens uses the term 'numerals' for what we describe as 'values'. For example, Gender is a common nominal variable with the values Man, Woman, Transgendered. Typically, the values associated with Gender cannot be ranked (but not always, see below).

Ordinal data is stronger because its associated values can be ranked. Ordinal variables appear in most surveys. For example, one online website that asks students to 'Rate My Professor' (using a non-probability form of convenience sampling, we should add) has the variable Helpfulness. Students are asked to tick one of five boxes for associated values that range from Useless to Extremely Helpful. Therefore these values can be ranked (e.g., Useless, Not Much Use, So-So, Helpful, Extremely Helpful). However, we cannot determine if the interval/difference between Useless and Not Much Use is less, the same, or greater than the distance between Not Much Use and So-So.

Interval data is stronger still because its values can be ranked and the intervals between them can be determined. For example, Years Attending School might be an example of interval data, perhaps with values ranging from '5 Years' to '15 Years'. Levels of Income, and Hours Accessing the Internet per Week are other examples of interval data. Each of these related variables can be associated with values that have defined or determined intervals. As a result, we can tell that someone who has 15 years of attending school has been there three times longer than someone with 5 years of attending school. Stevens

TABLE 6.4 Type of data and appropriate statistical analysis

Type of data	Type of statistical analysis
Nominal	mode, chi square
Ordinal	mode, chi square, median, percentile
Interval	mode, chi square, median, percentile, mean, standard deviation, correlation, regression, analysis of variance

(1946: 679) said: 'With the interval scale we come to a form that is "quantitative" in the ordinary sense of the word. Almost all the usual statistical measures are applicable here, unless they are kinds that imply a knowledge of a "true" zero point.' The issue of a zero point in the scale is too technical for this textbook. Many social science textbooks don't bother with a distinction between interval and ratio scales/data.

The differing data types in terms of scales of measurement allows for differing levels of statistical analysis. As noted, we won't discuss statistical analysis in any detail (see below for further reading suggestions). The relationship between type of data and the type of statistical analysis that can be used is simple – the stronger the data type, the fuller the range of statistics (see Table 6.4).

Statistical analysis: hypothesis-testing and the null hypothesis

Survey research allows for hypothesis-testing through statistical methods. There is an enormous range of these and we will mention only the most basic.

Much of the time hypothesis-testing using statistical analysis actually centres on disproving or proving the 'null hypothesis'. The null hypothesis is that there is no relationship or covariance between variables. Changes in the values of a hypothesised independent variable will result in no changes in the values of a hypothesised dependent variable. The concept of the null hypothesis acts like a 'double negative'. This is because statistical analysis generally can't prove that something 'is', but it can prove that something 'isn't'. If the null hypothesis is proved, then there is no covariance between variables. If the null hypothesis is disproved, then there is covariance between the variables – or, more precisely, a covariance that can't be accounted for by the operation of chance.

CONCEPTUAL CONCERN 4

Survey research relies on statistical analysis for hypothesis-testing. Much of this testing centres on disproving the 'null hypothesis'.

TABLE 6.5 Cross-tabulation: Income by education

	Low level of Education	Middle level of Education	High level of Education	Total
Low level of Income	95 (60)	65 (60)	20 (60)	180 (60%)
High level of Income	5 (40)	35 (40)	80 (40)	120 (40%)
Total	100	100	100	300 (100%)

Covariance can be measured by the comparison between what we would expect if the null hypothesis was proved (i.e., no relationship between variables) and by what is observed. The most popular way of showing differences in expected and observed results is a cross-tabulation. For example, imagine we were testing the hypothesis that there is a positive relationship between the independent variable Education and the dependent variable Income: as Education goes up (measured in some way) so does Income (measured in some way). The values we assigned to Education are: 'Low level of Education', 'Middle level of Education', 'High level of Education'. The values we assigned to Income are 'Low level of Income' and 'High level of Income'. Imagine we surveyed 300 people and the results are cross-tabulated, as shown in Table 6.5.

Each cell in the cross-tabulation has two numbers. The top number is the observed results. Thus, 95 people had a 'Low level of Education' and a 'Low level of Income'. The bottom number in that cell (in brackets) is (60). This is the number of people we expected to be in that cell if there was no covariance, i.e., if there was no relationship between Education and Income. The number is calculated by distributing all the people with a 'Low level of Income' evenly across the three values that measure levels of education.

Looking at the cross-tabulation suggests that there seems to be some sort of covariance. All of the cells have differences between observed and expected results. Furthermore, the patterning of differences suggest a covariance. In the cells 'Low level of Education'/'Low level of Income' and 'High level of Education'/'High level of Income' the observed results greatly exceed the expected results. Conversely, in the cells 'Low level of Education'/'High level of Income' and 'High level of Education'/'Low level of Income' the pattern is reversed. This is indicative of a linear relationship between the variables.

The differences in the cross-tabulations can be calculated by the chi-squared formula $X^2 = \sum (O\text{-}E)^2 / E$. This means that chi-squared is the sum of all the differences in all the cells of the cross-tabulation. The differences are squared as otherwise all the pluses and minuses would cancel themselves out. The score for the cross-tabulation is:

TABLE 6.6 Degrees of freedom and *p* values

Degrees of freedom	p value = 0.05 (5%)	p value = 0.01 (1%)
1	3.84	6.64
2	5.99	9.21
3	7.82	11.35
4	9.49	13.28
5	11.07	15.09
6	12.59	16.81
7	14.07	18.48
8	15.51	20.09
9	16.92	21.67
10	18.31	23.21

$X^2 = \Sigma \ ((95–60)^2 / 60) + ((65–60)^2 / 60) + ((20–60)^2 / 60) + ((5–40)^2 / 40) + ((35–40)^2 / 40) + ((80–40)^2 / 40) = 118.77.$

The larger the score for the chi-squared formula, the greater the covariance. Chi-squared results can also be used in terms of disproving the null hypothesis. A chi-squared table shows the score needed for cross-tabulations of various sizes to be able to disprove the null hypothesis (Table 6.6).

Degrees of freedom refers to the size of the cross-tabulation. The degree of freedom is one less than the number of cells. *P* value refers to the probability that the result is the product of chance or that the null hypothesis was proved (i.e., there is no relationship between the variables). The two main *p* values or levels of significance are 5% and 1%. Levels of significance at 1% require higher chi-squared scores than at 5%. *P* values and significance are analogous to confidence.

Our Income by Education cross-tabulation had six cells = five degrees of freedom. At the 1% level of significance we require a chi-squared score of 15.09 or higher to disprove the null hypothesis. Our score was 118.77, so we can say that the null hypothesis is disproven with 99% confidence and that the covariance exists between the independent variable Education and the dependent variable Income.

SOME ISSUES IN RESEARCH

In this section, our discussion of epistemology includes the importance of good questioning, relating this to the epistemological reasoning that frames survey research.

Epistemology and scales of measurement

Good questioning can transform some aspects of nominal data into ordinal and even interval data. This potential reflects that survey research is an interactive approach. Interaction between researcher and respondent creates data at its point of collection. Survey research is not alone in this. For example, in-depth interviewing (Chapter 2), ethnographic research (Chapter 4) and other approaches create situations, encounters and pose questions that would not otherwise exist in the social world (for a longer discussion about interactive research see Chapter 10 on secondary research).

PRACTICE POINT 4

Good questioning can transform some aspects of nominal data into ordinal and even interval data.

There are several epistemological issues around question design and scales of measurement. Epistemology is the theory of knowledge that informs how research is shaped in its broadest sense (see Chapter 1). The three main epistemological positions are positivism, social realism and social constructivism. Positivists have the greatest confidence in the ability of social scientists to reveal the truth. They stress the techniques of observation and measurement and the potential for scientists to form objective/unbiased understandings of the social world. Positivists downplay the uncertainties that other epistemologies raise about the impact of power, meaning and culture on doing science (some common social realist critiques) or more radical concerns about the logical impossibility of developing an objective scientific stance (the social constructivist critique of 'science').

Hopefully, none of the readers of this chapter will be surprised that the champions of survey research are positivists and, to a lesser extent, social realists. Positivists and social realists feel that a properly designed and implemented survey can reveal the social world. In contrast, social constructivists feel that a survey is more likely to construct aspects of the social world that are unique to the interaction between researcher and respondent. This means that social constructivists see the question-and-answer interactions of survey research (either interview-based or self-administered questionnaires – see Dillman, 1978, 2007) as generating results that cannot be generalised beyond that particular encounter. Positivists and social realists see such interaction as essential to revealing general patterns. For positivists, this is a fairly straightforward process and issues like validity and reliability are treated as merely technical components of statistical analysis. For social realists, survey research is more fraught in that they also query the objective status of statistical analysis.

CONCEPTUAL CONCERN 5

Survey research is unproblematic for positivist scholars. Textbooks about survey research are inevitably written from a positivist epistemology. This is an all-pervasive approach among the champions of sampling and statistics but is hardly ever made apparent. Emergent researchers should remember that research in the social world may not be as certain as most textbook writers suggest.

Question formats

Researchers who are interested in survey research as a way of finding out about the world agree on the centrality of good questions. Thus Gender is a common nominal variable with the values Man, Woman, Transgendered. The values directly associated with Gender cannot be ranked. But, some of the attributes, attitudes and behaviour indirectly associated with Gender can be. For example, respondents can be asked to express an opinion about some facet of Gender, and this question can be couched in ordinal terms. Generating interval data from nominal material like Gender is more problematic. There are four main positions on how to do this:

1. **The assignment of arbitrary interval values**: The most straightforward but least rigorous approach is to simply ask the monotonic or bipolar scale questions as if they were interval data. For example, respondents could be asked 'Please indicate your level of agreement with the following statement: Where on a scale of 1 to 5, where 1 equals "Do not agree", 2 equals "Very weakly agree", 3 equals "Weakly agree", 4 equals "Strongly agree", and 5 equals "Very strongly agree"....'

2. **The assignment of referent interval values**: Interval values can be assigned with reference to pre-existing, agreed-upon values. For example, if other surveys have asked a question previously, it can be acceptable to use their question format and assigned values. Obviously, in order to implement this approach the researcher has to have access to other reputable surveys.

3. **The assignment of combined interval values**: Interval values can be achieved by adding results across several similar questions. For example, respondents can be asked to rate agreement/disagreement (using Likert questions) to statements about how they 'approved', 'liked', 'enjoyed' and were 'satisfied' about something. Each individual question would then produce data on the ordinal scale, but if we combined the results for approved, liked, enjoyed and satisfied, we can generate interval data about a new, broader variable which we might label 'orientation'.

4. **The assignment of statistically confirmed intervals:** The approach to generating interval data that is considered most rigorous relies on subjecting the responses to ordinal questions to further statistical analysis. This analysis can involve regression or factor analysis. Perhaps the most straightforward approach is to take all the responses from a Likert question format in which Strongly disagree $= -2$, Disagree $= -1$, Neither agree nor disagree $= 0$, Agree $= 1$, Strongly agree $= 2$, and calculate an overall average. For example, say 100 respondents answered accordingly: $((20 \times -2) + (10 \times -1) + (10 \times 0) + (20 \times 1) + (40 \times 2))/100 =$ an average of 0.5. The variation of individual responses to the average in the overall sample can then be assessed in terms of interval data.

PUTTING THE APPROACH IN CONTEXT

Survey research epitomises a variable-centric, variable-first approach and is undoubtedly a form of hypothesis-testing. The researcher starts with a combination of relatively few variables and seeks a sufficient number of cases to test an argument. Like most of these approaches, survey research is more fixed than fluid in its framing of research. The process of research is sequential and there is little chance to move between data collection and analysis in order to improve on the hypothesis being tested or to rewrite questions after data collection has begun. This combination of hypothesis-testing, fixed framing, focus on quantitative research and reliance on statistical analysis has been the dominant form of social science for half a century, especially for sociologists interested in contemporary society (Savage and Burrows, 2007). It has played a (perhaps, the) major role in the quantification of research, by which we mean the representation of the world through numbers and statistics.

PRACTICE POINT 5

Survey research is fixed in its framing. In particular, once data collection has begun it is problematic, if not impossible, to change or add variables or values. For this reason, surveys are often evaluated by a focus group of field-tested with a pilot survey.

Oakley (1998) harks back to a time of the 'science wars' when positivist and quantitative research was criticised by feminists, radicals and a host of other non-positivists (social constructivists and social realists in our terminology). Survey research and other mainly positivist approaches (experimental research, content research, etc.) weathered this attack. In so far as the positivist stranglehold over the social sciences was loosened, allowing the proliferation of new approaches (semiotic analysis, autoethnography, etc.), no one seems to have told positivist researchers they lost the science wars. Survey research is very similar to content research (see Chapter 9) in that its champions, and certainly the authors of the leading textbooks, have very little to say about epistemology. These outright positivists are secure in their belief in the utility of survey research. Hence issues about reliability and validity are treated as technical issues within a statistical framework.

Oakley (1998, original italics) notes how the feminist critique of quantitative research in the 1960s and 1970s focused on 'The Three Ps: the case against *positivism*, the case against *power*, the case against *p values*'. Survey research combines all three. To recap:

1. **The case against *positivism***: Oakley (1998: 710) argues that positivist claims to objectivity, lack of bias and rules of inference are all considered problematic by non-positivists.

2. **The case against *power***: Similarly, Oakley (1998: 710–11) argues that positivist claims to objectivity and science assume a hierarchy of knowledge in which the knowledge of the researcher is privileged over the researched. Respondents, participants, samples and populations are reduced to objects of study.

3. **The case against *p* values**: This refers to the reduction of issues of reliability and validity to statistical measures of probability, significance, null hypotheses, etc. (see above for our passing discussion of statistical analysis). At the same time, it is a rejection that people and social relations can be properly represented by numbers. For example, 'Feminist qualitative researchers argue that the *p*s they are interested in do not concern the probabilistic logic of statistical *p* values, but the value of *people*, and this can only be deduced by construction a qualitative knowledge about them' (Oakley, 1998, original italics).

Survey fatigue and over-sampling

Survey fatigue is a problem confronting survey research. Most readers of this book will have been on the receiving end of a survey, probably via the telephone and often when engaged in eating the evening meal. This overuse of the survey creates survey fatigue – the population becomes less and less willing to participate. Such overuse of the survey was anticipated more than a century ago by one of psychology's founding fathers, William James:

> Messrs. Darwin and Galton have set the example of circulars of questions sent out by the hundreds to those supposed able to reply. The custom has spread, and it will be well for us in the next generation if such circulars be not ranked among the common pests of life. (James, 1890: 144)

The more surveys are considered a pest, the more difficult it is to properly conduct them. Increasingly, the institutions that commission survey research are stipulating minimum response rates and requiring the over-sampling of problematic sub-populations. These problematic sub-populations include the poor, the young, the highly mobile, recent migrants, ethnic minorities, the religious, etc. Over-sampling is extra-sampling. It requires stratified sampling (see above) and an effort to collect data from a subdivision of the sampling frame over and above that required for the overall sample. Over-sampling introduces a deliberate bias into probability sampling in an effort to improve response rates. It also requires quite sophisticated statistical analysis to retain the random or probability component.

PRACTICE POINT 6

Over-sampling introduces a deliberate bias into probability sampling in an effort to improve response rates.

Over-sampling also contributes to the problem it is trying to solve, in that declining response rates indicate that elements of the population, potential respondents, feel that they have already been 'over-sampled'. Indeed, this dilemma in over-sampling is actually a variant of what Hardin (1968) called 'The tragedy of the commons', in which the self-interest of individual actors combine to destroy a collective resource. In survey research, the commons or collective resource is the willingness of the population to respond positively to surveys.

CONCLUSION

Survey research is an approach that collects data through sampling from the population and uses statistical analysis to make inferences about that population. Survey research is a variable-centric approach; there are relatively few variables (questions) and many cases (people, respondents). The postal survey was the preferred means of delivery for some decades, although survey fatigue has largely put an end to that means of data collection. Telephone interviewing then became the most popular means of survey administration, later supplemented by computer programs, during which the interviewer enters the respondent's answers into the analysis software as the respondent gives them. In the last decade or so, self-administered surveys, in which the respondent enters data into the computer system, for example by clicking on a link to a website hosting the survey, have become popular (with researchers, if not with the public).

Like most variable-centric approaches, survey research engages in hypothesis-testing. Sample size and composition is crucial to the success of the survey. The sample should closely resemble the population the researcher seeks to describe. The randomness of probability sampling makes it the better option because it allows the use of more powerful statistical analysis, called inferential statistics.

The appropriateness of the variables (questions) and values (response options) is also crucial to produce useful data. For this reason, questionnaires are almost always tested with a focus group (see Chapter 5) and/or a pilot survey.

Savage and Burrows (2007) have a gloomy prognosis for survey research. For them, the approach has had its day as a foundation for social sciences:

> However, the sample survey is not a tool that stands 'outside history'. Its glory years, we contend, are in the past. One difficulty is that in an intensely researched environment, response rates have been steadily falling, and it is proving more difficult to obtain response rates of 80 per cent or more, which were once thought normal. People no longer treat it as an honour to be asked their opinion, but instead see it as a nuisance, or even an intrusion. These problems are, however, not overwhelming because survey statisticians have developed methods for estimating the attributes of 'the missing', and it still remains possible to generalize on the basis of biased samples. A second problem concerns the way that surveys rely for their sampling frame on the empty homogeneous space defined by national boundaries. The survey emerged as a key device for imagining the nation, and in a global era of mass migration, this also marks a serious limit. ... A third telling issue is the proliferation of survey research in private companies, especially in areas of market research. Such survey research now has very limited reference to academic expertise. (Savage and Burrows, 2007: 890)

This stands in stark contrast to the optimism of textbook writers and, specifically, those like Dillman, who see a bright new future for survey research. Dillman (1978, 1999, 2007) is optimistic that new technologies – arguably wireless technologies allowing access to the internet and the networking of personal digital assistants – will counter survey fatigue associated with the traditional mechanisms for delivering questionnaires, i.e., face-to-face, by mail and by telephone. There is no doubt that the internet and wireless technologies provide a fillip for survey research. Furthermore, probability sampling and statistical analysis allowing inferences about a population remains a parsimonious, cost-effective way of doing research. It is a remarkably cost-effective way of exploring general patterns in society, and should be included in the skill-set of all emergent researchers.

FURTHER READINGS

Dillman is undoubtedly the leading expert on self-administered questionnaires and his textbooks are essential for researchers contemplating mail, telephone or internet surveys (Dillman, 1978, 2007).

De Vaus's multi-edition textbook (we use the 1986 version because we bought it as undergraduates) is probably the best on survey research. It combines a comprehensive how-to-do and a great overview of statistical analysis.

De Vaus also edits the four volume set on *Social Surveys 2* (2007). This is a great reference work for researchers who need more depth on survey research.

REFERENCES

Curtis, B. 2007. Doing research. In: Matthewman, S., West-Newman, C. L. & Curtis, B. (eds.), *Being sociological*. London: Palgrave Macmillan.

De vaus, D. A. 1986. *Surveys in social research*. London: Allen and Unwin.

De vaus, D. A. 2007. *Social surveys 2*. London: Sage.

Dillman, D. A. 1978. *Mail and telephone surveys: The total design method*. New York: Wiley.

Dillman, D. A. 1999. Mail and other self-administered surveys in the 21st century: The beginning of a new era. *The Gallup Research Journal*, Winter/Spring, 121–140.

Dillman, D. A. 2007. *Mail and internet surveys: The tailored design method: With new internet, visual, and mixed-mode guide*. New York: Wiley.

Hacking, I. 1990. *The taming of chance*. Cambridge: Cambridge University Press.

Hardin, G. 1968. The tragedy of the commons. *Science*, 162, 1243–1248.

James, W. 1890. *The principles of psychology*. New York: Holt.

Kish, L. 1965. *Survey sampling*. New York: Wiley.

Marsh, C. 2007 [1982]. History of the use of surveys in sociological research. In: De Vaus, D. A. (ed.), *Social surveys 2*. London: Sage.

Oakley, A. 1998. Gender, methodology and people's ways of knowing: Some problems with feminism and the paradigm debate in social science. *Sociology*, 32, 707–731.

Ragin, C. 1994. *Constructing social research: The unity and diversity of method*. Thousand Oaks, CA: Pine Forge Press.

Savage, M. & Burrows, R. 2007. The coming crisis of empirical sociology. *Sociology*, 241, 885–899.

Stevens, S. S. 1946. On the theory of scales of measurement. *Science*, 103, 677–680.

Webb, E. J., Campbell, D. T., Schwartz, R. D. & Sechrest, L. 1966. *Unobtrusive measures: Nonreactive research in the social sciences*. Chicago: Rand McNally.

SEVEN

EXPERIMENTAL RESEARCH – IN THE LABORATORY AND BEYOND

CONTENTS LIST

Key words: experimental research – experiment – Lost Letter – Milgram – obedience – behavioural study – ethics

SUMMARY

An outline of experimental research in psychology, and the social sciences generally, as an approach with which causal relationships can be effectively measured, including: (i) a brief history of experimental research;(ii) the key themes; and (iii) the use of a classic example to provide an overview of the key concepts relevant to experimental research.

Experimental research has been a core method in psychology, including social psychology. In this chapter, we argue that while other approaches have become increasingly popular among social psychologists, experimental research has much to offer all social scientists. In particular, it is the only approach with which cause-and-effect relationships can be confidently measured. We'll begin with a brief history of the approach before working through our key themes, making use of a well-known classic experiment to provide examples of key concepts.

DOING DATA COLLECTION AND ANALYSIS

In the social sciences, experimental research has been largely confined to the discipline of psychology. When other social scientists do conduct experiments, the basis is often derived from psychology. For example, the 'Lost Letter Technique' (Milgram et al., 1965), which has been widely replicated, including by sociologists (e.g., Ahmed, 2010; Burwell, 1987; Tykocinski and Barcket-Bojmel, 2009), is based on the work of the extremely influential psychologist, Stanley Milgram.

THE LOST LETTER TECHNIQUE

This experiment involves leaving stamped and addressed envelopes in public spaces and tallying how many are picked up and posted. The purpose is to examine prejudice and altruism. In Milgram, Mann and Harter's original experiment (1965), the envelopes were addressed to four bogus recipients: either Medical Research Associates, Friends of the Communist Party, Friends of the Nazi Party, or an individual, Mr Walter Carnap. A total of 400 envelopes were dispersed across various locations (100 for each of the 'recipients'). As expected, frequency of return of the

(Continued)

(Continued)

envelopes was related to social desirability of the recipient (Medical Research Associates: 72%; Mr Carnap: 71%; 25% each for Friends of the Communist Party and Friends of the Nazi Party). That is, assumptions made about the supposed recipients of the letters 'caused' unwitting participants to decide either to post the letter, or not.

Variations conducted by other researchers have included envelopes or misdirected email messages to individuals who appear to belong to a particular ethnic group (for example, Bushman and Bonacci, 2004; Tykocinski and Bareket-Bojmel, 2009) or religious group (Kremer et al., 1986), and in another case, students and non-students (Burwell, 1987). In the latter case, additional variables included male and female names, different types of envelope, and type of location.

Note that the Lost Letter Technique is an example of an experiment being conducted in the field, rather than in a laboratory.

So why are experiments more popular among psychologists?

- Psychology initially developed from the 'hard sciences' – chemistry, biology and so on – in which the experiment is by far the preferred, if not the only, approach to empirical research.

- Psychology has traditionally taken the individual as the unit of analysis: experiments are relatively easy to conduct on individuals. In contrast, many of the social science disciplines take groups or societies as the unit of analysis, and it is far more difficult (though not impossible) to involve a large group in a robust experiment.

- Other disciplines have other well-established research approaches, such as unobtrusive research (see Chapter 8), secondary analysis (see Chapter 10), or (supposedly) more naturalistic approaches such as interviews and focus groups (see Chapters 2 and 5, respectively). It is worth noting that some of these social scientists – and including some social psychologists – have been highly critical of experimental research, as will be discussed in more detail later in this chapter.

PRACTICE POINT 1

Experimental research dominates psychology, but also has potential for use across the social sciences. It avoids some of the pitfalls of other forms of primary research through allowing the researcher a high degree of control, lessens reliance on the perceptions and honest disclosure of participants and allows conclusions about cause-and-effect relationships to be drawn.

Then why include experimental research in a book aimed at social science students in general, if most social science disciplines have tended not to use experiments? Because the experiment:

- can be, and has been, used to good effect across the social sciences, despite some limitations

- is arguably the best way of determining cause-and-effect relationships

- may avoid some of the pitfalls of other research approaches, such as participants saying what they think the researcher wants to hear, or the researcher misinterpreting social actions.

PRACTICE POINT 2

An experiment involves the manipulation and measurement of a variable (e.g., obeying orders, completing a task, demonstrating empathy). It is a variable-centric approach.

Origins of the approach

The first social psychological experiment is widely attributed to Norman Triplett (1898) – at least in texts published in the English-speaking world. Triplett appears to have been interested in cycle races, and this was the impetus for this early experiment. He had observed that cyclists go faster when being paced or riding with others, than when riding alone, even when racing against the clock alone. He hypothesised that the presence of others increases competitiveness and nervous energy. To test this hypothesis – the phenomenon which social psychologists now refer to as 'social facilitation' – Triplett had children wind in fishing reels as quickly as possible, either in pairs, or alone. Each child performed this task alone three times, and in a pair three times. Although there was some variation in the results, overall the children wound in the fishing reel faster when doing so as one of a pair, confirming Triplett's hypothesis (it's unclear why Triplett went from cycling to winding-in fishing reels).

There are, however, other contenders for the crown of 'first person to conduct a social psychological experiment'. The claim is contested in part because of difficulty in defining exactly what *is* a social experiment. For example, Binet and Henri (1894) published the results of an experiment on suggestibility four years earlier than Triplett's publication (1898) and Charcot published on suggestibility even earlier (1881), but his work is often considered to be of a clinical nature, rather than social. Another issue is that years may elapse between conducting an experiment and the results being published. Ringelmann conducted experiments on what is now called 'social loafing' between 1882 and 1887 but his work was not published until some years afterward (Ringelmann, 1913). (Many of you will have observed social loafing yourselves – the phenomenon in which members of a group get less work done than if they had worked individually. For example, five students working on a group assignment that is to result in a 5,000-word paper will typically put in less hours each than if each of the five is to write a 1,000-word paper.)

Regardless of who conducted the first social psychology experiment, there are several classic examples that are well known throughout the social sciences and beyond. Perhaps the most famous of all is Milgram's shocking study of obedience (Milgram, 1963).

MILGRAM'S 'BEHAVIORAL STUDY OF OBEDIENCE' (1963)

Milgram's work stemmed from a desire to understand the mechanisms by which humans obey the commands of others, in particular in regards to the obedience to commands that led to the death of millions in Nazi death camps during the Second World War. The participants in the original study were men aged 20–50, of various income levels. The experiment consisted of ordering participants to administer increasingly severe punishment to another person in the context of a learning experiment, the punishment apparently consisting of an electric shock. Each time the learner answered a question incorrectly he (all the participants and the 'learner' were men) was to be punished. In fact, the 'shock generator' was non-functional and the 'learner' was an actor. Of course, the participants were not aware of this and believed they were actually administering electric shocks, as marked on the machine from 'Slight' to 'Danger: Severe Shock', supposedly ranging up to 450 volts. The 'learner' was strapped into a chair, ostensibly to prevent movement while being shocked, and electrode paste was applied to the learner's skin to 'avoid burns'. The 'learner' and research participant were then put into adjacent rooms so that they were unable to see each other.

All of the participants continued administering shocks up to the 300 volt 'Intense Shock' level, although in many cases they questioned the need to continue and were instructed to do so by the experimenter, despite earlier complaints and requests from the 'learner' to stop. At the 300- and 315-volt levels the learner was heard to pound on the wall and thereafter failed to respond to questions. Participants were told to treat a non-response as an incorrect answer – in other words, to continue 'shocking'. Thirty-five of the 40 original participants continued beyond the 300-volt level, and 26 (65%) continued to the maximum shock level, although many participants exhibited signs of extreme stress. This point is worth emphasising – participants who continued did not appear to lack empathy, but this empathy was overridden by the need to be obedient.

We will return to this classic experiment throughout this chapter, to illustrate key terms, discuss controversies and, finally, in our discussion of ethics.

Hypothesis-testing

Deductive reasoning works from the general to the specific. It is top-down, starting with a theory for which confirmation is sought (see Chapter 1) via development of a hypothesis to be tested. It may be associated with objectivity and seeking patterns of causation.

Milgram's theory could be conceived as '… the individual who is commanded by a legitimate authority ordinarily obeys. Obedience comes easily and often' (Milgram, 1963: 372).

CONCEPTUAL CONCERN 1

The development of an experiment begins with a theory to be tested. It is a deductive approach (inductive approaches typically *end* with a theory).

When using experimental research, a theory is followed by a hypothesis, which is an explicit, testable prediction about the conditions under which an event or action will occur. A hypothesis takes the form 'If a, then b', thus in situation a, b will occur. For example, a hypothesis about Milgram's research may have been 'If 40 American men are placed in the experimental situation described above, less than 5% will obey commands to continue to the end of the shock series'. Hypothesis-testing is discussed in more detail in Chapter 1.

Once we have our hypothesis, the next step is to move from an abstract concept to develop operational definitions and variables. An operational definition states specifically how the variable will be measured, manipulated, or otherwise studied. One of the operational definitions that Milgram used (1963: 374) was that a participant who refuses to continue with the experiment before administering the thirtieth shock is deemed a defiant subject, while any participant who complies fully with the experimenter's commands is termed an obedient subject.

Variables in experiments

Experimenters make use of several types of variables:

Independent variables: The factors experimenters manipulate to see if they affect the dependent variable.

Dependent variables: The factors experimenters measure to see if they are affected by the independent variable.

Subject variables: Variables that characterise pre-existing differences among study participants.

The independent variables include the experimental setting itself, for example, the formality of a laboratory setting in a university with a man in a laboratory coat overseeing the experiment and urging the participant to continue, versus a less formal setting in an office block, with the experimenter dressed casually and leaving the room as soon as the experiment begins. There are many other potential independent variables, some of which have been used in further studies by Milgram and others, such as having the 'learner' in the same room as the participant and shock machine during the experiment (when the 'learner' was in the same room, the compliance rate dropped from 65% to 40% (Milgram, 1974)).

CONCEPTUAL CONCERN 2

Experimental research is a variable-centric approach. Following the development of the hypothesis, the key concern is the development of appropriate variables and ways of measuring these.

Milgram stated that the primary dependent variable was the maximum shock a participant administers. This was measured by noting the shock levels, from 0 (refusal to administer any shock at all) to 30 (willing to administer the maximum shock), and measuring the duration of shocks with timers. In addition, experiments were filmed and/or audio-taped, photographs were taken through one-way mirrors and notes of any unusual behaviours were kept. Finally, after the experiment, participants were interviewed using open-ended questions, projective measures and attitude scales (see Chapter 5 on focus groups and Chapter 2 on in-depth interviews for further discussion of these).

Subject variables include the gender of participants (in later experiments females were just as likely to administer the maximum shock as males), or education levels or social class.

CONCEPTUAL CONCERN 3

Experimental research is initially characterised by fixed framing. Once the key components of the experiment are decided upon – the hypothesis to be tested and the means for doing so – it is very difficult, if not impossible, to change them. In order to conduct statistical analysis, the conditions of the experiment must be the same in each case. However, it is common for variables to be altered in subsequent experiments, incorporating some fluidity. Consider Milgram's later variations conducted in an office building, with the 'learner' in the same room as the participant, with the experimenter in a different location, etc. These variations provide important additional insights.

Given the fixed framing of this approach, the validity of the variables is imperative. Validity refers to the extent to which the variables measure what they are intended to measure. With some other approaches this is quite straightforward. For example, when designing a survey the researcher makes sure the questions (variables) are easily understood and that the available answers (values) capture all possibilities accurately. This may be tested by discussing the questions in a focus group (see Chapter 5) or a pilot survey (see Chapter 6). However, in an experiment the question of validity may be more complex.

Validity and reliability in data collection

Validity and reliability refer to the robustness of the research – how likely it is that experiment 'works' and produces results that are accurate and meaningful beyond the experiment itself. They are often conceptualised as:

- *internal* validity, and

- *reliability* (or *external* validity).

The key concern of internal validity is 'How certain can we be that the independent variable caused the effects obtained on the dependent variable?' Thus, is the experiment itself valid? That is, do changes in the setting in which electric shocks are administered (e.g., from university laboratory to anonymous office) really cause changes in obedience, or is there some other reason changes occur?

Construct validity is a type of internal validity and is used to evaluate the manipulation (change) and measurement of variables. It refers to the extent to which the manipulations in an experiment really manipulate the conceptual variables (constructs) they were designed to manipulate, and the measures used in a study really measure the conceptual variables (such as obedience) that they were designed to measure. For example, is the strength of the electric shocks (the dependent variable) that someone is prepared to administer really an indication of how obedient that person is? Control groups may be useful for ruling out alternative explanations for results. In a variation on his original experiment, Milgram included a control group who were not given continuing commands. Once participants were given the initial instructions, they were left to decide at what point to cease giving shocks, in contrast to the experimental (non-control) groups who were continually encouraged to keep shocking. Less than 5% of control group members gave the maximum shock level, indicating that the ongoing commands (a manipulation of the independent variable) were an important aspect of continued obedience.

Reliability (or *external* validity) refers to the degree to which the findings can be generalised to other people and to other (external) situations, as opposed to behaviour that occurs in an experimental setting only. It also refers to the extent to which the results can be reliably produced at another time, or by another researcher (assuming all the conditions/variables are the same). Some key considerations are:

- Is the sample representative of the population as a whole?

- Is the setting in which the research is conducted likely to affect participants' behaviour?

Reliability may be measured by repeating the experiment with another sample of participants, to see if the same findings are achieved. If the samples are representative, you would expect to get the same results, providing the setting and other experimental conditions are the same. (Briefly, we say that a sample is representative when it largely reflects the composition of the population from which it is drawn – the same proportions of men and women, of various age groups, ethnicities, etc.) This type of repetition of an experiment is known as replication. We know that Milgram's original experiment was not representative of the population in so far as all the participants were men, therefore it was not possible to assume that women would behave in the same way.

Although the setting of Milgram's experiment was a laboratory, as opposed to a 'real world' setting, we can assume that the experiment had a relatively high level of realism in some respects; that is, participants really believed they were administering electric shocks. However, it is worth noting again that the results varied according to the setting. We cannot conclude that the 65% of participants who administered the maximum level of shock in the laboratory would also do so in other settings – the original experiment only tells us what people would do in a laboratory. Although participants were less likely to administer the maximum level of shock in later experiments conducted in more neutral settings, this is likely to have been due to the deliberate manipulation of the independent variable: the more casual atmosphere, and the experimenter therefore seeming to have less authority. It seems plausible that the experiment appeared real regardless of whether it was conducted in the laboratory or an office building. Experimental realism is achieved most readily in field experiments, as summarised in Table 7.1:

TABLE 7.1 Laboratory and field experiments compared

Laboratory experiments	Field experiments
Conducted in settings designed for the purpose.	Conducted in real-world settings.
• Advantages: The environment can be controlled; the participants can be carefully studied.	• Advantages: Realism; participants may feel more comfortable; participants are more likely to act naturally.
• Disadvantage: Participants may behave differently from how they normally would.	• Disadvantage: Experimenter has less control.
• Example: Milgram's 'Behavioural study of obedience'.	• Example: Milgram's 'Lost Letter Technique'.

Experimental realism is also discussed below, in relation to the use of technology – video games – in a study on prejudice.

Cases in experiments

Our discussion of data collection has focused on issues around variables. This is natural, as the experiment is a variable-centred approach. However, we have also discussed cases. In experimental research, the cases are the participants.

CONCEPTUAL CONCERN 4

As noted, experimental research is a variable-centric approach. Here the cases are participants in the experiment. The number of cases is relatively few compared to other variable-centric approaches (such as the survey). Like the survey, experimental research is primarily quantitative, with data analysed using statistics. However, there is often untapped potential for incorporating qualitative material, for example in debriefing the participants.

Figure 7.1 shows us the data from Milgram's original experiment, as it might look entered into a computer spreadsheet. There are only two variables showing: 'Participant Number' and 'Shock'. The rows represent the cases – the 40 people who took part in the experiment. The information within each of the cells in the column headed 'Shock' are the values, i.e., the possible 'answers' to the variable (question) 'What is the maximum level of shock a person is prepared to give in this experiment?' Because the cases have been entered in order according to maximum shock level, we can see that 26 people (65% of the sample) gave a maximum shock of 450 volts, one person refused to continue past 375 volts, and so on.

Compared to deciding on the variables, and appropriate ways of measuring them, determining the cases is relatively easy. The key question is whether it is desirable for the cases/participants to be representative of the population in general. Often the answer will be yes – you will want to be able to generalise your findings to the population at large. In this situation, your next concern is recruiting a representative sample. For example, how will you make your research known to people? Are there any incentives you can offer them for participating? Sometimes, though, you may wish to conduct your experiment with a particular group of people. For example, a repeat of Milgram's experiment with members of the armed forces may yield interesting results, especially given that this experiment came about as a result of Milgram's interest in the obedience of Nazi soldiers. Even in a situation such as this, however, you will

Participant Number	Shock (volts)
1	300
2	300
3	300
4	300
5	300
6	315
7	315
8	315
9	315
10	330
11	330
12	345
13	360
14	375
15	450
16	450
17	450
18	450
19	450
20	450
21	450
22	450
23	450
24	450
25	450
26	450
27	450
28	450
29	450
30	450
31	450
32	450
33	450
34	450
35	450
36	450
37	450
38	450
39	450
40	450

FIGURE 7.1 Word data matrix showing the variable 'shock' by 40 cases

probably want to be confident that your sample of soldiers represents the population of soldiers from which it is drawn, for example in terms of rank, gender, age and time served.

> ## PRACTICE POINT 3
>
> Generally speaking, it is better to have a large sample if you intend to undertake statistical analysis, as is usually the norm with experiments. You will want to be able to make some claims that your sample represents the population from which it is drawn, and that your results didn't occur by chance. If you only have five people in your sample, it is possible that they could all be unusual in some way, and you wouldn't have achieved the same results with another sample. If you have a sample of 50, it is likely that any individual idiosyncrasies will be averaged out, and is even more likely with a larger sample.

A final point to consider before we move on to discuss data analysis is that psychologists have often recruited participants from first-year psychology classes. This is convenient because psychology students are reasonably likely to be interested in psychology experiments, and they are often offered an incentive such as a credit of marks. What are some situations in which it may be desirable to recruit participants solely from this group? What are some situations in which it would be problematic?

Analysing experiments

Experimental data analysis is usually analysed using software such as SPSS. A thorough discussion of statistical analysis is beyond the scope of this text. However, we will introduce you to some core concepts regarding the analysis of experimental data. These basics include statistical significance, normal distribution and standard deviation.

Statistical significance

In order to be able to understand research findings that you are likely to encounter in the course of your studies, there are some key terms you should be familiar with. Chief among these is 'statistical significance'. This term refers to the likelihood that the results could merely have occurred by chance or coincidence. If a result has occurred five or fewer times in 100 possible outcomes, then it is considered to be 'statistically significant', i.e., it is unlikely to be a coincidence. This is often expressed in academic journal articles as a 'p value': $p < 0.05$ (the 'p' stands for probability, and 0.05 is another way of saying five in a hundred or 5%). The more zeros after the decimal point, the more significant the result: 0.0005 is much more significant than 0.05. However, a p value does not necessarily include a 5. In fact, although 0.05 (or 5%) is the general cut-off point for significance, you are more likely to see p values of <0.01 (or 1%, which is more significant than 5%) and <0.001 (which is the same as one in a thousand or 0.1%).

Normal distribution (also called the bell curve) and standard deviation

The normal distribution tells us how we would expect scores to be distributed, according to the mean (average) score for the sample. A standard deviation is used to demonstrate how much a score deviates (is different) from the mean. For example, imagine that the marks for your final examination have just been posted, showing that the mean was 56.3%, and that you scored 82%. It seems likely that you did well in comparison to your classmates, but you can't be sure unless you know what is within the normal range – in other words, how much your score has deviated from the norm. It could be that lots of people got scores above 80% (although this would also mean that a lot of people got very low scores since the mean is 56.3%). Figure 7.2 illustrates how these issues may be represented graphically. To the right of the graph is some basic information: the mean, the standard deviation, and the number of participants. You can see that your score was more than one standard deviation from the mean (56.3 + 16.9 = 73), so was unusually high. In fact, you are one of only three people out of the 42 who sat the exam to score above 80% (the vertical y axis is labelled 'Frequency' and indicates how frequent each score was – i.e., how many students scored within each range of marks – while the horizontal x axis shows the marks, with each bar representing a range of 10 marks, from 0–10, and so on). The line forming an upside-down U is the normal curve. We can see that the marks attained reflect the normal curve fairly closely. A few more people scored in the 50–60% and 0–10% ranges than the mean and normal curve would suggest, while the 30–40% and 40–50% are perhaps a little low, but only slightly.

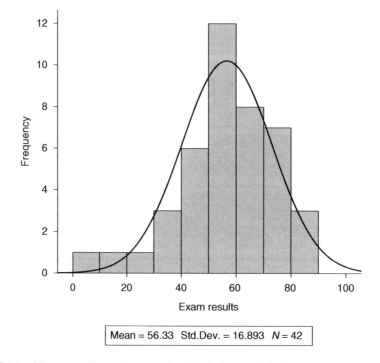

Mean = 56.33 Std.Dev. = 16.893 N = 42

FIGURE 7.2 Histogram illustrating standard deviation and distribution – exam results

TABLE 7.2 Frequency table – Milgram's experiment

Volts	Frequency	Percentage	Valid percentage	Cumulative percentage
300 volts	5	12.5	12.5	12.5
315 volts	4	10.0	10.0	22.5
330 volts	2	5.0	5.0	27.5
345 volts	1	2.5	2.5	30.0
360 volts	1	2.5	2.5	32.5
375 volts	1	2.5	2.5	35.0
450 volts	26	65.0	65.0	100.0
Total	40	100.0	100.0	

Let's look again at our core example for this chapter. A simple calculation tells us that the mean shock level administered by the 40 participants in Milgram's original experiment was 405 (in the 'Danger: Severe Shock' range). Table 7.2 gives us some basic information on the frequency of administration of maximum shock levels, while the graph in Figure 7.3 gives us some additional information, including the normal curve and the standard deviation. Both have been exported from SPSS.

The x axis (the one that goes across) represents the level of volts. The y axis (the one that goes up) represents the frequency at which participants stopped giving shocks – or, to put it another way, the number of people/cases who stopped at each volt level. So by reading across to the first bar on the left we can see that nobody stopped administering shocks before they reached 300 volts, but five refused to go on past that point. (We can also see this in the first line of Table 7.2.) Then four people stopped at 315 volts, etc. If we look across to the last bar on the right, we can see that 26 people stopped at the 450-volt level (the maximum). The gently curving line across the graph is the normal curve; it tells us what we could expect to happen if people conformed to the norm that is predicted by the mean – where we would have expected the tops of the bars to reach. It looks quite different from the normal curve in the graph of exam results (Figure 7.2), in which the normal curve is quite close to the tops of the bars. Given that the mean in Milgram's study is 405 volts, we would expect the highest bar to be located at the 400 point on the x axis, the next highest bars to be immediately to the left and right at 380, and so on, with the lowest bars being at either end. Instead, something interesting has happened. The actual height of the bars – the numbers of participants and the maximum shocks they were prepared to give – does not conform to the normal curve at all. The highest bar is at the extreme right, not the middle of the curve. This suggests that something very important has happened in this experiment.

It is also interesting to note that no one stopped between 375 volts, which had the additional notation on the machine of 'Danger: Severe Shock', and the maximum – people continued through 390, 405, 420 and 435 volts. Unfortunately, Milgram gives no explanation for this, but we will return to it later in the chapter.

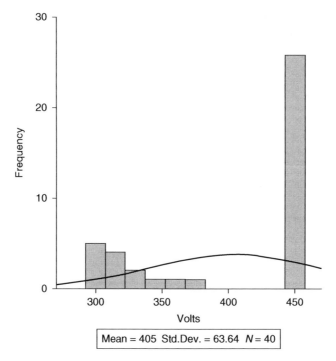

FIGURE 7.3 Histogram illustrating standard deviation and distribution – Milgram's experiment

SOME ISSUES IN RESEARCH

The use of experimental research in the social sciences has been highly criticised. In this section we discuss the key concerns: ethics and epistemology. We also consider the impact of the availability of resources.

Ethical issues

Researchers have a moral and legal responsibility to abide by ethical principles, based on moral values. Chief among these is the minimisation of harm, such that if there is a risk of distress, procedures must be in place to prevent this occurring wherever possible, and if it should occur, it should be dealt with as quickly and effectively as possible. To further minimise the risk of harm, 'informed consent' is considered paramount. Every participant should be clear about what the research will involve before agreeing to take part, and should be able to refuse to participate, or to stop participating at any time, without negative consequences. These strictures may seem quite sensible and straightforward at first glance, but consider how they apply to Milgram's experiment, in which deception was an essential ingredient and participants were very strongly encouraged to continue whenever they showed reluctance, with repeated exhortations to complete the 'learning task': 'It is absolutely essential that you continue' and 'You have no other choice, you *must* continue'. Indeed, Milgram used the phrase 'bring the subject [participant] into line' when discussing unwillingness to continue (1963: 374). As you can imagine, the use of deception such as this has caused particular concern in social psychology. Virtually every study now has to be evaluated for its ethical appropriateness by experienced researchers before the study can be conducted. Debriefing is generally considered a necessity whenever a deception has occurred as part of an experiment.

Debriefing refers to the process of discussing the research with the participants after completion of an experiment (or interview, etc.). It allows the participant to ask questions about the procedure, and for the researcher to explain, which is particularly important where deception has taken place. Milgram describes 'dehoaxing', or procedures to ensure that the participant would 'leave the laboratory in a state of well-being. A friendly reconciliation was arranged between the subject and the victim, and an effort was made to reduce any tensions that arose as a result of the experiment' (1963: 374). No doubt participants were greatly relieved that they had not, in fact, inflicted pain and suffering on anyone. However, it seems reasonable to assume that the experiment had ongoing consequences for at least some of the participants. How would you feel if you had behaved in a way that seemed to be causing someone great pain, even endangering their life, and you had continued to do so, despite their protests (even if you later found it had been a hoax)?

As mentioned above, moral values inform ethical practice. But do moral values affect science in areas other than ethical issues? Should values affect scientific inquiry? Traditionally, (social) psychologists strived for an objective, value-free approach to research. It was felt that one's personal values could impinge on research in a negative manner, resulting in unconsciously leading participants to behave in ways that justify the researcher's values or beliefs, or the misinterpretation of findings. However, can science be totally unbiased and objective? The experiment is based on a positivist approach, and the positivist would likely say that science can, and should, be value-free and objective. However, we can see that researchers' values are often inextricably intertwined with their research. Milgram's research was based on his desire to contribute to our understanding of some of the most reprehensible behaviour to ever occur. This is clearly based on a moral value. Further, social research is often undertaken with a goal of 'making the world a better place'. A major figure in the social sciences of the 1930s to 1950s, Kurt Lewin, argued that research should be applied to important, practical issues (Lewin, 1951). This in itself is a value-laden statement.

Despite a desire for scientific neutrality, our personal ethics and values often do contribute to the research process, through the research topics we find interesting to the application of findings in the wider community, whether through informing social policy or social service and health programmes. Many current researchers would argue that it is better to recognise personal positions and consider how they may contribute to our research.

CONCEPTUAL CONCERN 5

The experiment is firmly rooted in the positivist tradition. Developing from the hard sciences, experimenters attempt to apply scientific approaches to the understanding of society. Theories are formulated and tested with reference to measurable, quantifiable results.

While it appears to be unusual for experimenters also to use other research approaches, there is certainly the potential to do so. Again, Milgram provides an example. As mentioned above, he gathered various types of additional information, including notes of participants' behaviour, tape-recordings and photographs. Although the use made of these is quite limited, some illuminating observations are reported. For example:

> I observed a mature and initially poised businessman enter the laboratory smiling and confident. Within 20 minutes he was reduced to a twitching, stuttering wreck, who was rapidly approaching a point of collapse. ... At one point he pushed his fist into his forehead and muttered: 'Oh God, let's stop it.' And yet he continued to respond to every word of the experimenter, and obeyed to the end. (Milgram, 1963: 377)

Milgram also quotes some subjects who did not continue to the maximum shock level (remembering that *everyone* began at 15 volts and continued to 300 volts, with a minimum of 15 shocks administered):

> 'I think he's trying to communicate, he's knocking. ... Well it's not fair to shock the guy ... these are terrific volts. I don't think this is very humane. ... Oh, I can't go on with this; no, this isn't right. It's a hell of an experiment. The guy is suffering in there. No I don't want to go on. This is crazy.' (Milgram, 1963: 376)

Yet think how interesting it would be if we had information on how participants felt after the experiment, what their thoughts and feelings were, how they explained their obedience to themselves, both before and after they were told they had been deceived. Further interviewing may also have helped us to understand why all those who quit the experiment before the end did so between the 300-volt level (the top of the 'Intense Shock' range, at which point five people quit) and the 375-volt level. No one quit the experiment between 375 volts and 450 volts (there were four shock levels in between, at which participants could have refused to go on, yet no one did refuse). What was the reasoning of the individuals behind this distinct pattern? Similarly, we have no information on the longer-term impact of taking part. Issues such as these led to experimental research coming under increasing criticism from the 1950s to the 1970s.

The crisis in social psychology: a crisis in positivist epistemology?

The 1960s and early 1970s can be thought of as a time of questioning and consciousness-raising in western society in general, engendering both optimism and expansion, and crisis and debate. This extended to social psychology too, in particular the appropriateness of the dominant research method, the experiment.

Hepburn (2003) conceptualises the crisis in social psychology as consisting of three areas:

- Critique of method.

- Critique of individualism.

- Theoretical critique.

Together, they can be understood as a critique of the positivist standpoint on which experimental research was based.

The experimental/laboratory approach had been dominant in social psychology for decades, but by the 1950s it already had critics. These criticisms increased in the 1960s, particularly around the inadequacy of laboratory methods to understand cultural and historical significance and motivations. In addition, the experiment was criticised as mechanistic: the study of cause and effect treats people as machines without capacity for plans and options, while the artificiality of the laboratory meant (it was argued) that findings cannot be extrapolated to real life (this is why experimental realism is important). In some cases, there are only a certain number of possible responses. It is assumed that the researcher knows all the possible options and therefore the possibilities for alternatives are negated. Kenneth Ring stated that social psychological research treated important social issues as fun-and-games experiments (Ring, 1967).

In regards to individualism, concern was raised that social psychology was focused on social aspects of the individual, ignoring how the social environment impacts the individual. This is a one-sided view of human behaviour. For example, Lewin (1951) developed a set of fundamental principles for social psychology: (social) behaviour depends to a large extent on how we perceive and interpret the world around us; it is a function of the interaction between the person and the environment; social psychological theories should be applied to important, practical issues. His concluding statement may be seen in part as an indictment of the constraints of the prevailing research method: 'No research without action, no action without research' (Lewin, 1951: 193), while his emphasis on the interaction between the person and his or her social world points to the need to consider the social context as much as the individual. In Milgram's obedience experiment we can learn about a specific aspect of social behaviour in a specific setting – obedience in a laboratory. However, the broader social and historical context is ignored and the ability to use the findings for social action is limited. For example, we learn nothing about the impact of upbringing, or ethnicity, on participants' behaviour, or how the participants felt about their behaviour, either during or after the experiment. Nor do we learn anything about the 35% of people who did NOT continue administering 'electric shocks' to the maximum level. When the unit of focus in research is the individual, it is likely that solutions to social issues will be focused on changing individuals, such as behaviour, personality, or moral reasoning, rather than considering social structures and their impacts, such as inequality, income, (un)employment and social influences.

Traditional psychology places little value on theory, beyond a rather narrow focus on the specific topic. This lack of focus on wider applications of research was seen increasingly in the 1960s and 1970s as the result of an inappropriate emphasis on positivist epistemology. (We discuss epistemology in more depth in a number of chapters, particularly in Chapter 1.) The crisis in social psychology was evidence of a broader challenge to positivism and the positivist emphasis on observation and measurement, and the potential for scientists to form objective/unbiased understandings of the social world. In contrast, a number of approaches drawn from social realism and social constructivist epistemologies were advanced by a disparate group of critics. Thus phenomenology, ethnomethodology, structuralism, Marxism, feminism, and other critical theories offered new conceptions which claimed to be more appropriate for understanding social psychological behaviour and society and for improving them.

A major European social psychological work published at this time was Serge Moscovici's *The context of social psychology* (1972). Moscovici criticises the individualist and capitalist assumptions of traditional social psychology, arguing that they reinforce the political *status quo* by treating it as universal and inevitable. In contrast, Moscovici argued from a social realist stance that:

- Society both individualises and socialises: it teaches us how to behave.

- Behaviours only acquire their meaning according to the responses received and our interpretations of these responses, and this is regulated by our common history of norms and rules.

- Therefore, the study of social psychology must include the broader social context.

The 'crisis' strengthened psychology as a discipline, and furthered the rise of social psychology, particularly through the adoption of pluralism: that is, the acceptance of many approaches to research in addition to the laboratory experiment and the development of international and multicultural perspectives (Kassin et al., 2008). However, positivism has proven to be more robust in psychology than its sister disciplines in the social sciences. A cursory glance at almost any introductory psychology or even social psychology textbook will reveal that experimental research still dominates.

The resources required to conduct an experiment can vary enormously, from almost nothing but the experimenter's time, to extremely expensive equipment and the time of a technician and a multi-person research team.

Resourcing

Many experiments require little in the way of resources, beyond any single researcher's time and some office space. Consider the recent variations of the Lost Letter Technique, using email. In these experiments all that would be required is time and a computer with an email connection and statistical analysis software. In an experiment one of the authors participated in while an undergraduate student, all that was required was an office and a large bag of condoms (don't be alarmed – the experiment was on embarrassment and nothing untoward happened). In contrast, Milgram's original obedience experiment required rather more: a confederate (the 'learner'), three rooms beside each other (the room in which the 'learner' sits, the room with the shock machine and, on the other side of one-way glass, an observation room), the experimenter himself, at least one observer, the 'shock machine' and associated equipment, and recording equipment. As new technology becomes available, the potential for more complex and expensive experiments increases.

PUTTING THE APPROACH IN CONTEXT

While the availability of new technologies has certainly allowed experimenters to undertake innovative and complex work, it has also standardised the approach in some respects, particularly in regard to data analysis. In this section we consider the impact of new technology as both an aid to the development of experiments and as the impetus behind new methodological orthodoxies.

Experimenters have a history of adapting experiments and taking advantage of new technology as it becomes available. Milgram's 'shock machine' is an example of the use of the available technology in the 1950s being utilised, while his Lost Letter Technique has been adapted by others using electronic mail. Another example follows.

In an experiment on prejudice, participants played a video game in which a person popped up unpredictably, holding either a gun or another object (Correll et al., 2002). Sometimes the individual was white, sometimes African American. Participants were to 'shoot' the individual if he was holding a gun, or to press a different button if he was holding another object – and in either situation to respond as quickly as possible. Participants made mistakes equally often when the target was white – shooting at an unarmed target and not shooting the armed target. However, they were significantly more likely to shoot the unarmed African American target, and significantly less likely to fail to shoot the armed African American target.

In similar experiments that didn't involve video games (such as showing photographs: Judd, Blair and Chapleau (2004); Payne (2001)) a tendency to associate weapon use with African Americans was clearly displayed. Note that while these experiments do appear to indicate a tendency towards stereotyping African Americans as more likely to be dangerous, there is an important aspect of a 'good' experiment missing – realism. This lack of realism raises issues of generalisability, as discussed above. While participants were willing to 'shoot people' while playing, they were fully aware that they weren't really harming anyone and it is highly unlikely that they would so willingly shoot people in real life. While these experiments appear to tell us something about the frequency of prejudicial thinking, we cannot conclude anything about racist actions (in addition, they tell us nothing about the participants' underlying beliefs or attitudes, so are not a useful source of information for counteracting prejudice). On the other hand, experimental realism was an integral part of Milgram's electric shock experiment, but carried with it some major ethical concerns. Here are some points to ponder regarding Correll, Park, Judd and Wittenbrink's (2002) work:

- How might these experiments be adapted to heighten experimental realism – that is, to encourage the sense of a 'real life' situation rather than a game?

- What would be the ethical concerns with doing so?

- How might these ethical concerns be addressed?

We can see that the availability of computers and other electronic equipment has allowed experimenters to both update old experiments and develop new ones. The use of video games in experiments probably also adds an additional element of fun, and may well assist in the recruitment of participants through making the experience seem attractive.

An undeniable advantage of new technology is the availability of software that allows us to quickly and accurately undertake statistical analysis. Once data is entered, tables and graphs showing results can be produced in a matter of seconds – work which once would have taken hours or days. Note that the results shown in this chapter, including frequencies, norms and standard deviations, are merely the 'tip of the iceberg' in terms of the analysis it is possible to do. For example, if an experiment uses a control group and an experimental group, it would be usual to conduct an 'analysis of variance' to determine if any differences between the two groups are significant (are unlikely to have occurred by chance) or one may perform cross-tabulation analysis using chi-square to see if there were differences according to subject variables, such as gender. Such analyses are now considered standard, even necessary.

However, it is interesting to note that until fairly recently many of these analyses were not undertaken. The paper reporting the results of Milgram's Lost Letter Technique includes the percentages of letters returned only, broken down by the four addresses on the envelopes. We are left to draw our own conclusions about the fact that 25% of the letters addressed to 'Friends of the Communist Party', and to 'Friends of the Nazi Party' were posted, while 72% of the letters posted to 'Medical Research Associates' were posted. We are not told if these numbers are in any way significant. Similarly, Milgram tells us only the numbers of participants who stopped administering shocks at each level – he does not even give us percentages. He does tell us how many participants are in each of the three age groups, and in each of the three occupational groupings, but he does not tell us if there are any differences between the groups in terms of shocks administered. Of course, given that the sample is relatively small, if resulting differences are small it could simply be due to coincidence, BUT differences between the groups could be large (and therefore probably significant) – we simply do not know. We suspect that if a researcher were to submit a manuscript for publication that contained so little analysis now, it would be rejected. We suggest that the possibility of undertaking complex analysis quickly and easily has rendered it a necessity.

CONCLUSION

Experimental research has a somewhat checkered history in the social sciences – arguably it is over-utilised in social psychology and under-utilised in the other disciplines. Certainly, it has much to offer in terms of discovering cause-and-effect relationships and uncovering behaviour that may be difficult to investigate using other means. After all, if most people were asked 'If I put you in a room with an electric shock machine … (etc.) … would you give the "learner" a 450 volt shock that could seriously harm him or her?', we suspect they would say 'No!', yet we know that in some circumstances that is precisely what the majority of people will do.

The experiment is a variable-centric approach and fixed (once the experimental protocol has been decided upon and experiments begun, it is problematic to change it), so careful planning is essential. Experiments, like all research, can vary in their efficacy. In order to conduct a successful experiment, we must have clearly defined variables – it is a variable-centric, fixed approach, based on the positivist perspective, so it is imperative that variables do measure the thing we want them to measure – and a high level of realism, especially if deception is involved.

A well-designed experiment can tell us much about individual behaviour in specific circumstances. In addition, the high level of control the experimenter has and the straightforward analysis process means that it is a straightforward approach for emergent researchers.

However, experiments alone tell us little about participants' underlying thoughts and motivations, and nothing at all about the social context that lead to the development of those thoughts and motivations. Indeed, some of these experiments remind us of Ring's comment about trivialising important issues to 'fun and games' experiments. We may learn that people continue to hold racial prejudices, but experiments such as these, unless supplemented with other approaches, may be of limited practical use. Of course, one may argue that knowing that people hold prejudices (for example) is important for its own sake. Nevertheless, some researchers will want to apply their findings in practical ways – to respond to Lewin's call for 'action'. To do so, the application of other approaches, perhaps incorporated in a debriefing session, are required.

FURTHER READINGS

There are many texts which provide detailed discussion of the use of the experiment for social research. Your university library will probably have several of good quality. However, such texts tend to gloss the potential disadvantages. Ring's (1967), Gergen's (1973) and Helmreich's (1975) criticisms of social psychology, particularly the use of the experiment, are also instructive. Although dating from the time of the crisis in social psychology, many of the concerns of the day remain relevant.

Milgram's original account of his obedience experiment is worth reading in its entirety, both as an example of the approach as used 50 years ago and for the interesting quotes from participants.

REFERENCES

Ahmed, A. M. 2010. Muslim discrimination: Evidence from two lost-letter experiments. *Journal of Applied Social Psychology*, 40, 888–898.

Binet, A. & Henri, V. 1894. De la suggestibilité naturelle chez les enfants. *Revue Philosophique*, 38, 337–347.

Burwell, R. J. 1987. The lost letter experiment: A class exercise for research methods. *Teaching Sociology*, 15, 195–196.

Bushman, B. J. & Bonacci, A. M. 2004. You've got mail: Using e-mail to examine the effect of prejudiced attitudes on discrimination against Arabs. *Journal of Experimental Social Psychology*, 40, 753–759.

Charcot, J. M. 1881. *Oeuvres complètes*. Paris: Bureaux du Progrès Médical.

Correll, J., Park, B., Judd, C. & Wittenbrink, B. 2002. The police officer's dilemma: Using ethnicity to disambiguate potentially threatening individuals. *Journal of Personality and Social Psychology*, 83, 1314–1329.

Gergen, K. J. 1973. Social psychology as history. *Journal of Personality and Social Psychology*, 26, 309–320.

Helmreich, R. 1975. Applied social psychology: The unfulfilled promise. *Personality and Social Psychology Bulletin*, 1, 548–560.

Hepburn, A. 2003. *An introduction to critical social psychology*. London: Sage.

Judd, C. M., Blair, I. V. & Chapleau, K. M. 2004. Automatic stereotypes vs. automatic prejudice: Sorting out the possibilities in the Payne (2001) weapon paradigm. *Journal of Experimental Social Psychology*, 40, 75–81.

Kassin, S., Fein, S. & Markus, H. R. 2008. *Social psychology*. Boston, MA: Houghton Mifflin.

Kremer, J., Barry, R. & McNally, A. 1986. The misdirected letter and the quasi-questionnaire: Unobtrusive measures of prejudice in Northern Ireland. *Journal of Applied Social Psychology*, 16, 303–309.

Lewin, K. 1951. Problems of research in social psychology. In: Cartwright, D. (ed.), *Field theory in social science*. New York: Harper & Row.

Milgram, S. 1963. Behavioral study of obedience. *Journal of Abnormal and Social Psychology*, 67, 371–378.

Milgram, S. 1974. *Obedience to authority: An experimental view*. New York: Harper & Row.

Milgram, S., Mann, L. & Harter, S. 1965. The lost letter technique. *Public Opinion Quarterly*, 29, 437–438.

Moscovici, S. 1972. Society and theory in social psychology. In: Israel, J. & Tajfel, H. (eds.), *The context of social psychology: a critical assessment*. London: Academic Press.

Payne, B. K. 2001. Prejudice and perception: The role of automatic and controlled processes in misperceiving a weapon. *Journal of Personality and Social Psychology*, 81, 181–192.

Ring, K. 1967. Experimental social psychology: Some sober questions about some frivolous values. *Journal of Experimental Social Psychology*, 3, 113–123.

Ringelmann, M. 1913. Recherches sur les moteurs animés: Travail de l'homme. *Annales de l'Institut National Agronomique*, 2, 1–40.

Triplett, N. D. 1898. The dynamogenic factor in pacemaking and competition. *American Journal of Psychology*, 9, 507–533.

Tykocinski, O. E. & Bareket-Bojmel, L. 2009. The lost e-mail technique: Use of an implicit measure to assess discriminatory attitudes toward two minority groups in Israel. *Journal of Applied Social Psychology*, 39, 62–81.

EIGHT

UNOBTRUSIVE RESEARCH – STUDYING ARTEFACTS AND MATERIAL TRACES

CONTENTS LIST

Key words: unobtrusive – artefacts – material traces – non-interactive – non-participant observation – non-reactive – bias – deception – informed consent

SUMMARY

An exploration of sources of unobtrusive data including: (i) examples of unobtrusive data; (ii) the advantages and disadvantages of a lack of engagement with participants as it relates to social sciences; and (iii) potential ethical issues.

The previous chapters of this book have dealt with methods of conducting research directly with people, including interviews, life histories, focus groups, surveys and experiments. With this chapter we turn to look at non-interactive approaches. Unobtrusive research is 'non-reactive', that is, there is no direct interaction between the researcher and participants (Webb et al., 1966). Instead, data is drawn from existing (1) physical (material) traces, (2) existing records and (3) non-participant observation. The approach is similar in this regard to other non-interactive approaches such as content research, secondary research, semiotic analysis and auto/biographical research (see Chapters 9, 10, 11 and 12 respectively).

In this chapter we explore sources of unobtrusive data and review some examples. The advantages and disadvantages of this lack of engagement with people, as it pertains to social science, and potential ethical issues – an issue of some debate – will be discussed.

DOING DATA COLLECTION AND ANALYSIS

Throughout this textbook we use the concepts of variable-centric and case-centric research approaches as an organising principle and as a way into unpacking each approach. This is discussed in depth in Chapter 1. We argue that with variable-centric or variable-first approaches the researcher starts with an intuition or theory about variables and then has to find a suitable number of the right kind of cases for hypothesis-testing. This testing can take many different forms. In contrast, case-centric approaches begin with a case and the process of research is about developing variables and ending with a theory.

Unobtrusive research is a partial exception to this binary. We argue that unobtrusive research is only weakly variable-centric because of its 'supplementary character' and its reliance on found or serendipitous data sets – cases. In the 1960s Webb and colleagues argued that all research approaches have weaknesses, but that these may be overcome by combining approaches that have different methodological flaws, thereby countering the weaknesses in each and producing a more robust final data set – a process known as triangulation of research (Webb et al., 1966). According to Webb and colleagues, the use of unobtrusive research provides an opportunity to supplement and corroborate data gained via other methods, using measures that avoid collaboration with participants and the potential resulting weaknesses. We think this is a brilliant assessment of unobtrusive research and is actually a unifying element in the approach. The most obvious element of unobtrusive research is, of course, that it is unobtrusive to the participants. Another is this triangulation/supplementary focus. It is the latter that helps account for the eclecticism of the approach and makes it weakly variable-centric.

CONCEPTUAL CONCERN 1

The use of unobtrusive research provides an opportunity to supplement and corroborate data gained via other methods, using measures that avoid collaboration with participants and the potential resulting weaknesses.

Unobtrusive research is weakly variable-centric because it is so often used to supplement existing research or to provide another way of testing a hypothesis. Furthermore, more often than not the cases that are used to gather supplementary data are the result of happenstance. Serendipity often seems to play a role in unobtrusive research. In the examples discussed below, researchers: (1) are given access to a juvenile correctional facility just before it is demolished and take the chance to study graffiti; (2) analyse photographs of players in an old *Baseball Register*; and (3) attend criminal sentencing hearings. These three examples of the approach are also united by being weakly variable-centric and/or relying on 'found' cases.

CONCEPTUAL CONCERN 2

Unobtrusive research is weakly variable-centric because it is often used to supplement existing research or to provide another way of testing a hypothesis (that is, the variables have already been determined in or by the previous research which it supplements). In addition, because the data is often found, rather than created by the researcher, the ways in which the variables may be conceptualised will often be predetermined.

Unobtrusive research involves the assessment of actual behaviour rather than self-reported behaviour. Examples of material traces include graffiti, gravestones, or patterns of wear on a university library carpet. Existing records can include personal documents such as letters or diaries, medical records, newspaper articles or music videos. Non-participant observation may include recording the use of swear words by students in a university café, facial expressions during an undergraduate final examination or the behaviour of people walking alone late at night (Kellehear, 1993; Lee, 2000; Liamputtong and Ezzy, 2005; Webb et al., 1966). For example, through the use of unobtrusive time measurement, Nash (1990) found that writers often engage in procrastination-related behaviour such as tidying electronic folders on their computer in order to avoid the writing process – an example the authors of this book (and, we suspect, many of its readers) have personal experience of. *Participant* observation is discussed in Chapter 4, Ethnographic Research.

PRACTICE POINT 1

Unobtrusive approaches are non-interactive. There is no direct interaction between the researcher and participants. Instead, data is collected using one or more of three source categories: (1) material traces; (2) existing records; and (3) non-participant observation (Webb et al., 1966).

Unobtrusive research can be similar to experimental research (see Chapter 7) especially in regards to 'contrived observation'. Indeed, the blurring of the boundary between experimentation and observation has been the focus of debate and ethical concern. Webb and colleagues (1966) differentiate between 'simple' and 'contrived' observation. In the former, the researcher/non-participant observer has no control of the people or situation being observed. The observer is a seemingly passive bystander, no different from anyone else. In contrived observation, the researcher has actively structured a situation that appears natural, but then returns to the 'bystander' role. We regard a 'contrived' observation as an unobtrusive experiment. That is, unobtrusive research *may* include experiments provided there is no direct engagement between the experimenter and participants, and participants do not know that they are participating. For example, the Lost Letter Technique (Kremer et al., 1986; Milgram et al., 1965), discussed in Chapter 7, is an unobtrusive experiment. We will discuss the potential ethical issues involved in having people unknowingly participate in an experiment later in this chapter.

Origins of the approach

Unobtrusive research was popularised by Webb and colleagues (Webb et al., 1966) although there are certainly earlier published instances, such as LaPierre's work on the discrimination practices of restaurateurs (1934). Thomas and Znaniecki's analysis of a Polish man's personal letters was undertaken even earlier (1918). Going considerably further back in time in regards to the time the actions under investigation were performed, archaeologists reconstructed the day-to-day lives of the early Athenians via inscriptions on the walls of marketplaces, concluding that 'One of the earliest uses to which … handwriting was put … was sexual insult and obscenity' (American School of Classical Studies, 1974). Epigrapholologists have undertaken similar processes with regards to the ruins of Pompeii.

Webb and colleagues argued against the dominance of interviews and questionnaires in the social sciences. They argued that these approaches introduce a foreign element into the social settings they seek to describe, creating attitudes and eliciting atypical responses while also limiting data sources to those who are willing to co-operate. As noted, the aim of unobtrusive research is to examine what people actually do, rather than what they say they do. However, Webb et al.'s strongest objection is to the fact that these approaches are usually used alone.

PRACTICE POINT 2

A key advantage of unobtrusive approaches is that they allow us to study what people *actually do*, in contrast to what they *say* and what they *say they do* (Page, 2000; Webb et al., 1966). This is not to suggest that participants deliberately mislead researchers when interacting directly (though this is a possibility), but rather that people may be mistaken or react to the researcher.

Applications of unobtrusive methods

While Webb and colleagues argue for the use of unobtrusive approaches alongside other methods, Kellehear (1993) made the point that there are relatively few guides to undertaking unobtrusive research precisely because this approach (or more accurately, collection of approaches) draws on numerous disciplines which often have little in common, including musicology, photography, archaeology, and computer technology, among others. We consider this trans-disciplinarity to be a strength of the approach. Not only have unobtrusive approaches had a broad range of applications across disciplines, but they can also be readily used to supplement existing popular approaches within disciplines.

To some extent unobtrusive research fell out of favour due to ethical concerns, as discussed below. Despite this, the literature contains some fascinating examples of this flexible and wide-ranging suite of approaches. It is interesting to note that there are several topics that have been explored in various manners and/or across several disciplines. We mentioned graffiti above. This appears to have been a particularly popular data source, as Klofas and Cutshall (1985) further review, and as noted by Webb and colleagues (1981), who described it as the 'example *par excellence*' of accretion data (a form of material trace). It has been used to study public toilets as locations for gay rendez-vous; attitudes towards homosexuality; adolescent personality; gender subordination; gang identification; statements of rebellion, and more. We will return to Klofas and Cutshall's work below to explore further the practicalities of the use of graffiti for research.

Tattoos have also been useful sources of data, as discussed by Webb and colleagues (1966), Lee (2000), Klofas and Cutshall (1985) and others, and have been used to investigate allegiance to gangs; symbols of rebellion; reclamation of control of the body by sexual abuse victims; identification with a college sorority; and tribal allegiances. There are, of course, at least two potential difficulties inherent in the unobtrusive study of tattoos. First, the fact that tattoos may be on parts of the body not readily observed may be problematic, although the authors have noted that users of thermal pools appear to be good sources of data (people in swimming pools seem less likely to have tattoos and also the combination of being submerged much of the time and moving makes examination difficult, in contrast to the relatively stationary behaviour of those in hot pools). That brings us to the second issue: the observer may find it wise to be particularly careful to not be observed! This point raises an ethical issue which will be discussed below: is it ethically appropriate to 'use' members of the public as data sources without their knowledge?

As you will have gathered, unobtrusive measures have many applications. In part, this is because of the many possible data sets readily available, covering a diversity of topics, often informed by previous research in various disciplines. We shall turn now to review three examples of unobtrusive research.

CONCEPTUAL CONCERN 3

Unobtrusive methods can be applied to many research questions and disciplines within the social sciences, due to the readily available existing data sources on many topics.

Examples of unobtrusive research

First, let's review Klofas and Cutshall's (1985) detailed report on the use of graffiti to analyse the process of socialisation in a correctional facility. Graffiti is a form of material trace. Material (sometimes called 'physical') traces are often broken down into *erosion measures*, where the material being measured is wearing down, as in patterns of wear on a carpet, and *accretion measures*, or things humans have left behind – such as graffiti.

Klofas and Cutshall's study used content analysis (see Chapter 9) of graffiti found on the walls of a correctional facility which had been abandoned 13 years prior, supplemented by newspaper reports and interviews with former staff (the superintendent, a security master) and two former inmates. The graffiti

TABLE 8.1 Categories of graffiti in Klofas and Cutshall's study

Percentage	Category	Example
35.7	Personal Identifier	Initials, names, names and places
21.8	Romance	Poems, names, hearts, e.g. "BC & CC forever"
12.3	Miscellaneous	Cartoons, song titles
7.8	Criminal justice	Personal experiences, e.g. "Jail stinks"
6.6	Political activism	Peace symbols, clenched fists
2.5	Religious	Crosses, references to God

were transcribed verbatim from the walls of the institution, which was due for demolition (the article describes the institution in interesting if somewhat disturbing terms, noting staff assaults on inmates, long periods of solitary confinement, infestations of vermin and – unsurprisingly – a high suicide rate). The boys and young men confined in this facility ranged in age from 12 to 21, although the average was 15 years. Each 'unit' of graffiti was determined by handwriting, subject and writing tool. Each unit was then copied on to a card and categorised. The supplementary newspaper material and interviews were used to obtain information about the programme at the facility which may be of use in interpreting the data. For example, it was learned that because the facility had rarely been painted in its final years of operation, the researchers could argue that the data were a continuous record for a period of time.

A total of 2,765 graffiti were collected. The authors note that in contrast to public settings, such as outside walls and bus shelters, or semi-public settings such as public toilets, cell walls in this facility displayed a mixture of markings – some for audiences, but others only for the author, for example, 'Night after night, day after day, I just sit on my bed thinking about good times had with her "Paula"'. In addition, the topics addressed seem unusually diverse (Table 8.1).

Klofas and Cutshall note that nearly 50% of identifying graffiti also include the writers' home town or state, and there were 127 inscriptions of location alone, perhaps suggesting the importance of the 'outside world', for example, 'Jamaica Plains rules all'. Some of these also indicate conflict within the facility, such as this pair of graffiti: 'Leominster is Boss' and 'Fitchburg kicks Leominster's ass'. Unlike much public graffiti, only 1.2% denoted group identification. Another interesting finding was that only 1.3% of graffiti dealt with race. This appears to have been superseded by hometown affiliation. A further difference from public graffiti was the relative lack of sexual content (1%). The authors also note that the descriptions of personal experience with the criminal justice system provided an interesting elaboration of newspaper accounts.

Klofas and Cutshall's preliminary analysis was the calculation of percentages for graffiti themes, and also location. Statistically significant differences in location were found when calculated using chi-square. The most popular place for inscription was the front wall (38.7% of graffiti), near a window looking out on the corridor and other cells, and only 10% on the back wall, which had an outside-facing window. This suggests interest in others' activities and/or conversations carried on across the corridor. Much of the remainder was placed near the inmates' beds. This statistical analysis threw up some interesting findings about the content combined with the location. The graffiti on the front walls were most commonly personal or group identifiers or about sex. Time spent interacting with others appears to have evoked social (externalised) concerns. In contrast, graffiti near beds or desks was more reflective (internalised), centring on religion or experiences with the criminal justice system. Klofas and Cutshall also provide interesting analysis of the graffiti in terms of the six corridors, which appears to relate to the length of time spent in the facility.

Klofas and Cutshall (1985) conclude that the method employed has resulted in useful information, in particular regarding prison subcultures and inmate identities. However, they also point out some limitations to the use of unobtrusive measures in the study of graffiti. First among these is that it is impossible to know how many of the inmates left graffiti, and whether those who did are in some way different from those who did not. Therefore we cannot generalise information gleaned about the graffiti-writers to the whole facility inmate population – we do not know if this sample (the graffiti-writers) are representative of the whole. In addition, the graffiti does not contain the breadth of information that may be available by other methods, such as interviews. However, this points to the usefulness of combining approaches. Perhaps much could be gained if the authors had had access to inmate files and were able to match these up to some of the graffiti-writers (given the prevalence of identifiers) to further elucidate data from both sources. We can also add a note about specificity as a counter to generalisability issues. While we may not be able to be completely confident in generalising from the sample of graffiti-writers to the facility population overall, we can say quite a lot about this specific case (the correctional facility), given that there are 2,765 units of graffiti and 13 initial categories, further analysed by four walls in each cell and six corridors.

To summarise, the key elements of this research include:

- the main data source was a form of material trace
- supplementary data was gained from newspaper reports and interviews
- the units of graffiti were recorded on individual cards
- each unit was then categorised into one of 13 themes
- descriptive statistics were calculated – for example, the frequency and percentage of each category of graffiti, such as the finding that the most common categories were personal identifiers
- inferential statistics were also utilised, such as the finding that graffiti category varied as a factor of location within cells.

Abel and Kruger used statistical analysis to deduce their finding that intensity of smile (the predictor variables, as exhibited in photographs of baseball players) is positively correlated to longer life. These researchers used 230 photographs taken from the 1952 *Baseball Register* and rated them for smile intensity, using three categories (values). Five people rated each player's smile, and the photographs (which had been enlarged) were shuffled prior to rating to avoid a possible bias. Modal ratings were calculated for each player and entered into a database. Information on the death years of each player was obtained and longevity was calculated. Of course, longevity (numbers of years lived) can be affected by many factors, such as possible confounding variables. The authors therefore controlled for year of birth, body mass index, career length (a possible reflection of physical fitness), marital status and college attendance, using the Cox proportional hazards regression model. Not all of the players had died at the time the study was carried out, but of those who had, the average age at death was 72.9 for those who were not smiling in the photographs, 75.0 for those with partial smiles, and 79.9 for those exhibiting a full smile. Further examination using chi-square was performed to determine overall significance (with a result of $p = .012$). This analysis revealed that people who smile fully appear to live longer than people who don't, as has been found in various other studies mentioned by Abel and Kruger (2010).

In this study, the key elements are as follows:

- the hypothesis was that smile intensity predicts longevity

- the data source was an existing record (the *Baseball Register*)

- the variables to be measured were the smile intensities as shown in baseball players' photographs

- the values were the three levels of smile intensity, as rated by coders

- analysis was carried out using statistical software to calculate descriptive and inferential statistics.

A fascinating comparison of research methods that may be used in legal psychology is provided by Konečni and Ebbesen (1979), which includes the unobtrusive approaches of observation of legal hearings and archival analysis of sentencing files, as well as interviews, questionnaires and experiments. In these studies, the variables are the factors that may influence the sentencing decision, while the cases are the sentences imposed on each defendant.

The purpose of Konečni and Ebbesen's observational study of sentencing hearings was to break down the types of information to which judges are exposed in such hearings into a number of predictor variables and unobtrusively to code the values of these variables in live hearings (see Chapter 1 for further discussion of variables and values). Key questions that informed the development of hypotheses included:

- Do any of the variables that can be isolated from hearing content affect the sentencing decision?

- How well can the sentencing decision be predicted on the basis of the information available in the hearings alone (that is, excluding documents)? (Konečni and Ebbesen, 1979).

A time-sampling process was used to code the verbal exchanges in the hearings. Trained assistants observed and recorded every 10 seconds who was talking and the topic of discussion. The form on which observations were recorded consisted of a person by time-interval matrix. The observer recorded an appropriate content code at the end of each 10-second interval in the row representing the person who was speaking. This procedure produced a string of codes indicating who talked when, about what, and in response to whom (see Figure 8.1 for an example of such a coding sheet). Note that observers had a list of 70 possible content topic codes – they did not have to actually record words used or a summary of the topic.

So, for example, the hearing may open at 10.00 am exactly, with the judge (01) making some opening remarks about the type of crime (C5) in the first case. These comments are responded to in turn by the prosecutor (03) and the defence attorney (04). The assistant district attorney (02) then asks a question (at 30 seconds past 10.00 am) of the defence attorney. The defence attorney (03) responds to the clerk and in doing so introduces new topic (C7). The prosecutor then turns back to the judge (at 50 seconds past 10.00 am) and elaborates both topics (C5, C7). The judge then speaks further on these two related topics to the assistant district attorney and defence attorney, and continues to do so for some time – at least to the end of our coding sheet. In contrast to the impression one might gain from cases discussed in the media, these hearings were usually completed within five minutes.

Before the beginning of each hearing, the coders rated the appearance of the defendant (physical attractiveness, dress, etc.). After the hearing, the coders also

Time	Person speaking	Content code	Response to
10.00.00	01	C5	–
10.00.10	03	C5	01
10.00.20	04	C5	01
10.00.30	02	C5	03
10.00.40	03	C5, C7	02
10.00.50	03	C5, C7	01
10.01.00	01	C5, C7	02, 03
10.01.10	01	C5, C7	02, 03
10.01.20	01	C5, C7	02, 03

FIGURE 8.1 Example coding sheet for observational time-sampling

rated the defendant's grammar. Lastly, they indicated whether the defendant appeared indifferent or attentive during the hearing. In addition, demographic factors such as the defendants' race, sex, age, type of crime and criminal record were noted.

Following this, the relationship between the variables and the sentencing decisions made were statistically analysed, with the finding that *none* of the variables was significantly associated with the final sentencing decision. The single exception was the finding that judges tended to give lighter sentences in those cases in which the assistant district attorney and the defence attorney raised more positive than negative points. However, even this result was negated when the researchers controlled for the type of crime and the prior criminal record of the defendant. Konečni and Ebbesen (1979) argue that this is because the main function of sentencing hearings may be one of maintaining the public image that the criminal justice system is open to public scrutiny: little that occurs in the hearings seems to affect the sentencing. This raises the issue of the importance of documents related to the hearing, and also underlines Webb and colleagues' (1966) arguments about the importance of triangulation.

Konečni and Ebbesen (1979) next discuss an archival-analysis research approach to sentencing, in which four predictor variables that *are* significantly associated with sentencing decisions are described. These are: severity of the crime, prior criminal record of the defendant, whether the defendant was in jail or out on bail while awaiting trial, and the probation officer's recommendation. These significant predictors were rarely discussed in sentencing hearings. The probation officers rarely verbalised their recommendations and, in fact, very rarely spoke about anything: 'Only 3.2% of the duration of sentencing hearings we examined was spent on the probation officers' verbal contributions; in only 19.1% of 404 cases did the probation officers make at least one utterance; and the mean length of their utterances in these cases was only 8.2 seconds' (Konečni and Ebbesen, 1979: 58). The authors go on to note that hearings were carried out quickly in a noisy environment and that 'it is no wonder that even the predictors of the sentencing decisions that are available elsewhere (i.e., in the court files) do not emerge in these "public hearings", which are, for all practical purposes, merely a smoke screen for the actual decision-making process' (1979: 59).

The key features of this study are:

- the data sources were court hearings and the approach used was non-participant observation

- the hypothesis was that length of sentence could be predicted from variables such as probation officers' comments

- more than 70 variables were coded

- content research was carried out, including the percentage of time taken by speakers

- statistical analysis showed no significant results.

When reading about Konečni and Ebbesen's observational study and finding that there was no significant result found, you may have felt surprised or disappointed – but here's an important point to bear in mind: finding that there is NO significant relationship can be just as important as finding a relationship, as was the case in this study. In contrast, there were significant findings when archival analysis (of court files, in this case) was undertaken. Konečni and Ebbesen's reflection about the relative usefulness of the methods in this context, and in particular, the actual role of hearings as opposed to perceived role, are both valuable in themselves.

CONCEPTUAL CONCERN 4

A negative finding – that there is no relationship between two variables when one was expected – can be more important than finding the expected result. It will require careful consideration of the reasons why this occurred, for example, to ensure there is no bias present and that data was captured appropriately, but robust research will explore these issues anyway.

Let's turn briefly to the archival-analysis approach that was of use to Konečni and Ebbesen (1979). They found that typically the judge views a file that contains the probation officer's report and various other documents (information on the criminal record of the defendant, documents filed by the district attorney's office, a bail report, information about the plea, etc.) a day before the hearing. The instrument developed for the coding of these files was quite different from that used for observing and recording sentencing hearings (see Figure 8.2 for an example). Many items (variables) were coded, including the judge's name; the probation officer's name; demographic characteristics of the defendant; the charges on the arrest report; the charges of which the defendant was convicted; court-related data about prior custody, plea agreements and bail; aspects of the crime, such as witnesses and types of physical evidence; the defendant's statement; prior record; employment history; and medical and psychiatric history (Konečni and Ebbesen, 1979: 59).

Def'nt name	Def'nt sex	Def'nt age	Def'nt race	Charge	Plea	Bail	Judge	Probation officer
John Jones	M	22	B	Theft	NG	$5000	Roger	C. Robins
Paul Adams	M	50	W	Fraud	G	N	Wilson	P. Perry
Mary Smith	F	19	W	Theft	G	$8000	McIlroy	I. Mkawa

FIGURE 8.2 Example coding sheet for archival research

There were just four variables that accounted for almost all of the systematic variation in the sentencing decisions: the type of crime, the extent of the offender's prior criminal record, the status of the offender between his/her arrest and conviction (e.g., whether remanded on bail or in custody), and the probation officer's sentence recommendation.

Next, statistical examination of the relationship between the predictors was conducted. This revealed that the relationships of the four predictor variables to sentencing are independent of each other.

The key features of this research include:

- the data sources were court files, and the approach used was archival analysis

- the hypothesis was that length of sentence could be predicted from variables such as type of crime

- statistical analyses used four major sentence categories as the 'dependent measure':

  o prison

  o a period of imprisonment, followed by probation

  o probation alone and

  o all others (such as confinement in a mental hospital, a monetary fine)

  o variables that could be considered predictors of sentences were found.

PRACTICE POINT 3

The potential sources of data are limitless. In addition to those discussed in this chapter, official statistics are a key source, as are any public arena you can think of. A vital element, then, is careful consideration of the appropriate recording methods so that the data thus gathered can be analysed effectively. See Chapter 9 on content research for further discussion of recording and coding.

We have reviewed three studies, each using a different variant of the unobtrusive suite of approaches, and each on a different topic:

- Klofas and Cutshall's research (1985) using material traces – graffiti

- Abel and Kruger's study (2010) of smile intensity and longevity, using existing records

- Konečni and Ebbesen's non-participant observation (1979).

These studies have some features in common, such as:

- There was no interaction between researchers and participants. In two of the three cases the 'participants' (and we use the term loosely here) – the baseball players and graffiti-writers – were not even present.

- The research supplements other research:

    o in the case of Klofas and Cutshall's research some analysis of newspaper reports on the facility and interviews with former staff and inmates

    o Konečni and Ebbesen included analysis of existing archives and several other methods, such as surveys, experiments and interviews.

- Analysis of variables was carried out using statistical means (as is common to variable-centric, hypothesis-testing research).

- The framing of the studies was largely fixed.

In Abel and Kruger's (2010) work, the approach was clearly fixed (the variables were determined before the study began and there was no opportunity to change them) – there was one data source which could not be changed. Similarly, Konečni and Ebbesen (1979) had little opportunity to change their research process or variables of interest – the data they were using was reliant on the court processes, etc. However, Klofas and Cutshall's research (1985) was somewhat fluid. They used other materials for supplementary purposes, but they could have chosen to conceptualise the variables differently, or to focus on a particular aspect of the graffiti. However, once data collection had begun, it would have been problematic to change the process or variables – they would have had to start afresh. We argue, then, that unobtrusive research is usually fixed, but there may be exceptions.

CONCEPTUAL CONCERN 5

The framing of unobtrusive research is usually fixed, especially when used to supplement existing research. However, it is possible for it to be fluid in some circumstances, if it is to be 'stand alone' research.

In addition, the data is often found rather than created by the researcher, so the ways in which the research can proceed will be limited. For example, it would not have been possible for Klofas and Cutshall to decide to explore differences in graffiti according to the age of the writer because they simply did not have that information.

A TRIP TO HALIFAX

Halifax has one of the oldest cemeteries in Canada. Pictured below is an information plaque within the cemetery that contains some analysis of the gravestones, discussing the ways the pictures engraved on the stones has changed as thinking about death and mourning has changed. The author of the plaque notes that the depictions provide clues to the gravestones' age. Older stones show stylised images of death, such as skulls, bones and angels, but the images gradually changed from representations of death to bereavement, such as extinguished lamps and weeping willow trees. No information is provided on the process involved, so let's take this as an opportunity to review the key features:

What are the cases in this example? *(the gravestones)*
What are the variables? *(images inscribed on the gravestones)*
What are the values? *(the categories of images, such as death images (bones) and bereavement (weeping willows); another value category not shown could be religious images (crucifix, star of David))*

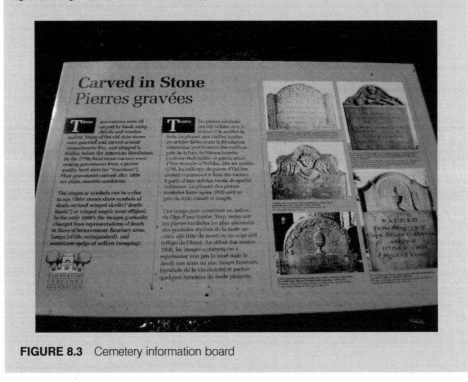

FIGURE 8.3 Cemetery information board

SOME ISSUES IN RESEARCH

In an earlier section of this chapter we mentioned that unobtrusive approaches have fallen out of favour due to methodological and ethical concerns. Let's explore these in more detail.

Methodological issues: observer bias

Although one of the key advantages of unobtrusive approaches is the reduction in the need for interpretation, a risk of error due to researcher bias remains. Webb and colleagues (1966) and Goffman (1976) argued that the observer is more likely to notice and therefore report on behaviour or physical characteristics that seem exotic or unusual – different from her/his own community or subculture. However, after a period of time those same behaviours cease to be seen as unusual and become, instead, unremarkable and therefore are not recorded. For this reason, a systematic approach that lists and classifies the behaviour to be recorded should be developed before data collection begins. While it *may* be possible to add unanticipated behaviours to this list as data collection progresses, items should not be removed simply because they are no longer perceived as unusual (or interesting). The possibility of observer bias may be reduced by having more than one recorder/observer, thereby introducing some of the benefits of triangulation (see Chapter 9 for a more detailed discussion of coding and reliability).

PRACTICE POINT 4

A well thought-out, systematic recording method will go a long way to reducing observer bias.

This error may be most likely to occur when undertaking simple observation, as opposed to contrived observation. By 'contrived observation' Webb and colleagues refer to the introduction of non-human recording devices. The use of these tools mean that no unconscious decisions are made to omit a behaviour or characteristic because it has become 'normal' and they may be more permanent and therefore more readily checked for observer or interpreter bias and reliability. Among the most common examples are audio- and video-recordings. Devices to measure pupil dilation (an indicator of both fear and sexual attraction – not necessarily at the same time!) were also popular around the middle of the twentieth century. Other variants are described in the next section, on the use of new technologies.

Methodological issues: bias within the data

As discussed above, the data used in unobtrusive research is often 'found' or pre-existing; at the very least the researcher will have very little control over the data source. This raises the possibility of biases within the data source, such as simple recording errors in existing records. Social conventions and politics may also lead to what we term 'data bias' or periodicity (see Chapter 6 for a discussion of periodicity within survey samples). For example, up until very recently (and perhaps currently in many societies) men would generally have more ornate and detailed gravestone inscriptions than women. This could have consequences for researchers seeking to understand attitudes to death and bereavement, as illustrated in the example given above. There may also be a social class and/or cultural contaminant as these factors impact both mortality rates and the desirability of inscriptions. Similarly, letters to the editor may be subject to bias, as many newspapers cater for particular audiences, differentiated on class or political lines – see Chapter 9 (Content Research) for further discussion of these issues. Though these issues are potentially very important, if they are taken into consideration in the design of the research and factored into analysis (for example, by including material from several newspapers, or explicitly analysing men's and women's gravestones separately and comparing the results), they need not be an impediment to robust research and may in fact add another dimension.

PRACTICE POINT 5

Researchers should consider the possibility of bias in pre-existing data.

Ethical issues: defining 'unobtrusive'

Kellehear (1993) and others have argued that research was considered unobtrusive if participants are unaware the research is taking place. Remember that a key strength of unobtrusive approaches is that participants are unlikely to change their behaviour out of a concern to behave in the way they think the researcher expects. Therefore validity is enhanced. *However*, says Kellehear, the approach is intrusive if the research does cause unwitting participants to do something they otherwise wouldn't have done. This may seem of little ethical import if all the participants are doing are finding a letter (or receiving an email) and forwarding it on. Even so, is it ethical to observe and record people's behaviour without their knowledge? Or to examine, analyse, and write about someone's diaries and personal papers, or internet postings, without their knowledge? These questions and the search for appropriate answers had a major impact on unobtrusive approaches. It is interesting to note that the second edition of Webb and colleagues' book dropped the word 'unobtrusive' from its title, replacing it with 'non-reactive' (Webb et al., 1981).

CONCEPTUAL CONCERN 6

Ethical issues coalesce around the related topics of:

- informed consent
- deception
- debriefing.

These are also discussed in Chapter 1.

Ethical issues: informed consent

Unobtrusive research offers the possibility of research without ethical concerns if the research is confined to material traces or archival materials. However, there is the potential for ethical concerns to arise in the case of observation or experiments in which the participant is unaware that they *are* participating, such as the Lost Letter Technique (Burwell, 1987; Kremer et al., 1986; Milgram et al., 1965; Tykocinski and Bareket-Bojmel, 2009; see also Chapter 7).

A key concern that contributed to the decrease in popularity of unobtrusive approaches, particularly observation, is that of ethics, especially with regard to informed consent. As discussed in Chapter 1, informed consent is generally considered an essential requirement of ethical research, in the context of minimising the risk of harm (and, a cynic might say, the risk of lawsuits). However, gaining informed consent is not always practicable, especially where deception is used.

Clearly, the usual steps of voluntary recruitment and gaining consent are not possible in the vast majority of instances of unobtrusive research. Yet, as Page (2000) notes, ethical and good practice guidelines have increasingly frequently stipulated that 'good' research is 'with participants' who are collaborators rather than 'on subjects'. In contrast, in Webb and colleagues' philosophy of unobtrusive approaches, collaboration was a potential source of data contamination and was therefore to be minimised (Webb et al., 1966).

This brings us to the issue of deception in research. This often applies to pretending that an experiment is about something different from what appears to be the case. Here we also use the term to refer to pretending that an experiment is a naturally-occurring, real-life event – for example, pretending that a deliberately planted letter has been accidentally dropped to see whether someone will post it or discard it.

Ethical issues: deception

Newman and Krzystofiak (1979) asked whether deception is ever warranted, in the context of deception as it usually applies to unobtrusive research – a lack of awareness that one is engaging in research – and find that the answer to this question is yes, in some circumstances. Newman and Krzystofiak argue that because we seek to present ourselves in a positive manner, self-reports may be 'distorted'. Therefore, deception may be required in order to produce accurate results. However, they cite three criteria for consideration, as discussed by Kelman (1972):

- The degree of deception involved balanced by the probability of harmful consequences.

- The importance of the research topic.

- The availability of other data collection strategies that are both capable of producing similar information and are deception-free.

CONCEPTUAL CONCERN 7

Concerns about ethical issues had a major impact on the practice of unobtrusive approaches. Concern focused on the informed consent of participants and the use of deception. These concerns have also arisen with regard to experiments (see Chapter 7).

Ethical issues: debriefing

Debriefing is rarely possible with unobtrusive approaches. First, the researcher may not know who the participants are (e.g., people who wrote graffiti some time earlier, or people who did or did not post a letter) and they may not be contactable if the researcher does know who they are (e.g., baseball players who have died) or it may be impractical to do so (if they are random passersby or thousands of people watching a sporting event). In addition, one could question the value of debriefing with people who did not know they were being observed in the first place.

Ethical issues: where to from here?

We have raised a number of issues that may have left you questioning the possibilities for ethical unobtrusive research. However, in the majority of cases, the dilemma is readily resolved.

First, the approach most likely to raise concern at first consideration is observation. However, the general consensus is that observation carried out in public settings does not contravene the usual social and ethical boundaries of appropriate behaviour. This is because when we are in public we know we are under scrutiny and the researchers' observations are not significantly different from those of any other member of the public (Kellehear, 1993; Lee, 2000). Although it is possible that a person may become annoyed if they realise they are being systematically observed, it is highly unlikely that the observation itself would result in any harm. Nonetheless, we suggest you seek permission from relevant authorities – for your own protection as much as anyone else's – before conducting observational research in semi-public places such as university campuses, playgrounds, outdoor events (e.g., music festivals, sports fixtures) or public toilets, though we note that all of these have been popular data sources.

As stated at the beginning of this chapter, unobtrusive research is usually based on found data or material that is readily available. The same principles about observations in public settings apply here: if material is publicly available, then using it for research purposes is unlikely to pose ethical issues.

PRACTICE POINT 6

Material that is publicly available may generally be considered appropriate for research use.

Second, we agree with Kelman's analysis and believe that these three factors can be broadly applied to unobtrusive research. That is, the ethical concern is minimal or non-existent if:

1. There is little or no possibility of harm.

2. The research is on an important topic.

3. There are few or no other means of capturing similar data by non-deceptive means.

Of course at least the first two of these three points are a matter of opinion, and in all probability researchers would be required to undergo an approval process from a suitable body.

PUTTING THE APPROACH IN CONTEXT

Webb and colleagues (1966) indicated that the greatest value of unobtrusive research is the use of independent sources of data; these are particularly useful for supplementary or triangulation purposes, but can be extremely useful in their own right, as we have seen in the examples given.

Unobtrusive approaches have several advantages over most other forms of empirical research. They analyse actual behaviour, do not require the co-operation of participants, are usually easily checked and repeated, and are inexpensive. They are also ideal for longitudinal studies, for example, comparing census statistics over time, or criminal sentencing patterns, or the presence of graffiti, or tattoos.

There are, of course, some potential disadvantages. The original data sources may be distorted or difficult to interpret, particularly for members of different (sub)cultures, or there may be intervening or confounding variables. This is true of most research. More directly relevant to unobtrusive research is the difficulty in determining the intentions or motivations that influence people's actions, or biased recording or interpretation (Kellehear, 1993).

The use of new technologies

We have earlier discussed the use of recordings as a way of reducing researcher error. Consider also television shows such as the classic *Candid Camera* or

Ashton Kutcher's variant, *Punked*. In these shows, there is certainly a degree of contrivance – in fact, often a very large degree of deception – while we, the audience, get to play the role of passive observer. At first these may seem like rather inappropriate examples given the level of contrivance. However, they are not particularly removed from many of the experiments categorised as unobtrusive by Crosby, Bromley and Saxe (1980). Though obviously not designed as social research, it would certainly be possible to make some interesting observations if it were possible to access the unedited film. Fortunately for Kutcher, the ethical constraints of scientific research do not apply to the making of television.

The internet, as Murray and Fisher (2002: 5) put it, has been 'a virtually untapped tool for research'. Though writing some years ago, we believe this statement holds true today, particularly in regards to unobtrusive approaches. As discussed by Kraut and colleagues (2004), the internet provides a vast amount of potential data on a huge range of topics and this information is very readily available via public fora such as chat-rooms. Much of this information would be difficult to access by other means, both in terms of the topics discussed, but also the production of this information, that is, the social processes that people engage in when using the internet. Unfortunately, there are practical issues involved, such as:

- Sample biases (Are people who use the internet representative of the wider population?).

- Differences between public and private behaviour (Do internet users behave in a less inhibited way if their interactions are anonymous? If so, does this mean that their thoughts, beliefs or actions thus reported are more or less 'accurate' than if this information was collected by another method?).

- The ethical issues discussed in an earlier section, though some researchers argue that people who post to public online fora should have no more expectation of privacy than people on the street.

CONCLUSION

Unobtrusive approaches continue to be somewhat overlooked by researchers, yet they offer several advantages over many other methods, including the wide range of possible topics and applications, the availability of data sources, the relative cost, and the ease of replication.

Unobtrusive research consists of a suite of non-interactive approaches, gathering data using one or more of three source categories: material traces, existing records and non-participant observation. It was popularised by Webb and colleagues (1966), who argued against the dominance of interactive methods in the social sciences because they introduced a foreign element into the situations researchers seek to explore. In contrast, unobtrusive research involves the assessment of actual behaviour rather than self-reported behaviour. However, Webb and colleagues' strongest objection to other approaches is that they are usually used alone. They argue that all research methods have weaknesses, but that these may be overcome by combining approaches that have different methodological flaws.

A key concern that contributed to the decrease in popularity of unobtrusive approaches is the matter of ethics, particularly with regard to informed consent. The unobtrusive approach renders the consent process impossible. This notwithstanding, the potential sources of data are limitless. We consider unobtrusive research to be weakly variable-centric, although unobtrusive methods can be used in either variable or case-centric approaches. Unobtrusive research is often used to supplement existing research or to provide another way of testing a hypothesis utilising fixed variables. The cases that are used to gather unobtrusive data are often the result of happenstance, and are pre-existing or naturally-occurring. This means that the framing of the research is usually fixed whether by the previous research or by the available data. A vital element, then, is careful consideration of the appropriate recording methods so that the fixed data can be analysed effectively.

Coding sheets are frequently used to record data obtained by unobtrusive means. We refer readers to the chapters on secondary research and content research for further examples, and to the chapter on interviews for further discussion of the collection and analysis of case-centric material.

Finally, the use of new technology, such as the internet, as a data source offers great potential for unobtrusive researchers.

FURTHER READINGS

Crosby, Bromley and Saxe (1980) provide an interesting review of unobtrusive studies of racial discrimination and prejudice. They discuss a variety of methods, including experiments. Several of the latter are variations on Milgram's Lost Letter Technique (Milgram et al., 1965), while participants in others were aware they were taking part in an experiment, but deception was used, so that (for example) participants did not realise that the emergency situation they found themselves in, or that the unexpected request for assistance, was part of the experiment.

Goffman has undertaken several classic studies of interest to unobtrusive researchers. In his book *Gender advertisements* (1976), he provides a fascinating discussion of photographic advertisements of the period and gender display in general. Although he discusses the strengths and weaknesses of his study, unfortunately there is little mention of his analytical process. Nonetheless, this book is highly recommended, particularly for those interested in the use of archival information (or, as Lee puts it, 'observation by proxy' (2000)). In *The presentation of self in everyday life* (1956), Goffman uses observation to explore the performance of the self.

Those of a more macabre bent may enjoy Alison, Snook and Stein's discussion of the use of police information as a source of unobtrusive measurement in the world of forensic research (2010). For example, they point out the generalisation of erosion measures, a form of material trace measurement classically discussed with reference to wear patterns on flooring, to human body decomposition, and the examples of archival information include extortion (blackmail) letters.

REFERENCES

Abel, E. L. & Kruger, M. L. 2010. Smile intensity in photographs predicts longevity. *Psychological Science*, 21, 542–544.

Alison, L. J., Snook, B. & Stein, K. L. 2010. Unobtrusive measurement: Using police information for forensic research. *Qualitative Research*, 1, 241.

American School of Classical Studies 1974. *Graffiti in the Arthenian Angora*. Princeton, NJ: Princeton University Press.

Burwell, R. J. 1987. The lost letter experiment: A class exercise for research methods. *Teaching Sociology*, 15, 195–196.

Crosby, F., Bromley, S. & Saxe, L. 1980. Recent unobtrusive studies of black and white discrimination and prejudice: A literature review. *Psychological Bulletin*, 87, 546–563.

Goffman, E. 1956. *The presentation of self in everyday life*. Edinburgh: University of Edinburgh Social Sciences Research Centre.

Goffman, E. 1976. *Gender advertisements*. London: Macmillan.

Kellehear, A. 1993. *The unobtrusive researcher: A guide to methods*. St Leonards, NSW: Allen & Unwin.

Kelman, H. D. 1972. The rights of the subject in social research: An analysis in terms of relative power and legitimacy. *American Psychologist*, 27, 989–1016.

Klofas, J. M. & Cutshall, C. R. 1985. The social archeology of a juvenile facility: Unobtrusive methods in the study of institutional cultures. *Qualitative Sociology*, 8, 368–387.

Konečni, V. J. & Ebbesen, B. B. 1979. External validity of research in legal psychology. *Law and Human Behavior*, 3, 39–70.

Kraut, R., Olson, J., Banaji, M., Bruckman, A., Cohen, J. & Couper, M. 2004. Psychological research online. *American Psychologist*, 59, 105–117.

Kremer, J., Barry, R. & Mcnally, A. 1986. The misdirected letter and the quasi-questionnaire: Unobtrusive measures of prejudice in Northern Ireland. *Journal of Applied Social Psychology*, 16, 303–309.

LAPierre, R. 1934. Attitudes versus actions. *Social Forces*, 13, 230–237.

Lee, R. M. 2000. *Unobtrusive methods in social research*. Buckingham, UK: Open University Press.

Liamputtong, P. & Ezzy, D. 2005. *Qualitative research methods* (2nd edn). Melbourne: Oxford University Press.

Milgram, S., Mann, L. & Harter, S. 1965. The lost letter technique. *Public Opinion Quarterly*, 29, 437–438.

Murray, D. M. & Fisher, J. D. 2002. The internet: A virtually untapped tool for research. *Journal of Technology in Human Services*, 19, 5–18.

Nash, J. E. 1990. Working at and working: Computer fritters. *Journal of Contemporary Ethnography*, 19, 207–225.

Newman, J. & Krzystofiak, F. 1979. Self-reports versus unobtrusive measures: Balancing method variance and ethical concerns in employment discrimination research. *Journal of Applied Psychology*, 64, 82–85.

Page, S. 2000. Community research: The lost art of unobtrusive methods. *Journal of Applied Social Psychology*, 30, 2126–2136.

Thomas, W. I. & Znaniecki, F. 1918. *The Polish peasant in Europe and America: Monograph of an immigrant group*. Chicago: University of Chicago Press.

Tykocinski, O. E. & Bareket-Bojmel, L. 2009. The lost e-mail technique: Use of an implicit measure to assess discriminatory attitudes toward two minority groups in Israel. *Journal of Applied Social Psychology*, 39, 62–81.

Webb, E. J., Campbell, D. T., Schwartz, R. D. & Sechrest, L. 1966. *Unobtrusive measures: Nonreactive research in the social sciences*. Chicago: Rand McNally.

Webb, E. J., Campbell, D. T., Schwartz, R. D., Sechrest, L. & Grove, J. 1981. *Non-reactive measures in the social sciences*. Boston, MA: Houghton Mifflin.

NINE

CONTENT RESEARCH – CODING AND COUNTING

CONTENTS LIST

Key words: content research – coding – counting – messages – codebook – coding form – sampling

SUMMARY

The historical development and current purposes of content research and the practicalities of the approach, such as (i) design and use of coding forms; (ii) deciding on what constitutes a case; (iii) sampling issues; and (iv) various forms of reliability and internal validity.

Content research is quite different from the approaches discussed in the foregoing chapters in so far as it does not involve interacting with research participants in any way. Instead, data is collected from existing (usually written) sources, although voice and audio-visual sources may also be used.

We begin this chapter by defining content research, elaborating the idea that it entails identifying patterns and interpreting communications. We briefly trace the origins of the approach, from 'muckraking journalism' to the current purposes which include identifying underlying patterns of bias or propaganda in messages; comparing messages, in particular to reveal how different authors may share views; and demonstrating changes in messages over time. We discuss the practicalities of the approach, such as design and the use of coding forms, deciding on what constitutes a case, sampling issues, and various forms of reliability and internal validity. A practical example is given in the form of an evening's television viewing.

DOING DATA COLLECTION AND ANALYSIS

Content research (also called content analysis, although it does have a research component) is an approach that collects and analyses data from messages that are communicated by a variety of means. Klaus Krippendorff describes the approach as 'a research technique for making replicable and valid inferences from texts (or other meaningful matter) to the contexts of their use' (Krippendorff, 2004 [1980]: 18). This inference means identifying patterns and interpreting what is being communicated by authors in messages to their audiences. These sorts of messages were once printed in newspapers, books and in the speeches of politicians, but are now communicated primarily through broadcasting and narrowcasting in printed and digital forms.

PRACTICE POINT 1

Content research is an approach that collects and analyses data from messages that are communicated by newspapers, books and other physical media and increasingly by digital forms of communication.

The approach can be applied to visual and physical media and its range extends across the social sciences and journalism into literary and art criticism. Content research has come a long way from its origins in journalism when it was used by radical writers to prove the biases of newspapers and their editors (Babbie, 1979).

CONCEPTUAL CONCERN 1

Content research is primarily concerned with the manifest or overt elements of messages. These are elements that can be readily coded for and counted. Uncovering the latent or covert elements of messages is not a strength of this approach (see Chapter 11 on semiotic analysis).

Origins of the approach

Berelson (1952) provides a nice history of content research that shows how the approach was championed by journalists and then adopted by social scientists for more generalised research. Krippendorff (2004 [1980]) also provides an overview. Content research was the creation of newspaper journalists, in particular of 'muckraking journalists' who played an important and progressive role in the United States between the 1890s and 1920s. Muckraking journalism was made possible by the rise of the mass circulation daily newspaper in the urban United States. These newspapers tended to be owned by powerful families, who were able to use a media monopoly to advance their vested interests (see the opening chapter in Bagdikian, 2000). Newspaper oligarchs used city-wide monopolies to advance the interests of big business and corrupt politicians. Content research was a technique that muckraking journalists used to demonstrate bias in news coverage and editorials. It involved the counting of 'column inches' to demonstrate the skewed coverage of political and social issues. A column inch was the common measurement of space in newspapers.

A crucial, legitimating, component of the approach was its focus on numbers. Numbers – the measurement of column inches of news and editorials – were regarded as a scientific and value-free way of showing bias. While the subject of content research has broadened considerably in the last century, the ethos of objectivity and quantitative analysis remains at the core of contemporary content research.

Similarly, the use of content research has broadened beyond those of innovative journalists. Content research is now used:

1. To show how messages are constructed or encoded by their authors (Hall, 1980 [1973]).

2. To identify underlying patterns of bias or propaganda in messages.

3. To compare messages, in particular to reveal how different authors may share views.

4. To determine the authorship of disputed or anonymous messages.

5. To demonstrate changes in messages over time.

Looking at a coding form

We will work through the more or less sequential steps of data collection and analysis below. However, it is useful to start this discussion mid-way through the process and to look at some results of a content research. This helps in making sense of the various stages of research.

PRACTICE POINT 2

Coding forms are the mechanism by which all data is collected in content research. Content research can only be as good as its coding form and supporting documentation (the codebook).

The exercise we will use is a coding form (or coding scheme) for a piece of content research from an hour's viewing of advertisements on a television station (Figure 9.1).

The coding form helps show how content research results in a quantitative output. This doesn't mean strictly numerical values in the first instance, although recoding and then analysis of the coding form allows for a statistical use of frequencies and correlations and more sophisticated techniques like regression. Rather, content research allows the distillation of observation into numbers or other forms of notational 'shorthand'. In this example, 60 minutes of television programming has been reduced to a number of counts across some key variables and the use of some related values. The key variables are shown in the column headings: 'No.' (unique number for advertisement), 'Programme/Type' (the name of what is on air and its classification), 'Time' (the advertisement started), 'Duration' (of the advertisement), 'Product' (being advertised), 'Types' (of humour used in advertisement). The variables have associated values. For example, 'Types' has seven categories (as well as combinations of types, allowing for 49 humour values). The basic humour values are: C = comparison, E = exaggeration, L = language (puns), P = personification, R = ridiculous, S = sarcasm, U = unexpected (see Catanescu and Tom, 2001). Further information on the codes is given below.

PRACTICE POINT 3

It is important that coding forms are comprehensive but also easy for the coder to complete in the allotted time.

No.	Programme/Type	Time	Length	Product	Types
001	Shortland Street/Soap Opera	1909	15 sec	Movie: Predator 3	
002.1			30 sec	Telco: 2 Degrees	ELR
003			15 sec	CD: Adam Lambert	
004			15 sec	Jenny Craig	CR
005			15 sec	DVD: Kids TV Series	
006			15 sec	Greggs: spices	
007			15 sec	CD: NOW 33	
002.2			30 sec	Telco: 2 Degrees	ELR
	Station Promo: Hell's Kitchen	1920	15 sec		
	Shortland Street/Soap Opera	1920	15 sec	Guthries: paint	
008			15 sec	CD: Groove Armada	
009			15 sec	Oust Air-freshener	E
010			30 sec	Government: Quitline	
011			30 sec	Burger King	ER
012			15 sec	Movie: Karate Kid 3	ERS
013			15 sec	GE Money: loans	
014			15 sec	Nestlé: baby food	
015			15 sec	CD: Glee 3	
016			30 sec	Government: Road safety	
	Station Promo: Private Practice	1932	15 sec		
	Station Promo: Shortland Street	1932	15 sec		
	Hell's Kitchen/Reality TV	1932	15 sec		
017			15 sec	Farmers': Toy sale	
018			15 sec	Telco: NZ Telecom	
019			15 sec	Toilet Duck	PR
020			15 sec	Rebel Sport: Sale	
021.1			60 sec	Hyundai: IX35	ER
	Station Promo: Undercover Boss	1952	15 sec		
	Station Promo: Troy	1952	15 sec		
001			15 sec	Movie: Predator 3	
022			15 sec	Exit Mould	
023			15 sec	100% Electrics: Sale	E
024			15 sec	Glade scent candles	S
025			15 sec	Valentines Restaurant	
026			15 sec	Warehouse: CD sale	
027			15 sec	Lemsip Max: Cold cure	EP
021.2			60 sec	Hyundai: IX35	
	Station Promo: Cougar Town	1955	15 sec		
	Hell's Kitchen/Reality TV	1955	15 sec		

FIGURE 9.1 Example of a content research coding form

The practicalities of using a coding form are important. If the observation is taking place in real time this imposes severe restrictions on what an observer/coder can do. In this example, your authors have to confess to being under-prepared and the resulting coding form ended up a ratty piece of paper that had to be rewritten before anyone else could understand it. This was primarily the result of a lack of preparation and the short duration of the advertisements – the norm was only 15 seconds. In this time the observer/coder had to:

1. Allocate a number to each advert, while remembering any repeats and noting different adverts for the same product.

2. Record the programme and determine its type (its value).

3. Note the time of the first of the adverts in the 'ad breaks'.

4. Check with his watch for the length of each advert and note that.

5. Record the advert details.

6. Judge what combination of humour (if any) was being used.

And do all this up to ten times in three minutes.

Hypothesis-testing

Content research is one of a number of variable-centric approaches. Like all variable-centric approaches, content research is centred on hypothesis-testing. A hypothesis provides the formulation of a provable relationship between variables. The movement from an initial insight to the use of a research instrument to test a hypothesis is often called operationalisation.

- **Insights have multiple sources**: A researcher begins with an insight about some aspect of the social world. The insight might be an original idea or someone's theory that the researcher wants to test empirically through scientific means. The insight can come from many sources: a response to a social problem, personal experience or from secondary research – a literature review may have thrown up a theory that deserves further attention (see Chapter 10 on secondary research). For example, after watching a lot of television and reading about the subject, the researcher might feel that there is some sort of relationship between the use of humour and advertising. In particular, it may appear that advertising aimed at men uses humour more often that advertising aimed at women. Often the humour used in male-focused advertisements appears to be ironic or sarcastic.

- **Converting an idea into a series of propositions**: The researcher then has to convert an insight into a hypothesis. The researcher will probably generate more than one hypothesis from an initial idea. For example, the hypothesis that 'TV adverts aimed at men tend to use humour more than those aimed at women' and 'TV adverts aimed at men tend to use exaggeration and sarcasm' and 'TV adverts that aim to build a brand are more likely to use humour than one-off advertisements'. These statements are propositions. They are something that can be tested and proven or disproven. But we have to make two caveats. First, in their current, underdeveloped form the propositions are not very testable. In order to become testable the variables 'humour', 'adverts aimed at men', and 'adverts aimed at women' have to be developed and made measurable (assigned values). Second, the process of developing a testable hypothesis is a branching one. An initial idea will generate multiple starting hypotheses; each hypothesis will generate multiple propositions; and propositions will require multiple variables and values to be made measurable. While most of this branching and iteration is necessary in developing a testable-hypothesis, not all of the results will be used in the actual research.

- **Developing mutually exclusive and collectively exhaustive values**: Variables are conceptualised as ways of capturing what is interesting about cases. Variables are made measurable by the assignment of values. The assignment of values to specific variables is not a random or hit-and-miss process. It requires considered decision-making that should be informed by a thorough understanding of similar or related research on the topic. The most important guiding principle of this research design is that of being *mutually exclusive and collectively exhaustive* (MECE). The set of values assigned to a variable are mutually exclusive (and there is no conceptual overlap) when only one value can be allotted to any aspect of that variable. The set of values are collectively exhaustive when they describe all the possible aspects of the variable. For example, in our hypothetical content research the variable 'Types of humour' is assigned seven main values (comparison, exaggeration, language, personification, ridiculous, sarcasm, unexpected). Our confidence that this assignment of values is both mutually exclusive and collectively exhaustive comes from reading the literature on types of humour and in particular the review article by Catanescu and Tom (2001) 'Types of humor in television and magazine advertising'.

CONCEPTUAL CONCERN 2

Content research is a variable-centric approach. There are few variables and many cases. The researcher begins with a problem or an intuition or some secondary research that focuses on some variables or sets of variables.

Deciding on what is a case

Variable-centric approaches like content research face the task of finding a sufficient number of cases to make the research worthwhile. This process always involves deciding on what is a case, although sometimes the choice is seemingly so

No.	Programme/Type	Time	Length	Product	Types
002.1	Shortland Street/Soap Opera	1909	30 sec	Telco: 2 Degrees	ELR
002.2		1911	30 sec	Telco: 2 Degrees	ELR
021.1	Hell's Kitchen/Reality TV	1934	60 sec	Hyundai: IX35	ER
021.2		1955	60 sec	Hyundai: IX35	

FIGURE 9.2   Coding form – modified extract

straightforward that it obscures the element of choice. Cases can be coded to reflect some of their context. For example, in the content research coding form (Figure 9.1) above, all of the TV adverts were given unique numbers, but those that were part of a campaign for a brand were given an additional marker in the form of a decimal place. This additional marker is intended to aid data analysis: it makes the case multidimensional. Among other things, it would allow the researcher to make comparison between one-off adverts and campaigns (see Figure 9.2).

The primary focus of the case might be individual TV adverts but a careful conception and coding of the cases can mean that they can be aggregated or disaggregated in different ways. For example, individual adverts can be aggregated to take account of advertising campaigns. Similarly, individual adverts can be disaggregated to perhaps focus on more fine-grained details such as lines of dialogue. With modern software it is a simple process to aggregate/disaggregate cases as long as they have been sensibly defined on the coding form prior to data collection.

Krippendorff (2004) provides five sets of boundary conditions to determine cases. We have substantially modified and simplified his discussion. He, like most textbook writers, uses the hideous term 'unitizing' for deciding on a case. In this jargon a case is called the 'unit of analysis'. Before going on to list the ways in which a case can be constructed, it is useful to stress that content research is always improved by having some idea about what the research may reveal before data collection has begun. This knowledge of the context of messages/communications isn't always possible and when it is, it doesn't fit neatly with a sequential or step-by-step way of understanding research. What we mean here is an appreciation of the context of the production and distribution of the data. Knowing some context directly impacts how researchers decide on what is a case. For example, setting up a content research of the speeches of Winston Churchill would be greatly aided if the researcher knows something about the statesman's career and the circumstances of his speeches. As a rule of thumb, the more a researcher knows about the context of messages, the more likely she/he will want to explore their 'textual elements' and to construct cases around rules of grammar. By textual element we mean the extent a message (and it can be pretty much anything) was either intentionally or unintentionally made to be read by an audience. In our discussion of semiotic analysis (the study of signs and their meaning), we insist that an appreciation of a basic grammar or set of language rules is a prerequisite for doing this research (see Chapter 11). We are not so insistent here, but an understanding of the grammar (the study of the rules of language in its broadest sense) and/or an appreciation of the context(s) in the production and distribution of messages is very helpful.

Keeping the benefits of 'context' in mind, here are some ways in which cases can be constructed. We move from simple to more complex approaches:

- **A focus on individual authors as cases:** It is common for content research to focus on the individual authors of messages, whether they are newspaper editors, novelists, politicians, movie directors, video-game producers or installation artists. When the focus is on individual authors it is important to allow the aggregation or disaggregation of messages. For example, by type (speeches or articles, etc.), or over time, or even in terms of the intended audience (public or private documents), and so on.

- **A focus on sets of authors, institutions or the channels of broadcasting and narrowcasting:** This is probably more common than an individual focus. Often the focus can be on the channels or mechanisms by which messages are produced and distributed. Returning to our hypothetical study of TV advertisements, this might mean that the cases/units of analysis are the TV stations or the networks that broadcast these messages. Furthermore, the author of the content can be thought of as a corporation, institution or even a set of vested interests. For example, this approach to deciding on what is a case can be used in a content research to compare the media statements on gay marriage of the US Republican and Democratic parties.

- **Using the physical and/or temporal separation of cases:** Deciding on what is a case is more problematic for content research than it is for the run-of-the-mill survey because its focus on messages introduces a textual element. Nevertheless messages have a physical and/or temporal separation which can be the basis of a case. Physical separation is most obvious in the printed media. For example, books, speeches and newspapers are physically distinct – as are chapters, sections and features within them. Indeed, this use of physical separation and distinction was used by the founders of content research when they measured column inches in newspaper editorials and opinion pieces. Digital media also has separation, but this tends to be determined by time rather than by space. For example, 15, 30, 45 and 60 second slots for TV advertisements or station promos. We record some of these examples in the coding form (see above).

- **Using grammar to determine cases:** The advantage of a focus on individual or sets of authors, and on spatially or temporarily distinct messages, is that they are very easy to do. Indeed, these decisions around the units of analysis seem to reflect what is occurring *naturally*. That is, a book appears to be an object that we should normally and naturally appreciate as a distinct thing. A book invites us to engage with the messages it contains without thinking about the mechanisms of production and distribution behind it. But there is a huge body of writing that stresses how messages are not naturally occurring and may be deliberately constructed to give the impression of naturalness.

Stuart Hall (1980 [1973]) famously noted that all messages are encoded by their authors and decoded by their audiences. This lack of naturalness is another way of stating the textual element of messages and the need for forms of decoding or deconstruction in their analysis (see Chapter 11 on semiotic analysis). Krippendorff (2004) doesn't use the term 'grammar' as we do, but talks about syntax – which we think can be used interchangeably here. Krippendorff uses the term 'syntactical distinctions' in his review of 'unitizing'. Syntax is, strictly speaking, the study of the rules of sentence construction and it is important to remember that content research can and should be applied to a far wider range of messages than written ones. We assert that it can be applied to an analysis of all types of message.

Using grammar to determine cases means that the cases, the units of analysis, become the building blocks of a message. For example, the cases in the study of a piece of writing could be the sentences that make up the writing. This would facilitate a very fine-grained sort of research that shares a boundary with semiotic analysis. But, to reiterate, messages don't have to be written. For example, dance could be studied in this way. Perhaps the researcher might have a hypothesis about different uses of male and female bodies in contemporary dance. In this example, the cases – used in making a comparison – could be the building blocks of dance and codified in various choreographic schemas (see the choreographic notation provided by Saskatchewan Education Instructional Resources Unit, 1996).

PRACTICE POINT 4

There are several ways of deciding on what is a case or unit of analysis. These include a focus on individuals or institutions or the separation of cases, and include more sophisticated textual approaches that focus on grammar or themes.

- **Using themes to determine cases**: Using grammar to determine cases results in the 'natural' forms of messages and communication being broken up or subdivided to allow a fine-grained analysis and/or to better capture the context of their production and distribution. As we noted above, this sort of reworking of the 'natural' forms of messages tends to require the researcher to have an appreciation of content/grammar – perhaps gleaned from thoroughgoing secondary research (see Chapter 10). Using themes to determine cases takes this process a step further by assuming that there are themes or propositions in the messages (data) and making these the focus of attention. Of course a researcher has to be confident that such themes do exist before making them the focus of their attention. If the researcher is confident in the existence of themes, they are a powerful way of constructing cases. Indeed, many researchers link the development of a hypothesis with deciding on what is a case through this use of themes or propositions. For example, in the first coding form (Figure 9.1 above) we used temporal separation to determine our cases. Each TV advertisement was a case. But we could also use themes as our basis of case. For example, each humour type and combination of types could be a theme and the basis of a case. This would mean that the unit of analysis would be types of humour and this would allow a more fine-grained sort of hypothesis, such as: 'Sarcasm and language (puns) forms of humour are rarely used in combination because they appear too intellectual for a general audience.' If we were going to test this sort of hypothesis we would also need to develop variables about the appeal of advertisements. For example, cute, obnoxious, factual, sexy, etc. could be variables. We might also need variables about the sort of audience being targeted. For example, general, youth, retired, yuppie, etc.

Coding: develop a codebook, design a coding form, train the coders

Coding is the process in which an observer (the coder) or a number of observers complete a coding form while observing a predetermined event. Observation normally takes the form of watching or hearing, but we can also include the other senses of smell, taste, touch or any possible combination. Coding requires a series of acts of judgement on the part of the observer/coder when faced with various stimuli. The development of a codebook, design of a coding form and training of observers/coders are all intended to make coding as reliable (consistent, repeatable, standardised) and valid (sensitive, accurate, truthful) as possible.

First an aside: Content research shares many features with survey research. For example, because it is a variable-centric, variable-first approach, there is an initial focus on developing variables that are mutually exclusive and collectively exhaustive (see above). The choices in sampling are also more or less the same (see below). Further, developing a coding scheme is a lot like developing a questionnaire, at least in terms of 'scales of measurement'. Better results can be generated if coding is for ordinal and interval rather than nominal scales (see Chapter 6 on survey research).

When nominal data is assigned a variable, the variable acts as a label only. The variable/label shows only that the data belongs to a certain category of thing: happy/sad/angry or fluffy/spiky/lumpy or male/female. The variables of nominal data have no related values other than versions of 'present/not present'. Nominal data is the least useful for statistical analysis. For example, central tendency can only be measured by mode, i.e., the most common variable/label. For example, if after 100 observations there are 62 instances of fluffy, 20 instances of spiky and 18 instances of lumpy, the mode for this coding is 'fluffy'. However, careful work in coding often allows for the creation of ordinal options. Ordinal data have variables with meaningful values. We can tell if a variable has more or less of something. The term for this is rank order. For example, occasionally, generally and highly fluffy gives us a ranking of fluffiness. As a result, the central

TABLE 9.1 Types of data, with statistical analysis and coding options

Type of data	Type of statistical analysis	Type of coding instruction
Nominal	Mode, chi-squared	Is the speech conservative, liberal or radical?
Ordinal	Mode, chi-squared, median, percentile	Is the speech occasionally, generally or highly conservative, liberal or radical?
Interval	Mode, chi-squared, median, percentile, mean, standard deviation, correlation, regression, analysis of variance	How many agreed upon examples of conservatism, liberalism or radicalism are in the speech?

tendencies for fluffy/spiky/lumpy can all be generated using the median. Interval data is better still. It has a label (categorical value) and rank ordering can be assigned using real numbers: 1, 2, 3, 4 … Interval data lets us know precisely how fluffy something is observed to be.

PRACTICE POINT 5

Carefully thought-out coding allows for the use of ordinal and interval data rather than nominal data. This improvement in the scales of measurement allows the use of better statistical analysis (see Chapter 6 on survey research).

Table 9.1 shows some differences in scales of measurement and coding options. Scales of measurement are also important when it comes to measuring for reliability and validity. We will discuss reliability and validity in more detail after we have reviewed the components of coding: develop a codebook, design a coding form, train the coders.

- **Develop a codebook:** Developing a codebook means putting together a sensible notation for the variables and values that have been generated in operationalising a hypothesis. The codebook must explain this notation to coders and any other researchers. As a result, the codebook can be quite a long document and contains some discussion about the variables and values, perhaps even including good examples used in other published studies.

Kimberley Neuendorf's *The content analysis guidebook* (2002) has a handy companion website (http://academic.csuohio.edu/kneuendorf/content/) with a number of codebooks and coding forms. We have modified one of her

---

An analysis of humour in TV advertising

Case/Unit of Analysis: Individual TV advertisements, (1) including governmental or related advertisements but (2) excluding TV station promotions.

No. = Give each TV advert a unique 3-digit number beginning with 001 and proceeding upward, with the following exceptions: (1) TV adverts for the same product or the same company should be allocated a unique 2-digit number after the decimal point. Subsequent but different adverts in the campaign should be allocated the proceeding number after the decimal point; (2) repeated adverts are allocated the number given to the first airing. The range of possible advert IDs is 001.00 to 999.99.

Programme/Type = (1) Programme: Name of the programme in which the TV advert was screened or describe station promotion. (2) Type = The type of programme being screened. Determine the type of programme from the following list. Select only one option from the list: Comedy, Documentary, Drama, Game show, News, Reality TV, Soap Opera, Sports.

Time = The time in hours and minutes when the programme, promotion or advert was screened. Use 24-hour notation.

Length = Record the length of each TV advert.

Product = Record the name of the product and if possible the name of its maker. There is no coding scheme for this, use open coding.

Type = Type of humour used in the advert: Indicate the type of humour used. There are seven main categories: C = comparison, E = exaggeration, L= language (puns), P = personification, R = ridiculous, S = sarcasm, U = unexpected (see Catanescu and Tom, 2001). Record all combinations of humour. For example, exaggeration and sarcasm and unexpected = E, S, U. If humour is not used leave blank.

FIGURE 9.3   Extract from our hypothetical codebook

examples to fit our hypothetical investigation of humour and TV adverts (Figure 9.3).

- **Design a coding form:** We provided a hypothetical coding form for a piece of research that took place one evening in the Curtis family living room (see above). A crucial component of the coding form is that it is easy to use. The codebook should have provided the coder(s) with a complete understanding of how to complete the observation.

- **Training the coders and the problem of imagination:** In all but the smallest scale content research, the researcher relies on others (observers/coders) to complete the coding form. This means that coders must be trained in the process of observation and coding. Becoming familiar with the notation and rationale in a coding scheme is an important part of training. Speed and accuracy in coding an observation are essential, especially if it is a real-time event. But coding from observation is also an act of imagination and the most important component of content research is getting harmony (or standardisation) between coders and across time in making this act of imagination.

The act of imagination in coding from observation reflects the interpretive part of the process. Coders have to interpret what they are seeing and find the best way of recording this in terms of the notation available to them on the codebook. Any ambiguities in the codebook or the coding form will cause major problems for coders and will result in flawed data. This is why Neuendorf (2002: 133) states: 'Three words describe good coder preparation: Train, train, and train.' Training focuses on minimising differences between coders. There are no short-cuts. The more coders can practise and be reviewed on the process of observation and coding, the more reliable their results are likely to be.

PRACTICE POINT 6

Neuendorf (2002: 133) rightly states: 'Three words describe good coder preparation: Train, train, and train.' The minimum criteria for training coders are: (1) That coders should practise one or more dummy runs of the observation, be evaluated and receive feedback prior to doing the real thing; and (2) Wherever possible the observations by coders should overlap. This means that coders should double-up on some work/observations.

The minimum criteria for training coders are:

1. That coders should practise one or more dummy runs of the observation, be evaluated and receive feedback prior to doing the real thing; and

2. Wherever possible the observations by coders should overlap. This means that coders should double-up on work.

Of course the more overlap between coders the greater the opportunity to check on the reliability of coding (this is termed inter-coder reliability), but the greater the costs.

Drawing a sample

Researchers doing content research have the same options for sampling as those doing a survey. Sampling can be a non-probability sample (cluster, quota or convenience) or a probability sample (simple random sampling, systematic sampling, stratified sampling). The key difference between a non-probability and probability sample is that in the latter all potential participating cases have an equal chance of being selected. We discussed sampling in depth in Chapter 6 on survey research and won't rehash it here. We will focus on the distinctive aspects of sampling for content research. What is most distinctive is that the cases (units of analysis) in content research are typically an aggregation or disaggregation of messages.

A sampling frame is a list of all the cases/units of analysis in a population. Probability sampling (random sampling) is only possible when the researcher has access to a sampling frame. Probability sampling is important because it provides a better platform for statistical analysis than non-probability sampling. Probability sampling allows inferential statistics, which lets the researcher make inferences about the *population* from patterns observed in the sample. Certainly most textbook writers see the purpose of content research as making inferences from the sample about the population. See Krippendorff's comments at the start of this chapter as an example. Non-probability sampling allows for descriptive statistics only. Descriptive statistics can only describe patterns in the *sample*.

Decisions about sampling – about generating a frame and selecting a strategy – should be made concurrently with those about 'what is a case?'. There is no point in designing research, identifying the ideal units of analysis and so on if there is no potential sampling frame or way of accessing the data.

PRACTICE POINT 7

It is crucial not to get fixated on the sequence or steps of doing research: hypothesis-testing, defining a case, drawing a sample, and so on. There should always be common-sense circuit breakers in the process. For example, decisions about sampling – about generating a frame and selecting a strategy – should be made concurrently with those about 'what is a case?'

SOME ISSUES IN RESEARCH

Epistemology and claims for validity and reliability

Reliability and validity are at the core of research approaches that make claims to being scientific. Reliability measures the extent to which the analysis of data yields results that can be repeated or reproduced at different times or by different researchers. Validity measures the extent to which the research is accurate and the extent to which claims can be made based on the research.

For content research the measurements of reliability focus on intra- and inter-observer differences in coding and the comparison of research coding with known standard of codings – on inter-coder reliability. Krippendorff (2004) posits three levels of confidence about reliability: stability, reproducibility and accuracy.

- **Stability**: Stability refers to the measurement of intra-observer consistencies in coding. Testing for stability is the most simple form of gauging reliability. Intra-observer inconsistencies refer to the mistakes or errors in coding made by individual observers. This is determined by 'test-retest': a single observer is asked to code the same observation twice (or more times) and the results are compared. The research is said to be stable when the consistencies in coding shown up by test-retest are satisfactory. This is the lowest acceptable level of reliability. It shows that observers, operating as independent observers, have learnt consistency in coding.

- **Reproducibility**: Reproducibility refers to inter-observer differences in coding. Testing for inter-observer differences involves comparing the codings of multiple observers who are coding the same or very similar events. The testing strategy is called 'test-test' and involves the comparison of coding by different observers. Testing for reproducibility provides a higher level of confidence about reliability than does testing for stability because it captures both intra- and inter-observer mistakes. The test-test strategy is the most common approach used in content research.

- **Accuracy**: Accuracy refers to an even higher level of confidence in reliability than stability and reproducibility. The strategy here is 'test-standard'. This involves comparing the codings of multiple observers with an accepted set of results for coding (the 'standard'). Acceptable levels of test-standard measurements indicate that intra- and inter-observer mistakes (i.e., single and collective coding errors) are satisfactory and, more importantly, that the content research is generating the expected data. Of course using the test-standard strategy is absolutely reliant on the availability of a standard, a generally agreed-upon set of results from previous research. It is often the case that there is no agreed-upon standard available to researchers and so this level of reliability cannot be assessed or attained.

Testing for inter-coder reliability in research focuses on the process of data collection and analysis. There are multiple statistical tests for reliability that focus on differences between actual and expected observations, or the quantification of differences between sets of observations (applied in test-retest, test-test and test-standard settings). The most basic of these comparisons is the 'percentage agreed'. This simply involves comparing codings of the same event (over time, or between observers, or to a standard) and calculating the percentage of agreement, for example, 20% of observers or observations agreed. Low percentage agreement suggests low reliability. High percentage agreement suggests high reliability. But, what is an acceptable percentage for reliability? The rule-of-thumb seems to be better than 80% agreement (using a variety of tests). What is also missing from the simple calculation is an assessment of chance. What percentage of agreement is the result of luck? The more sophisticated measures of inter-coder reliability try to factor in the chance component, such as Scott's pi, Cohen's kappa and even Krippendorff's alpha. They do so by including expectations about actual and expected observations. These more sophisticated measures also try to use the more robust data generated by ordinal and interval coding rather than nominal coding (see above). We suggest that you check out the very extensive statistical sections in Neuendorf (2002) and Krippendorff (2004 [1980]).

Low reliability (the research is unreliable) is usually associated with low validity. It is commonly agreed that research which cannot be replicated (i.e., it produces different results each time) is not valid, and is therefore not a good basis for making truth claims. It is interesting to note that Krippendorff, in describing 'accuracy', blurs the line between reliability and validity, seemingly suggesting a straightforward correlation between high reliability and high validity. Neuendorf (2002) makes a similar connection in her assumptions about the ease of coding from manifest (i.e., obvious) content. Many social scientists would challenge the notion that any social situation is manifest or easy to understand. We think the textbook writers are overly optimistic. High reliability guarantees consistency, but it does not measure whether the research is consistently correct or consistently incorrect. It is true that if content research is tested and found to be reliable, then we can be confident that it is, in all likelihood, a well thought-out and executed piece of research. But this is not the same as proving that it is revealing the truth (that it is valid).

There is no single test or series of tests for proving/disproving the validity of research and truth claims. Where writers suggest that there are such tests, they are engaging in wishful thinking. Both Neuendorf (2002) and Krippendorff (1980, 2004) are guilty of this. Our perspective is that it is impossible to have certainty about validity and truth claims. There are no statistical tests or heuristic devices that can guarantee validity. But there are weaker 'tests' that can provide some confidence about validity: reliability or external validity, internal validity, content or construct, face or instrumental validity, peer validity (see also Chapter 12 on autoethnographic research).

- **Reliability or external validity**: This relates to the use of reliability as a gauge for validity. However, we more modestly include reliability as an indicator of validity only in so far as the more reliable a piece of research the more likely it is to be well thought-out and executed (see also Chapter 7 on experimental research).

- **Internal validity**: This refers to measures of correlation and causality between variables. We refer here to statistical measures. For example, strong measures of correlation and significance are weak indicators of validity. So are tests to reject the null hypothesis. However, validity cannot be reduced to an issue of statistical measurement because the variables used in the tests are products of the researcher's imagination. Variables (and values) are not independent of the research project and may indeed be the cause of flaws.

- **Content or construct validity**: Whereas internal validity refers to statistical measures of the relationship between variables, content or construct validity focuses on the comprehensiveness of the variables used. The argument is similar to that used in testing for accuracy in reliability (see above). It assumes the existence of an agreed-upon standard, which in this example details all the variables and values needed to describe some objects of research. The core of content validity is the existence of such a standard, for example, a standard that shows all the dimensions of humour, or of personality traits, or of attractiveness. In practical terms, this approach can only be used when there is a body of very similar research that is well documented and peer-reviewed.

- **Face or instrumental validity**: One of the proofs for validity is found in the often-quoted notion of 'face validity'. This is an appeal to common sense, that 'on the face of it' the research looks truthful. Does the research seem to work? Is it instrumental or helpful to other researchers?

- **Peer validity**: This assessment of validity is made by peer review. We discuss peer review as the basis of 'quality assurance' in the social sciences in Chapter 10 on secondary research. Whereas face validity relies on the opinion of the researcher, peer review relies on the opinions of a community of academics and other researchers. Peer validity carries with it the notion that a content research will be judged in comparison with others, both in terms of process and results.

The confidence demonstrated by textbook writers in the capacity for content research to be reliable and, more significantly, valid in its truth-claims is evidence of an underlying positivist, epistemologically and concomitant certainty in 'doing science'. We have discussed epistemology in depth elsewhere – in Chapter 1, in the discussion of survey research (Chapter 6), in secondary research (Chapter 10) and in semiotic analysis (Chapter 11) in particular. Epistemology is the theory of knowledge that informs how research is shaped in its broadest sense. The three main epistemological positions are positivism, social realism and social constructivism. The proponents of content research are securely positivist in their orientation.

Positivists have the greatest confidence in the ability of social scientists to reveal the truth. They stress the techniques of observation and measurement and the potential for scientists to form objective/unbiased understandings of the social world. They tend to downplay the uncertainties that other epistemologies raise about the impact of power, meaning and culture on doing science and on reliability and validity (some common social realist complaints) or more radical concerns about the logical impossibility of developing an objective scientific stance (the social constructivist complaint). Of all the research approaches covered in this text, content research has the most unreflexive proponents. The textbooks say much about how to do content research as a series of unproblematic techniques, but say very little about epistemology.

The definitions provided by textbook writers shows this epistemological blind spot. Alongside the quote from Krippendorff used in the introduction to this chapter (2004: 18), Neuendorf (2002: 10) states:

> Content research is a summarizing, quantitative analysis of messages that relies on the scientific method (including attention to objectivity, intersubjectivity, a priori design, reliability, validity, generalizability, replicability, and hypothesis testing) and is not limited as to the types of variables that may be measured or the context in which the messages are created or presented.

In short, content research seems to have been largely untouched by the debates about reliability and validity, epistemology and methods that dominated much of the social sciences since the 1970s. This of course doesn't render the approach invalid, but emergent researchers are cautioned that the highly positivist framing of science and research fore-fronted by the writers of content research textbooks may not be the dominant position in other arenas. It also means that content research remains an important vehicle for privileging numbers over words and 'making qualitative into quantitative research' (see Chapter 1).

CONCEPTUAL CONCERN 3

Textbooks about content research are inevitably written from a positivist epistemology. This is an all-pervasive approach among the experts on content research, but is hardly ever made apparent. Emergent researchers should remember that research in the social world may not be as certain as most content research textbook writers suggest.

PUTTING THE APPROACH IN CONTEXT

Content research is a variable-centric, variable-first approach and ultimately a form of hypothesis-testing. The researcher starts with a combination of relatively few variables and seeks a sufficient number of cases to test an argument. Like most of these approaches, content research is more fixed than fluid in its framing of research. The process of research is sequential and there is little chance to move between data collection and analysis in order to improve on the hypothesis being tested, for example. But the scale of the research is an important factor here. The smaller scale the content research, the more it is possible to be fluid in framing the research – which is code for saying the easier it is to go back and fix your mistakes. The most important scalable aspect of content research is the training of coders. This is a resource-heavy (time, money and personnel) part of the approach. In short, the more coders there are to train, the more fixed and sequential is the process of research.

CONCEPTUAL CONCERN 4

Like most variable-centric, variable-first approaches, content research has a fixed framing of research. Very small-scale content research is surprisingly fluid. There are possibilities for iteration and correcting earlier mistakes. However, as the scale of research increases, the approach rapidly become fixed and sequential in the process of research. This is primarily because of the importance of training coders/observers.

This fluid framing is a major draw card for emergent researchers. While it doesn't free them from the constraints imposed by deadlines and resourcing and supervisors, it does allow mistakes made in designing a hypothesis or query to be easily rectified or approached iteratively. Of course where secondary research is being undertaken as a precursor to field research or primary research, the demands of sequential decision-making and of fixed framings are reintroduced.

Content research is, at least conceptually, very similar to survey research, but whereas the latter is considered the domain of quantitative social scientists (predominantly men who like numbers, statistics and computer programs), the former is far more attractive to researchers with a qualitative bent (an interest in words, rich descriptions, etc.).

Strinati (2004: 160–201) recalls the feminist scholars – some of the fiercest critics of positivism and quantitative research in the 1960s and 1970s – who have both used and criticised the approach (see also Oakley, 1998). Content research has been a powerful analytical tool used by feminist researchers to highlight the enduring patriarchal and sexist characters of popular culture. For example, Betty Friedan (1963) devoted a large part of *The Feminine Mystique* to content research of women's magazines and advertising. The gender stereotypes documented by her, in which women are presented as objects of (male) sexual desire, domestic labourers or otherwise ridiculed and marginalised, have been reaffirmed by numerous other studies since. Feminists, like the muckraking journalists that preceded them, found the quantitative, science-like aspects of content research very helpful in appearing objective and unbiased when making what at the time were very contentious claims.

This use of content research began at the time feminist scholars were criticising positivism and quantitative research for being 'malestream' and tending to discount the experiences of marginalised peoples. If nothing else this demonstrates the power of numbers and of quantitative research as an aid to making claims (Best, 1987). In this way, content research was important in a trend towards the 'quantification of research' (by which we mean the representation of the world through numbers and statistics) (see Chapters 5 and 6 on focus groups and survey research, respectively). Nevertheless, feminist scholars developed a thorough-going critique of content research (Strinati, 2004: 160–201) – we produce a brief rejoinder:

1. **Content research is atheoretical**: Content research is fundamentally about counting the number of times some things appear in a message. The approach lacks any engagement with theory. This is pertinent because the approach is often used to research aspects of the media and popular culture, but the focus on counting means it lacks any explanation for the production and consumption of messages/texts. In its defence, we should note that there is nothing preventing the integration of content research with a theory of the social world. Indeed, this is what hypothesis-testing is about. Thus, content research might provide the means for collecting and analysing data but it can and should be informed by an overarching theoretical framework.

2. **Content research lacks qualitative discrimination**: This criticism is a variant of one made of all quantitative approaches, which generate results in numerical form. There is no doubt that some content research suffers from a 'thinness' in its data. Describing a complex event – an advert, a speech, a book, a film – through a series of numbers can be to miss much of its richness. There are two dimensions to this criticism. First, content research tends to focus on manifest or overt elements, things that are apparent, obvious and can be coded for and counted. This inevitably downplays the latent or covert elements. The part of a message or text that audiences have to decode is often not at all obvious (Hall, 1980 [1973]). Second (2004: 175), it is claimed that content research cannot distinguish between levels of meaning. Strinati notes that: 'This criticism owes much to other theories such as semiology and Marxism which argue there are covert or hidden levels of meaning which lie behind and give rise to the overt or superficial meanings which content research deals with'. This means that the approach may capture an aspect of something (e.g., the increasing number of female newsreaders) while missing a more important counter-tendency (e.g., the increased use of stereotypically attractive newsreaders). However, content research can be very sophisticated and, as noted above, can and should be aligned with some theoretically-informed hypothesis.

3. **Content research is merely descriptive**: This criticism follows on from those made above. It follows that because content research is (1) atheoretical and (2) blind to covert elements, then it cannot hope to explain social relations but merely to describe them. This seems overly harsh and is based on a confusion of the roles of theory and method. Even if we accept the above criticisms, it seems misguided to require that content research (or any other approach or method) should be able to explain social relations or wider society. There are some approaches, predominantly case-centric ones such as life history research (see Chapter 3) or ethnographic research (see Chapter 4) that provide very rich accounts, using many variables, that border on explaining a life or a group in its total. But even in these examples, the role of method, of data collection and analysis are guided by theoretical and epistemological assumptions. Even the most positivist champions of content research make modest claims about the capacity of the approach to make inferences from messages. In short, this criticism of the approach is unfair and unsound.

PRACTICE POINT 8

Content research can be criticised for being atheoretical and 'thin' in its numerical analysis of data, and merely descriptive. However, the approach is a cost-effective way of generating data as long as its limitations are understood.

CONCLUSION

Content research is an approach that collects and analyses data from messages. It involves identifying patterns and interpreting what is being communicated by authors or speakers in messages to their audiences. These messages once primarily consisted of newspapers, books and political speeches, but are now increasing communicated through broadcasting and in digital forms.

Content research was a technique used by 'muckraking journalists' to demonstrate bias in news coverage and editorials. It allows the distillation of observations about the printed or spoken word into numbers or other forms of notations.

As a variable-centric approach, hypothesis-testing is a key feature. This involves converting an idea into a series of propositions, developing mutually exclusive and collectively exhaustive values. To some extent, determining what makes a case is a secondary (though essential) concern.

There are several ways in which cases can be constructed. These include focusing on individual authors as cases; using the physical separation of cases (e.g., book chapters) or temporal separation of cases (e.g., the time-defined slots for TV advertisements); or using themes to determine cases (assuming that there are themes or propositions in the messages and making these the focus of attention).

Coding is the process in which an observer (the coder) completes a coding form while observing some predetermined event. For content research the measurement of reliability focuses on inter-coder reliability – the degree to which coders agree. Krippendorff (2004) suggests three levels of confidence about reliability: stability, reproducibility and accuracy. There are no statistical tests that can guarantee validity, but there are weaker 'tests' that can provide some confidence about validity: reliability or external validity, internal validity, content or construct validity, face or instrumental validity and peer validity.

Content research has one particular benefit for emergent researchers in that carefully following the instructions found in a variety of textbooks can generate useful data. This isn't to say that content research is easy, but it is conceptually and logically straightforward. Further, content research has the benefit for the emergent researcher of not requiring a thorough grasp of the grammatical requirements in order to decode/deconstruct a text, and it is flexible. If your interest is primarily on the manifest or overt aspects of messages/texts in visual or physical media, then the approach is very attractive. Because it can be undertaken in scaled-down format (relying on the lone researcher), it is an ideal platform for the empirical component of dissertations or theses across the social sciences.

FURTHER READINGS

The textbooks by Klaus Krippendorff (2004) and Kimberly Neuendorf (2002) are comprehensive. The Neuendorf reader has a very useful, open-access companion website at: http://academic.csuohio.edu/kneuendorf/content/resources/car.htm. This provides links to other content research websites and related articles.

The textbook by Berelson (1952) was one of the first in the field. It has none of the technical material about reliability, validity, sampling, etc., but is a far more enjoyable read than many comprehensive and 'up-to-date' textbooks. Berelson focuses on the logic of content research and combines this with an easy writing style.

REFERENCES

Babbie, E. R. 1979. Content analysis and the analysis of existing data. *The practice of social research*. Belmont, CA: Wadsworth.

Bagdikian, B. 2000. *The media monopoly*. Boston, MA: Beacon Press.

Berelson, B. 1952. Content analysis in communication research. New York: The Free Press.

Best, J. 1987. Rhetoric in claims-making: Constructing the missing children problem. *Social Problems*, 32, 101–121.

Catanescu, C. & Tom, G. 2001. Types of humor in television and magazine advertising. *Review of Business*, 22, 92–96.

Friedan, B. 1963. *The feminine mystique*. Harmondsworth: Penguin.

Hall, S. (1980 [1973]). Encoding/decoding. In: Hall, S., Hobson, D., Lowe, A. & Willis, P. (eds.) *Culture, media, language*. London: Hutchinson.

Krippendorff, K. 2004 [1980]. *Content analysis: An introduction to its methodology*. Thousand Oaks, CA: Sage. (Originally published 1980).

Neuendorf, K. 2002. *The content analysis guidebook*. Thousand Oaks, CA: Sage.

Oakley, A. 1998. Gender, methodology and people's ways of knowing: Some problems with feminism and the paradigm debate in social science. *Sociology*, 32, 707–731.

Saskatchewan Education InstructionaL Resources Unit 1996. Planning in the dance strand.

Strinati, D. 2004. *An introduction to theories of popular culture*. London: Routledge.

TEN

SECONDARY RESEARCH – MORE THAN LITERATURE REVIEWS

CONTENTS LIST

Key words: secondary research – literature review – search engines – Boolean – Google – meta-analysis – quality checks

SUMMARY

An outline of the importance of secondary research as the platform for science, considering the issue of quality assurance and the practical aspects of using search engines and meta-analysis.

The previous chapter, Content Research, discussed an approach centred on the examination of messages, gleaned from written and audio-visual sources such as newspapers and public speeches. Secondary research involves the collection and analysis of a different type of message: academic writing. It is closely linked to documentary research and the literature review.

In this chapter we discuss the importance of secondary research as the platform for science. Secondary research deals with what has gone before in science and the social sciences, and it constitutes the logical starting point for emergent researchers. Although the approach may at first look very different from other variable-centric approaches, the principles of variable-centric, variable-first research remain the same. A researcher begins with an insight or observation about the social world. This observation is transformed into variables which guide the choice of literature that is examined.

Social science is always conducted in terms of distinct goals: researchers do research for a specific reason. In regards to secondary research, this entails finding gaps in and running with or against the literature to understand what is currently known about the topic at hand and to assess the quality of the material available. We discuss the issue of quality assurance, which is paramount for secondary researchers; the critical assessment of material is a vital component, but one which emergent researchers sometimes overlook or struggle with.

We include the practical aspects of using search engines to examine online holdings – this entails Boolean and Google queries. We also précis the meta-analysis – a process that goes beyond the literature review to collect and synthesise results from studies to develop an overall finding.

DOING DATA COLLECTION AND ANALYSIS

Secondary research is an approach that collects and analyses data sourced from the writings of social scientists and other authors. Secondary research often takes the form of a literature review (Becker, 2007) or as a means of triangulating or verifying other research (see Chapter 3, Life Histories). Secondary research accesses data that is physically located in libraries, archives and other public and private collections while an ever increasing share of knowledge is found online on the internet, in local area networks (LAN) and on stand-alone databases.

PRACTICE POINT 1

Secondary research is an approach that collects and analyses data sourced from the writings of social scientists and other authors. It is sometimes called a literature review.

The technologies or media for storing and retrieving data are diverse and can be bewildering for researchers. It is unlikely that any researcher could hope to search all databases. Nevertheless it is possible to conduct secondary research across physical and online databases and to be confident about the results. In this respect, the most important aspects of secondary research are (1) developing strategies or searches to collect data, and (2) developing strategies to analyse the findings, in particular to contextualise the data. In both examples, knowing as much as possible about the relevant database(s), the rules underlying its organisation and the techniques for searching are immensely helpful. We strongly recommend that one of the first things an emergent researcher does when starting secondary research is to ask their librarians for help. Librarians are experts in both physical and online holdings and combine an appreciation of the contents and expert knowledge in how to access the data.

PRACTICE POINT 2

One of the first things anyone starting secondary research should do is 'ask a librarian'.

Origins of the approach

Secondary research is the bedrock of western science. Isaac Newton famously talked of 'dwarfs standing on the shoulders of giants' in this regard. Because secondary research, often called a literature review, deals with what has gone before in science and the social sciences, it constitutes the logical and pedagogic starting point for emergent researchers.

Secondary research is a subset of what some textbooks designate as 'documentary research' (see the comprehensive four-volume set edited by John Scott, 2006a). Documentary research is broader than secondary research in one respect: it involves both the public and private worlds of writing. For example, in his introduction Scott (2006b) divides researching documents into three branches looking at:

1. [Private world documents of] personal documents (autobiographies, letters and photographs).

2. Published sources, the mass media and cyber documents.

3. Official records, reports and statistics.

We think the distinction between public and private worlds is an important one and in this chapter we focus on the former. We regard secondary research as mainly about the latter two types mentioned by Scott (2006b) (i.e., published sources and official records). We include a discussion of the private world of personal documents in our chapter on autoethnographic approaches (Chapter 12). Also, we wish to focus on using written documents as opposed to photographs, postcards, mementos, etc., which are more often simply 'found' in the public domain (e.g., studying artefacts – material traces, see Chapter 8 on unobtrusive research). Documentary research is narrower than secondary research in that it typically deals with physical documents rather than online materials.

Search engines

Online holdings and queries are probably where most emergent researchers will start. In this respect secondary research can be erudite and lead the researcher into unexpected domains, but it is also a common everyday activity. Most readers will be familiar with secondary research through doing online searches.

Online queries use search engines, which appeared first in 1993, just after it became impossible to comprehensively map the distribution and content of the internet. Early successes were Lycos and WebCrawler. The name of the latter gives a good idea of how search engines work; they crawl across the internet and operationalise a search algorithm seeking out the words entered into the initial query. In the majority of queries search engines refer to records of previous searches and report on that. So when a search engine reports back there are normally two components – a link to a live website and a cached/familiar site. The cache is the copy of the website the search engine recorded at some earlier point. Often there will be a difference between the cached website and the newer, live website. Minimising this difference is one of the biggest challenges for search engine designers.

The distinction between live websites and caches is presented here to underline that all search engines are imperfect and have limitations in their design. This problem also confronts researchers in the world of libraries, archives, etc. It is extremely unlikely that any one technique for searching will be sufficient in either online or physical contexts. This isn't a decisive problem in so far as the emergent researcher is aware of it and uses the most appropriate combination of techniques.

Search engines Yahoo, Bing and Google provide annual lists of the most popular searches. These show that mainstream search engines are most often used to find out about celebrities (especially recently deceased or disgraced ones), youth-focused movies and games, social networking sites, and an increasing number of queries about non-English search engines. You can enter 'most popular searches' into your preferred search engine and see what pops up.

The focus on popular culture indicates that Google etc. weren't designed for academic research but to facilitate everyday use of the internet in lieu of any systematic classification of its content (although at the time of writing Google and its main competitors do offer more academic, focused search engines). One of the reasons for the appeal of Google and its competitors is that the algorithm used in their search engines includes a component that selects for and reports back on 'popularity'. Popularity is measured in terms of hypertext links pointing to websites and the number of times websites are visited. The owners of search engines keep their search algorithms secret, which means it is impossible to tell what the overall influence is for reporting back on sponsored websites (i.e., the owners of websites pay the owners of search engines to highlight their sites) or on not reporting back on websites sponsored by their competitors, or on websites barred by various government agencies (e.g., websites deemed subversive or offensive by the government of the jurisdiction from which the search is instigated).

The search engines most available on our computers and mobile devices are designed to be user-friendly, if not too sophisticated. In most examples queries are handled as key word searches, so if you type in the phrase 'Why do people use public transport?' the algorithm that organises the search is able to pick 'public transport' as the key and base its search around that. Most of the more popular search engines can also identify questions by the use of why, what, where, etc. in the query and point to webpages with model answers. On the other hand, if the phrase is bracketed or placed in quote marks (" ") most search engines will attempt to find exact matches. The use of quote marks tends to focus and reduce the number of hits to any query.

Search engines also support functions to improve searches. The easiest of these are wildcards. You can enter 'using wildcards' into your search engine to get the specifics, but generally an asterisk (*) operates as a wildcard. (Please note that at the time of writing Google was very poor in allowing the use of wildcards). Wildcards can be substituted for a letter in a query. This allows for alternative spellings. The use of a wildcard at the end of word means most algorithms will search for all possible spellings of the word from the point where the asterisk* is inserted. A search for 'scien*' will throw up results for science, sciences, scientific, scientism, scientist and others, and will probably include close matches for terms like scene and scenic. Finally, a wildcard can be used as a substitute for an entire word. If the query 'Why do people use public transport?' is changed to 'Why do people use public *?' most search engines will conduct a key word search focusing on the phrase 'public *' – in other words, public something. This is likely to include hits on public baby-changing rooms, public libraries, public roads, public static (a programming rule) and many others as well as public transport. It is possible to use more than one wildcard in any query but as the number increases the accuracy and significance of the search results diminish.

Search engines are a reasonable and convenient starting point for much secondary research. What is crucial is to know the limitations of commercial software, how best to use it, and be able to identify alternative techniques. Emergent researchers will be well served if they start with Google but then move beyond it.

PRACTICE POINT 3

Mainstream search engines are a reasonable place to start secondary research. Emergent researchers need to be aware of the limits of this commercial software and be able to move beyond them.

Boolean searches

Searching the internet, local area networks (LAN) and stand-alone or subscription databases can be greatly enhanced by an appreciation of Boolean strategies. Boolean refers to the use of the conjunctions AND, OR and NOT in joining searched terms for the purpose of improving a query. The logic of Boolean searches – of broadening, narrowing and excluding what is searched for – applies more generally to all forms of research.

Boolean searching can be used on Google and most of its competitors, although the precise rules differ. Try typing in 'Boolean searches on [name of search engine]' to find out the rules. Boolean searching is also the most common and effective way of refining searches for specialist search engines. Greg Notess (2009) provides a nice table showing how Boolean algebra can be adapted for use on Google (Table 10.1).

Table 10.1 shows the notation of conducting a search for the terms 'A' and 'B' and using the conjunctions AND, OR and NOT. For example, say you were interested in black cats. Thus 'black' can be term A, and 'cats' can be term B. If you wanted to write a Boolean search you would have to type in black AND cats. The search engine would then report back only on those websites (or documents in a database) that included both terms. However, if you typed black OR cats the search engine would report back on a far bigger number of websites that include either term as well as both terms. You might get referrals to a wiki article on the

TABLE 10.1 Boolean algebra adapted for Google

Boolean	*Google*
A AND B	A B
A OR B	A OR B
A NOT B	A – B

TABLE 10.2   Example search term options

Query	Boolean	Venn diagram
black AND cats	A AND B	the area A n B
black OR cats	A OR B	the area A u B
black NOT cats	A NOT B	the area A\B
cats NOT black	B NOT A	area B\A

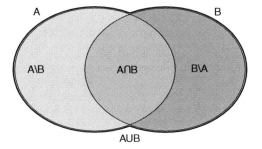

FIGURE 10.1   Venn diagram of search term options

colour black, websites about the 2005 movie *Black*, the Black Sabbath official website and a host of references to cats, as well as to both black and cats. If you typed in black NOT cats the results would include all the references to black excluding all those about cats. If you typed in cats NOT black the results would include all the references to cats excluding all those about black.

These possible combinations can be shown using a Venn diagram. Venn diagrams use the notation n = AND, u = OR, \ = not. So the simple searches above for versions of black cats has the notation shown in Table 10.2.

These areas are shown in Figure 10.1.

Boolean algebra allows for the use of brackets which facilitates quite complicated search algorithms (similar to maths formulae). Using brackets means Boolean searching is more flexible than the workaround offered by Google, etc. Further, most secondary research is going to involve more complicated conjunctions and terms than 'black AND cats'. Notess (2009) provides some further combinations (see Table 10.3).

TABLE 10.3   Boolean and Google search formats

Boolean	Google
(a OR b) AND (c OR d)	a OR b c OR d
a AND (b OR c OR d)	a b OR c OR d
a AND (b OR c) AND d	a b OR c d
(a AND b) NOT (c OR d)	a b -c -d
(a AND b) OR (c AND d)	no known option

Hypothesis-testing

All this flexibility in designing and refining searches using commonsense and Boolean algebra has to have some point. Dropping terms and conjunctions at random into a search algorithm isn't the most effective way to do secondary research. The point is to uncover what social scientists and others have said before about a particular topic and variables, and like other variable-centric approaches a version of hypothesis-testing is the key to secondary research.

CONCEPTUAL CONCERN 1

Secondary research is a variable-centric approach. There are few variables and many cases. Often a hypothesis provides the formulation of a relationship between variables. The cases which researchers seek are earlier arguments and 'facts' found online or in libraries, etc.

Secondary research is effectively about hypothesis-testing. This may not be apparent as the approach looks very different from other variable-centric approaches, including conducting a survey, or content research or experimental research. But the principles of variable-centric, variable-first research remain the same. A researcher begins with an insight, suspicion or observation about some aspects of the social world. These aspects are transformed into variables with associated values in the process of developing and writing a hypothesis and then the researcher engages in the process of testing, which centres on finding a sufficient number of cases to make the results valid and reliable (see Chapter 1). In secondary research, the cases the researcher must find are physical or online documents and, more pertinently, the arguments they contain.

Secondary versus primary research

Secondary research has phases of data collection and data analysis. Data is collected and then analysed. This data/analysis two-step is common to all research. However, secondary research differs from primary research. Primary research means the collection of data for the first time or the transformation of raw data into new forms as a precursor of analysis. Indeed, all the other approaches covered in this textbook are forms of primary research. Secondary research does not generate new data or novel forms. It reuses or revisits the primary research of other research projects, most commonly in the form of a literature review (see below).

Primary research has two variants: interactive and non-interactive. The interactive is easy to grasp. It means the creation of data at the point of its collection. Interactive research requires exchanges between researcher and research participants in the process of collecting data. In-depth interviewing (Chapter 2), ethnography (Chapter 4) and surveys (Chapter 6) create situations, encounters and pose questions that would not exist otherwise. For example, unless a researcher is posing questions, most people do not spend their days telling strangers about their preferences for public transport, etc.

On the other hand, non-interactive research is usually primary research because the researcher substantially transforms the raw data. For example, unobtrusive research (Chapter 8), content research (Chapter 9), semiotic analysis (Chapter 11) and autoethnographic approaches (Chapter 12) are all primary research in that raw data and source materials (physical traces, media outputs, diaries, etc.) intended for one purpose or audience are systematically reworked and recreated by the researcher. This sort of primary research can transform data into forms that may be unimagined by their authors. Semiotic analysis (Chapter 11) provides a good example of non-interactive primary research, in which a photograph produced for one reason can be endlessly deconstructed by a researcher.

When primary researchers transform raw data such as photographs, or the patterns of wear on a carpet, or the content of diaries, they are using the images, material traces and written words in ways that were not thought of by the authors of these data (e.g., the photographer, the folk who walked across the carpet, the diarist). In contrast, secondary research tends to use the data it collects in ways that were imagined by their authors and – with scholarly articles or monographs – explicitly intended by them.

This is not to say that secondary research has no relationship with primary research. Often a variant is undertaken as a precursor to fieldwork. This isn't strictly speaking secondary research as the purpose is to inform the subsequent primary research rather than the literature review being research for its own sake. However, research prior to fieldwork is essential (notably the literature review). Prior research is probably the most important thing an emergent researcher can do to ensure that he or she does not look stupid in front of research participants or the rest of the research team. This sort of research generates findings such as 'Research participants will expect a small gift on first meeting with the research team'. A literature review is also the normal basis for developing hypotheses to be tested in the field.

PRACTICE POINT 4

Secondary research is a rare approach that does not undertake primary research, neither creating nor reconfiguration data. Instead it relies on previous research.

Finding gaps in, and running with or against the literature

Howard Becker's little masterpiece *Writing for social scientists: How to start and finish your thesis, book, or article*, first published in 1986 with a second edition in 2007, is a must-read for all emergent researchers. Becker provided the gold standard for a generation of scholars moving into independent research. Certainly, since Becker, almost every discussion of doing a literature review focuses on 'finding gaps', which is a dumbed-down version of what he said (we don't think he used this term). Becker's writing is nuanced and the dumbing-down of his writings is a salutary lesson to all emergent researchers: secondary and further reinterpretations of the 'classics' almost always miss the sophistication and complexity of the original.

There are very useful guides on literature reviews scattered across libraries and the internet. Many universities will have an online research site, as do some departments. Most commonly these discussions urge the emergent researcher to 'look for gaps in the literature'. It is unfortunate that a lot of this sage advice is left unread by its intended audience. We reproduce the following bullet points from the Deakin University (2010), *The literature review*:

> There are good reasons for spending time and effort on a review of the literature before embarking on a research project. These reasons include:
>
> * to identify gaps in the literature
> * to avoid reinventing the wheel (at the very least this will save time and it can stop you from making the same mistakes as others)
> * to carry on from where others have already reached (reviewing the field allows you to build on the platform of existing knowledge and ideas)
> * to identify other people working in the same fields (a researcher network is a valuable resource)
> * to increase your breadth of knowledge of your subject area
> * to identify seminal works in your area
> * to provide the intellectual context for your own work, enabling you to position your project relative to other work
> * to identify opposing views
> * to put your work into perspective
> * to demonstrate that you can access previous work in an area
> * to identify information and ideas that may be relevant to your project
> * to identify methods that could be relevant to your project.

In short, a 'finding the gaps' approach to secondary research has the dual benefits of avoiding duplication of other researchers' work while facilitating incremental improvements on it. More prosaically, it is impossible to be taken seriously in scholarly circles if a thesis, article, book or research project is not buttressed by a decent literature review.

However, it is important to note that finding the gaps is by no means a straightforward process. Becker stresses that 'the literature' (e.g., data sourced from the writings of social scientists and other authors) is produced in an antagonistic environment. This means that all arguments and presentations of 'facts and figures' are produced in an environment of disputation. All of the material generated and used by social scientists are truth-claims that are subject to challenge and dispute. This disputation may not be acknowledged explicitly but it is ever-present. The differences between epistemologies and goals of social research are identified above. These provide arenas for dispute. The realm of social theory is even more complex and fraught.

The gaps in the literature can be thought of as primarily theoretical or methodological. First, let's look at the theory. The aim here is to explore an under-theorised area of social life or to improve on outdated theories. This comprehensive secondary research often involves a discussion of various traditions or schools. Second, methodology. The aim here is finding ways of doing the research. This research can be undertaken to inform subsequent fieldwork. In many respects this is a broader brief than contextualising social theory, depending on whether the researcher wishes to replicate existing studies or use what might be novel methods in the exploration of a particular area of social life.

The process of looking for theoretical or methodological 'gaps' forces the emergent researcher to confront a literature that is structured by explicit and implicit disputes ranging across epistemology, research goals, theory and method. This antagonism is important. We augment the ubiquitous bullet points around doing a literature review (see above) while keeping this antagonistic environment in mind. Our focus is on the practical steps an emergent researcher can take:

- Identifying gaps in the literature requires an appreciation of context.

- An appreciation of context is easiest to achieve when the researcher understands his/her own position.

- An emergent researcher should begin with an interrogation of his/her position. Where does he/she stand in terms of epistemology, goals of research, theoretical understandings and methodological preferences? (One way of thinking about this is that when a researcher is able to elucidate and justify his/her own position, he/she is demonstrating an understanding of context and an appreciation of any gaps in the literature.)

- Contextualising the literature is primarily about agreeing or disagreeing with the material uncovered. This means researchers will inevitably run with or run against the tenets of an argument, presentation of facts, etc.

- Running with and running against are both potentially useful. The former provides a platform for applying a theory to a new area, or incremental improvement, or as evidence for a novel position. The latter is probably more interesting in that by providing the basis for debate it opens up more possibilities for research.

- There are two key resources that are particularly useful at the beginning of secondary research: overviews and classic texts.

- Finding overviews provides ways into understanding how the literature is structured. Overviews used to be the domain of review articles in journals and introductory textbooks.

- Overviews generally provide references to the classic texts. These are foundational writings that may have started a debate or school of thought. The classic texts are the touchstones of later work and are usually pointed to in the references of later writings. A search of articles by references alone can throw up pointers to the classic texts.

- Emergent researchers should use mainstream search engines to begin their exploration. These searches can be very useful in identifying introductory texts or overviews.

- However, the best secondary resources are not readily available on the internet but are located behind portals. These are portals into local area networks (LAN), subscription-based databases and all the holdings of libraries and archives. In order to best use portals, emergent researchers should always ask a librarian about their research. Doing so is likely to provide massive shortcuts both in locating data and in analysing it.

PRACTICE POINT 5

Finding gaps in the literature is a key to secondary research. It is equally important to use the research process to develop your own scholarly position.

Meta-analyses: combining and testing results

A meta-analysis collects and synthesises results from previous research and calculates overall effects. It goes beyond the parameters of a literature review, which assesses existing literature, to actually perform calculations based on the results collated, thereby coming up with new results. It therefore has the potential to be extremely powerful, though carefully evaluating the quality of the studies included and making adjustments if necessary are absolutely essential.

Briefly, the process of meta-analysis involves:

- deciding on outcome variables
- conducting literature searches
- assessing the material found, using best practice
- coding the variables in the suitable material
- calculating overall effects.

We will use the example of Anderson and colleagues' work on the effects of violent video games to work through this process (Anderson et al., 2010).

Deciding on outcome variables: Anderson and colleagues focused on six outcome variables used in previous research on the topic. These were: physically aggressive behaviour, aggressive cognition (thoughts), aggressive affect (mood), physiological arousal (increased heart rate, blood pressure, etc.), prosocial (helping) behaviour and empathy/desensitisation.

Conducting literature searches: Two key academic online databases were searched for relevant material, PsycINFO and MEDLINE, using the terms (video* OR computer OR arcade); (game*); (attack* OR fight* OR aggress* OR violen* OR hostil* OR ang* OR arous* OR prosocial OR help* OR desens* OR empathy), as well as a search for Japanese material. (We are somewhat surprised that they did not include 'pro-social' in their search, as the hyphenated term seems fairly common.) Anderson and colleagues also searched the reference sections of previous reviews, and included dissertations, book chapters and unpublished papers, *and* contacted published authors to see if they had other work that had not been published. This last point is important. In order to avoid publication bias, researchers must conduct a search that is thorough, systematic, unbiased and well documented. This requires striving to include all material that meets the criteria for inclusion regardless of format. By not including all available material in the initial assessment, the researcher risks missing important work that has not been published in the usual academic sources, for example, reports prepared for government departments, or graduate dissertations that are not submitted for publication for various reasons but nonetheless contain important findings that may be at odds with published material (see Duval and Tweedie, 2000, for a discussion of publication bias and its avoidance). Anderson and colleagues retrieved 130 items that included a total of 130,000 participants. This gives us an indication of the potential power of the meta-analysis.

Assessing the material found, using best practice: The next step was to assess the material gathered. A number of the studies had methodological weaknesses, or were not appropriate for inclusion, such as not differentiating between violent and non-violent video games. Anderson and colleagues elected to include only studies that reflected best practice. Their article details the best practice inclusion criteria they developed, along with examples of criterion violations. We will not include all the criteria here in the interests of space, but it consisted of items such as 'The compared levels of the independent variable were appropriate for testing the hypothesis' and 'The independent variable was properly operationalized' (Anderson et al., 2010: 159).

Coding the variables in the suitable material and calculating overall effects: At this point coding and statistical analysis was undertaken of the collected data, beginning with the calculation of effect size. We will not go into the intricacies of these calculations here – this is, after all, a text for emergent researchers and although these calculations are not particularly difficult, they do require some specific knowledge of statistics. Rather, our purpose is to introduce you to the key elements of the approach and to encourage you to study a little further, or make friends with a slightly more experienced researcher if you wish to pursue this further.

The effects of violent video games are the topic of some debate among the general public. We have enjoyed reading student essays that have argued that playing violent video games is a harmless pastime (we suspect these students are game-players), and other essays that argue the opposite. Based on the work of Anderson and colleagues, and others (see Kassin et al., 2008, for a further discussion) it would appear that the secondary research techniques of those who found the playing of violent video games to be harmful are correct. Anderson and colleagues found that exposure to violent video games is significantly related to increases in aggressive behaviour, aggressive thoughts, aggressive mood, and to a lack of empathy and a lack of prosocial behaviour. This fits with Bushman and Huesmann (2001) finding that the link between media violence (which also includes television and movie violence) and aggression is almost as strong as the link between cigarette smoking and lung cancer.

The variable-centric, hypothesis-testing nature of this form of secondary research should be obvious. Meta-analyses usually have a fixed frame in so far as once the variables to be analysed are decided upon, searches undertaken and analysis begun, it is likely to be problematic to change those variables – or at least it will result in a lot of extra work. However, it is certainly possible to add more variables, and in fact this may be desirable if it is found that the initial scope of the project is too narrow.

SOME ISSUES IN RESEARCH

In this section we apply the three epistemological positions we have discussed throughout this textbook to secondary research. Each of these epistemologies carries with it a set of political assumptions about what does and does not constitute science. These assumptions will influence the researcher's assessment of material.

Epistemology and goals of social research

Gaining an appreciation of the literature and the context in which documents are produced is a difficult task. Emergent researchers may well be more savvy about the techniques of online or archival searches than their supervisors or colleagues but often don't have as great an understanding of the relevant literatures. Becker discusses how researchers can be terrorised by the literature (2007 [1986]). We suggest that one way of gaining insights into social theory and methodology, the arguments and presentations of facts uncovered by secondary research, is to have an appreciation of the issues of epistemology (Hindess, 1973) and the goals of social research (Ragin, 1994). Every article, book or table of data produced within the social sciences or of interest to social scientists was done so within an epistemological position and for a purpose. Epistemology refers to the theory of knowledge that informs how research is shaped in its broadest sense (see Chapter 1). Often the epistemology and goals are not made explicit and are buried beneath levels of assumption and bias that even the authors may not be aware of. However, spending a little time considering both is a useful way to start unpacking the material thrown up by secondary research.

Many scholars argue that epistemology influences the nature and focus of arguments in the social sciences. Some have tried to show, with mixed success, that epistemology determines methodology. For example, Blaikie (2007) identifies six epistemological positions and four 'logics of inquiry' that are nested across and within them. Our approach is a more modest three epistemologies (that we have taken from the material covered by Engeström (2000)). Rather than seeing epistemology as determining research, we think it informs it. This is a looser connection than that taken by Blaikie. The three epistemological positions outlined in this textbook have differing approaches to doing social science and what might be considered scientific (see Chapter 1). In each case these are political as well as philosophical positions:

1. **Positivism**. Positivists have the greatest confidence in the ability of social scientists to reveal the truth. They argue that social reality exists independently of our perceptions of it. Positivists stress the techniques of observation and measurement and the potential for scientists to form objective/unbiased understandings of the social world. This is an important political statement in the broadest sense (even though positivists often seem reluctant to accept it as such), and as a result positivism is commonly accused of ignoring issues like power and cultural relativism as determinants of what is accepted as good science. Instead, positivists spend most of their time perfecting a narrow methodology, as if it existed independently of the social world it aims to explore. They are highly critical of approaches that, among other things, adopt fluid framings of research and use iterative approaches to refine data collection and analysis. For example, a positivist is unlikely to accept participant observation or unstructured interviewing as good science, regardless of its context.

2. **Social realism**. Social realists also believe in an external and measurable social reality, but one that exists through the mediation of our perceptions of it and our actions. Social realists argue that revealing the social world is far more problematic than suggested by positivists. For social realists, doing science is a legitimate goal, but it is understood as a project that is limited by factors that social scientists have great difficulty in controlling for or being objective about. Where positivists strive for objectivity, social realists emphasise subjectivity and the appreciation of factors like power, meaning and the need for researcher reflexivity (or self-awareness). Any search for truth is always clouded by, among other things, the ways in which researchers and institutions

impose bias. Controlling for institutional and researcher bias becomes an important component of socialist realist efforts at doing science, whereas positivists, in their narrow focus on methods, tend to discount these political underpinnings of science.

3. **Social constructivism.** Social constructivists take the political-philosophical criticism of positivism further than their social realist colleagues, to the point where it challenges the notion of science as a legitimate concept. They don't accept social reality as an independent phenomenon, or straightforward ideas of truth or science. They have no faith in science as a project that generates anything resembling universal rules, laws or theorems. Social constructivists believe it is impossible to differentiate truth-claims based in social science, or folklore, or commonsense, or metaphysics because individuals or actors create the social world and at the same time all the possible measures of that social world. They argue that it is impossible to have a scientific stance – meaning an objective position outside the data and its analysis (if you are a positivist), or to control/filter the subject effects of power, meaning and bias (if you are a social realist).

These epistemologies are not just abstract notions in so far as each carries with it a set of political assumptions about what does and does not constitute doing (social) science. The epistemologies are antagonistic and as a result the social sciences are occasionally dominated by what some authors have called 'science wars', for example, debates regarding the status of feminist and radical scholarship in the 1970s (Oakley, 1998) and, more recently, of postmodernity (Matthewman and Hoey, 2006). Even in times of relative peace, arguments about epistemology are just as likely to shape what gets published in academic journals as those of social theory or method.

We believe that different sets of arguments or, to use Ragin's (1994) phrasing, 'goals of social research' are more likely to be expressed within different epistemologies. Ragin argues that social science is always conducted in terms of distinct goals, that is, researchers do research for a specific reason (Curtis, 2007). Ragin identifies six goals:

1. **Identifying patterns:** The first goal involves research where the aim is to measure social relations or phenomena. This form of research tends to focus on the behaviours, attitudes and beliefs of the general population or some designated sub-group. Such research is often undertaken at the behest of agencies of government or corporate sponsors (e.g., on ways of travelling to work).

2. **Making predictions:** This is closely linked to the first goal and involves the extrapolation of identified trends (e.g., on predicting the winner of an election). The results of the first and second goals of social research are often used to inform the policies of sponsoring organisations.

3. **Testing theories:** This centres on versions of hypothesis-testing (e.g., on the hypothesis that decriminalising marijuana will result in reduced anti-social

behaviour). The impact of theory testing is almost always incremental to social theory (as opposed to providing a paradigmatic shift in scholarly opinion).

4. **Developing theories:** This goal moves beyond the more conservative conventions of testing social theory. It challenges existing social theory and advances alternative perspectives (e.g., the notion that some powerful transnational corporations have a vested interest in advancing or checking the debates around global warming).

5. **Interpreting events:** Just as testing theory (goal 3) and advancing theory (goal 4) differ in that the latter is inherently more radical or challenging to prevailing assumptions, a focus on interpreting events also moves beyond simply identifying patterns (goal 1). Identifying patterns is useful for finding out what is typical and normal. Interpreting events tends to focus on happenings or sets of behaviours that are not assumed to be normal and may indeed be highly atypical (e.g., on the psychology of serial killers).

6. **Giving voice:** This goal of social research moves even further from the normative or socially conservative assumptions associated with the first three goals. Giving voice includes the task of advocacy (including being 'biased' in reporting). Its mission is of representing the margins of society and of taking the part of outsiders or excluded groups.

We think it is useful to chart the patterns between the six goals of social research and the epistemologies that inform them. We argue that there is indeed a pattern here, that the more conservative goals of research (goals 1, 2, 3) tend to cluster around the more conservative epistemological framing of science (primarily positivism). Similarly, the more radical goals of research (goals 4, 5, 6) tend to cluster around the more radical epistemologies of social realism and social constructivism.

CONCEPTUAL CONCERN 2

All of the literature, the subject matter of secondary research, is authored in an antagonistic environment. Authors inevitably contest the truth-claims of their contemporaries and predecessors. These conflicts pertain at every level: epistemology, goals of research, theory and methodology. This can make the process of engaging with the literature fraught for the emergent researcher.

This relationship is a pattern, a correlation only. It does not suggest the determination of research goal by epistemology or vice versa. It is logically possible for any combination to exist. For example, a proponent of positivist science may indeed want to give voice to marginal peoples. However, this is not a good practical

TABLE 10.4 Correlations between epistemology and goals of social research

	Positivism	*Social realism*	*Social constructivism*
Identifying patterns	Usual	Occasional	Unusual
Making predictions	Usual	Occasional	Unusual
Testing theories	Usual	Usual	Unusual
Developing theories	Occasional	Usual	Usual
Interpreting events	Unusual	Usual	Usual
Giving voice	Unusual	Usual	Usual

fit because the positivist emphasis on developing objective and unbiased under-standings of the social world (and therefore foregrounding issues of rigour and validity and sampling, etc.) is not conducive to gaining understandings of members of oppressed, or small, or outlier groups. Rather, an ethnographic approach is probably needed (see Chapter 4). The practical steps required to ensure that the requirements of positivist science are met, including using structured interviewing and an objective stance, are not the tools a researcher would normally choose to talk with rough sleepers or methamphetamine users or neo-Nazis. On the other hand, it is difficult to see how a champion of social constructivism could set about identifying patterns using the tried-and-true techniques like a large-scale survey (see Chapter 6). Perhaps as a result of this sort of disconnect between goal and epistemology, techniques such as semiotic analysis and deconstruction have enjoyed an upswing in popularity, precisely because they allow social constructivists the opportunity to comment on behaviours, attitudes and beliefs of the general population without having to engage in forms of positivism (see Chapter 1).

Table 10.4 is intended as a starting point only for contextualising the findings of secondary research. Emergent researchers are encouraged to ask questions such as 'What is the goal of this research, article, report, etc.?' and 'What is the epistemology of the author?'

PRACTICE POINT 6

Understanding the sometimes explicit but more often than not implicit epistemology and goals of research is a very useful way of contextualising research. These two dimensions are present in every piece of writing. They can provide a way into understanding an article or presentation of facts.

PUTTING THE APPROACH IN CONTEXT

Secondary research is a variable-centric approach and ultimately a form of hypothesis-testing. The researcher starts with a combination of relatively few variables and seeks a sufficient number of cases to test an argument. We have noted that hypothesis-testing, which is the core of this approach, can take a number of forms ranging across research prior to fieldwork, research informing fieldwork and what we designated as comprehensive secondary research. The last variant eschews all forms of primary research.

For example, Steven Seidman (1994) provides a wonderful account of the rise of feminist social theory and the continuities and breaks between liberal, socialist, radical and postmodern feminists. He does so purely through secondary research. We could argue that Seidman is providing evidence for a hypothesis that social movements like feminism have their origins in the rapid transformation of the social world. He starts by noting that the contemporary women's movement developed in response in post-second World War America. He then goes on to note the main strands of feminism (liberal, radical, socialist and postmodernist variants) and their major theorists. Seidman argues in his preface that the major variables affecting the women's movement were the natural and social aspects of gender, gender as a form of explanation for behaviour, the origin of male dominance, the relations between private and public worlds, the nature of domination and resistance (Seidman, 1994). He generates a powerful account solely from the literature, while providing exactly the sort of overview emergent researchers should seek in their own research (see above).

Most variable-centric approaches are associated with fixed framings of research. This means the process of research is strictly sequential and there is little chance to move between data collection and analysis in order to improve on the hypothesis being tested, for example. Large-scale survey research is probably the most fixed in its framing in that once a questionnaire has been implemented there is no real opportunity to go back and revise the decisions made regarding the hypothesis, or variables and values, or questions, etc. However, true secondary research (at least) has a fluid framing. There is plenty of scope for the research to move between data collection and analysis. This is because the approach is focused in the literature exclusively and does not involve primary research at all. The partial exception to this is meta-analysis, discussed above.

CONCEPTUAL CONCERN 3

Unlike most variable-centric, variable-first approaches, secondary research enjoys a fluid framing of research. This fluidity is the result of an absolute reliance on the writings of social scientists and other authors. It frees the secondary research from the need for strict sequential steps in collecting and then analysing data.

This fluid framing is a major draw card for emergent researchers. While it doesn't free them from the constraints imposed by deadlines and resourcing and supervisors, it does allow mistakes made in designing a hypothesis or query to be easily rectified or approached iteratively. Of course, where secondary research is being undertaken as a precursor to fieldwork or primary research the demands of sequential decision-making of fixed framings are reintroduced.

PRACTICE POINT 7

Because of its fluid framing it is relatively easy to move from data collection to analysis and vice versa when doing secondary research. This helps make the approach attractive to emergent researchers as a hypothesis or search strategy can be improved on an iterative basis.

Issues in quality assurance

The internet, particularly the Web 2.0 version (post-2004), and related mobile technologies have transformed data creation, storage and retrieval. Abbott (1998) talks about an information overload and the challenges and opportunities it poses for librarians. Abbott draws attention to both the massive influx of data resulting from the internet and the ongoing absence of protocols for storing and accessing holdings. More than a decade later, the internet remains a chaotic place for any emergent researcher and the chief challenge is that of assessing quality or quality assurance.

Twenty years ago secondary research meant working in libraries and archives, reading material printed on paper and taking notes with a pen. The issue of quality assurance was resolved primarily through a reliance on peer review. Researchers could be fairly confident that the journals and monographs they were accessing had been subjected to scrutiny and approval by other academics. Non-scholarly material (archival holdings, reports and other publications) could be assessed by tried-and-true methods in the realm of documentary research (Scott, 2006a).

The problems of quality assurance in secondary research were considered more or less solved, certainly for scholars operating from a positivist epistemology. The rules of the academic game were well understood. Scholars wanting to advance their careers or gain credence as researchers abided by the norms of anonymous peer review, referencing protocols, codes of ethics, and acknowledged the all-important gatekeepers who edited journals or commissioned monographs. While there were some notable iconoclasts, the vast majority of academics and researchers abided by the rules of the game, regardless of their epistemological positions. This may well have been a grudging respect on the part of social realists and social constructivists, who saw in the norms of peer review and documentary research a massive potential for bias and for shutting out the voices of others. Nevertheless, the commonalities between academics in terms of their everyday practices in research and publishing should not be understated (Halsey, 1992)

The internet has made things more problematic. While peer-reviewed journals (most of which are now available online), monographs and forms of documentary research remain the bedrock of academic practice in the social sciences, the massive influx of data and of forms of publishing made possible by the internet have disturbed the rules of the game. For example, academics, who spend most of their time teaching the next generation of academics and researchers, are increasingly concerned with issues of plagiarism among their students. On the other hand, students and emergent researchers seem far less concerned with the strictures of referencing and plagiarism than their teachers and supervisors. We can understand this in part as a generational shift. Marshall McLuhan (1911–80) long ago noted that new technologies force new norms and patterns of behaviour in how people relate to each other (McLuhan, 1964).

From an epistemological point of view, the internet seemed to realise the hopes of social constructivists for an end to positivist stifling of other voices (e.g., women, youth, radicals, post-colonial peoples, to name a few). Certainly with blogging and social networking there are a lot of voices, and most of the primary research approaches are realigning themselves to take advantage of this. For example, Don Dillman's essential textbook, *Mail and telephone surveys: The total design method* (1978), has become *Mail and internet surveys: The tailored design method: With new internet, visual, and mixed-mode guide* (Dillman, 2007) (see Chapter 6). In secondary research (i.e., the approach that collects and analyses data sourced from the writings of social scientists and other authors) there appears to be something of a lag. The positivist and social realist concerns about what constitutes doing science or good science remain in play. There is a definite reluctance to accept all internet-mediated authors as 'equal'.

CONCEPTUAL CONCERN 4

The development of the internet and mobile, digital technologies seems to provide a realisation of the hopes of social constructivists for all voices to be heard. However, the problem of quality assurance remains and is made more central by the mass of online data and fora. From the perspective of the social sciences as a profession, not all voices are treated equally and it is crucial for emergent researchers to continue to play the academic 'game' of referencing, peer review and 'good science'.

Regardless of generational and epistemological divides, the issue of quality assurance is paramount for secondary researchers. Four dimensions of quality described by Scott (2006c) are oriented to documents and the offline-world (see below). They are a touchstone for secondary research, where the focus is the arguments conveyed by online and offline 'documents':

1. **Meaning: literal and interpretative understanding**. Most documentarians rely on hermeneutics to gain an understanding of documents. Hermeneutics is a process that tries to understand the concepts underlying the production of texts through successive approximations which start with trying to interpret the worldview of the author. This is a literary concern rather than a social sciences one (although there is some overlap with semiotics – see Chapter 11). Further documentarians are interested in historical or private documents, and hermeneutics is the process by which they undertake primary research. Secondary researchers are typically more interested in contemporary and public debate and (as noted above) the approach does not generate new data or novel forms. Nevertheless three moments identified by Scott (2006c) in the movement of the text from author to audience are pertinent to achieving a nuanced reading:

   • Intended content is the meaning the author intended to convey to an audience.

   • Received content is the meaning constructed by the actual audience(s).

   • Internal or interpretative content are the multiple meanings that can be constructed by possible audiences. Studying interpretative content or internal meaning is the domain of content research (Chapter 9) and semiotic analysis (Chapter 11).

2. **Authenticity: soundness and authorship**. This dimension relates to whether a document is what it purports to be. For documentarians this revolves around whether the text is an original or a copy, and how to deal with errors that occur through copying. For secondary researchers, copying is an important issue. Digital texts and the ability to cut and paste means that mistakes can be spread across the internet very quickly and in part because the main search engines are skewed towards reporting on popularity. The internet is full of forgeries and bad science. Determining the soundness and authorship of the literature is important. Emergent researchers should treat with utmost suspicion any argument or presentation of facts where authorship is ambiguous or anonymous. And, where authorship is attributed it is always wise to double-check.

3. **Credibility: sincerity and accuracy**. This dimension acknowledges that all documents and the arguments they convey are authored in conditions that may be unknown to the reader. These conditions can affect credibility. This is much the same as saying that epistemological arguments are political as well as philosophical positions (see above). What documentarians identify as 'sincerity and accuracy' translate into explicit and implicit biases for secondary researchers. All authors have biases. These range from (1) scholarly concerns around epistemology, social theory and methodology to (2) practical constraints around implementing policy, protecting personal and institutional reputations, intellectual property and copyright, and (3) self-interest and outright prejudice. Emergent researchers must be aware that biases are both explicit (stated in the argument) and, more often, implicit (and unstated).

4. **Representativeness: survival and availability**. Scott makes the point that in order to survive and be available for analysis a document has to be deposited or held somewhere. This issue of representativeness is a defining issue for historians and for practitioners of autoethnographic approaches (see Chapter 12). Even with an excess of one hundred million websites on the internet and still larger holdings located in libraries, archives and other institutions, representativeness remains an issue. The central question that secondary researchers must address isn't so much 'How representative is this?' but its follow-up 'What is not represented here?' Whether it is within the context of a single document or across a particular literature, or in any representation of society or facet of life of interest to social scientists, emergent researchers should assume non-representation rather than representation. This is a more far-reaching concern than scholarly issues of credibility. The issue of representativeness reflects the patterning of power across the world (where an excess of one billion people go to sleep hungry each night) and where all but a small power-elite are in some way disadvantaged. The appropriate starting point of analysis is, then, that some ideas and voices will be systematically excluded. Emergent researchers should expect that revolutionary or radical positions are underrepresented, as are those which are held to be sacrilegious or distasteful, or simply those representing the views of the so-called 'silent majority'.

PRACTICE POINT 8

All of the literature has implicit, unstated assumptions and was authored in an antagonistic environment. The sensible starting point for all researchers confronting the literature is to be suspicious – to question what is presented and to expect bias, omissions and misrepresentation.

CONCLUSION

Gaining expertise in secondary research has a strong experiential component. This reflects the importance of gaining a comprehensive understanding of the literature(s) and developing and refining a personal perspective. There is no real short-cut to an immersion in the literature and self-reflection. Secondary research becomes easier and more effective with experience. It is a daunting task for any emergent research on first-time secondary researcher to confront a literature (i.e., all the data sourced from the writings of social scientists and other authors), and be asked to separate the wheat from the chaff.

We have offered some insights on how a search might be organised and some basics in starting analysis. All of these will be moderated by the substantive topic of the secondary research and the disciplinary focus being used. The good news for emergent researchers is that secondary research is a focused version of what at high school is called 'critical reading'. In *The complete idiot's guide to critical reading* (2005: 4) Amy Wall and Regina Wall describe it as:

> Critical reading is a way of looking at a book and analyzing what the author is saying and the methods the author is using to communicate a message or idea. Your analysis is complete when you have formed your own interpretation of the author's intentions.

This is good news because most emergent researchers will already have the basic skills from high school. The challenge is to upgrade these skills because secondary research is both a powerful research approach and it demands an engagement with the literature, the bedrock of academic life.

FURTHER READINGS

The four-volume set, *Documentary research*, edited by John Scott (2006a), contains considerable overlap with secondary research.

For readers who really want to go back to basics there is a wealth of high-school or junior college level material on critical reading. After all, the core of secondary research is a high level critical reading of the literature. *The complete idiot's guide to critical reading* by Wall and Wall (2005) is exactly that.

At the other end of the spectrum, many years ago Barry Hindess (1973) wrote a small monograph, *The use of official statistics in sociology*, in which he suggested that an understanding of epistemological issues was paramount in reading official statistics. This still provides a fascinating insight into critical reading at the most advanced level. It is a challenging but rewarding read for emergent researchers.

REFERENCES

Abbott, A. 1998. Professionalism and the future of librarianship. *Library Trends*, 46, 430–443.

Anderson, A. A., Shibuya, A., Ihori, N., Swing, E. L., Bushman, B. J., Sakamoto, A., Rothstein, H. R. & Saleem, M. 2010. Violent video game effects on aggression, empathy and prosocial behavior in eastern and western countries: A meta-analytic review. *Psychological Bulletin*, 136, 151–173.

Becker, H. S. 2007 [1986]. *Writing for social scientists: How to start and finish your thesis, book, or article* (2nd edn). Chicago: University of Chicago Press.

Blaikie, N. 2007. *Approaches to social enquiry: Advancing knowledge*. Cambridge: Polity Press.

Bushman, B. J. & Huesmann, L. R. 2001. Effects of televised violence on aggression. In: Singer, D. G. & Singer, J. L. (eds.), *Handbook of children and the media*. Thousand Oaks, CA: Sage.

Curtis, B. 2007. Doing research. In: Matthewman, S., West-Newman, C. L. & Curtis, B. (eds.), *Being sociological*. London: Palgrave Macmillan.

Deakin University 2010. *The literature review*. Available at: www.deakin.edu.au/library/find out/research/litrev.php [Accessed 10 May 2011].

Dillman, D. A. 1978. *Mail and telephone surveys: The total design method.* New York: Wiley.

Dillman, D. A. 2007. *Mail and internet surveys: The tailored design method: With new internet, visual, and mixed-mode guide.* New York: Wiley.

Duval, S. & Tweedie, R. 2000. A nonparametric 'trim and fill' method of accounting for publication bias in meta-analysis. *Journal of the American Statistical Association*, 95, 89–98.

Engeström, Y. 2000. Activity theory and the social construction of knowledge: A story of four umpires. *Organization*, 7, 301–310.

Halsey, A. 1992. *The decline of donnish dominion.* Oxford: Clarendon Press.

Hindess, B. 1973. *The use of official statistics in sociology.* London: Macmillan.

Kassin, S., Fein, S. & Markus, H. R. 2008. *Social psychology.* Boston, MA: Houghton Mifflin.

Matthewman, S. & Hoey, D. 2006. What happened to postmodernism? *Sociology*, 40, 529–547.

McLuhan, M. 1964. *Understanding media: The extensions of man.* New York: McGraw-Hill.

Notess, G. R. 2009. Showdown analysis: Boolean searching on Google. Accessed at: www.searchengineshowdown.com/features/google/googleboolean.htm [Accessed 10 May 2011].

Oakley, A. 1998. Gender, methodology and people's ways of knowing: Some problems with feminism and the paradigm debate in social science. *Sociology*, 32, 707–731.

Ragin, C. 1994. *Constructing social research: The unity and diversity of method.* Thousand Oaks, CA: Pine Forge Press.

Scott, J. (ed.) 2006a. *Documentary research (4 vols).* London: Sage.

Scott, J. 2006b. Editor's introduction: Documentary research. In: Scott, J. (ed.), *Documentary research.* London: Sage.

Scott, J. 2006c. Assessing documentary sources. In: Scott, J. (ed.), *Documentary research.* London: Sage.

Seidman, S. 1994. *Contested knowledge: Social theory in the postmodern era.* Oxford: Blackwell.

Wall, A. & Wall, R. 2005. *The complete idiot's guide to critical reading.* New York: Penguin.

ELEVEN

SEMIOTIC ANALYSIS – STUDYING SIGNS AND MEANINGS

CONTENTS LIST

Key words: semiotic analysis – signs – Derrida – structuralism – post-structuralism – grammar – signifier – signified paring – polysemy – synonym – discourse analysis

SUMMARY

A discussion of the origins of semiotic analysis, linking anthropological and sociological research, and the use of grammar as the key mechanism by which variables are recognised from signs as well as the popularity of semiotics in contemporary society and the impact of new technological developments on the approach.

Researchers who engage in semiotic analysis – semioticians – are interested in the meanings people attribute to signs and how they might use them in constructing other signs and sets of meanings. These signs are the outputs of various forms of media. They include such obvious signs as traffic signals as well as more complex and subtle images. Our attention in this chapter is primarily on semiotic *analysis* rather than data *collection* as social semiotics doesn't have a unique way of collecting signs, instead relying on found material and using approaches that we discuss elsewhere in this textbook, such as ethnographic approaches (see Chapter 4). For non-interactive approaches to data collection the relevant sections of two chapters in this textbook are useful: unobtrusive research (see Chapter 8) and content analysis (see Chapter 9).

In this chapter we discuss the origins of the approach, which is linked to anthropological and sociological research. We then use the example of a magazine cover to demonstrate the use of grammar as the key mechanism by which variables are developed from signs and meanings become values. We also develop an argument that semiotic analysis is unable to support a standardised approach, drawing from Derrida to illustrate this apparent lack and its epistemological or philosophical justification.

We argue that the popularity of semiotics reflects developments in contemporary society, in particular the increasing media saturation of the social world. Researchers are enmeshed with new media, new technologies and new channels of communication in their everyday life and these are also mechanisms for accessing and constituting signs and sign systems for study.

DOING DATA COLLECTION AND ANALYSIS

Semiotics is the study of signs and their meaning. Umberto Eco famously claimed that 'semiotics is concerned with everything that can be taken as a sign' (Eco, 1976: 138–41). Eco regarded things as diverse as a kiss or musical notation as signs (1976: 9–13). Our focus is the social sciences – a little narrower than what Eco was talking about – and Hodge's (2008) notion of 'social semiotics' is a very useful short-hand for the sorts of signs and meanings we might explore. Hodge defines social semiotics as:

> A broad, heterogeneous orientation within semiotics, straddling many other areas of inquiry concerned, in some way, with the social dimensions of meaning in any media of communication, its production, interpretation and circulation, and its implications in social processes, as cause or effect. (Hodge, 2008: 1)

The signs we are interested in are the outputs of various forms of media and inputs for further constructions. We are interested in the meanings people attribute to these signs and how they might use them in constructing other signs and sets of meanings. Our attention in this chapter is primarily on semiotic *analysis*. We don't talk much about data *collection* as we feel that social semiotics doesn't have a unique way of identifying and collecting signs, but uses approaches that we discuss elsewhere in this textbook (Manning and Cullum-Swan, 1994).

Origins of the approach

One strand of social semiotics is drawn from anthropological and sociological traditions of ethnographic research or fieldwork. In this approach the data collection phase of semiotics is the same as that discussed in ethnographic approaches – studying groups in natural settings (see Chapter 4). A good example of ethnographic-based social semiotics is Barley's observation and interpretation of funeral work, in particular what undertakers do to make death seamless with the lives and routines of mourners (Barley, 1983a, 1983b). Barley undertook ethnographic fieldwork that was indistinguishable from other non-semiotic inspired work. Where he diverged from the more traditional ethnographic approach was in his analysis; he undertook semiotic analysis.

The most important strand of social semiotics is linked to media research. Discussions of media research also give a priority to data analysis rather than to data collection (for an exception, see Deacon et al., 2007). Semioticians often are not all that interested in how they collected their data/signs. The discussions of methods in media research typically regard signs as exemplars of things, artefacts or traces simply found in the public domain. The data for analysis – signs from a movie, a TV series, a website, an advert – are found, in fact they are broadcast into researchers' living rooms. As a result, many semioticians rely on forms of non-interactive or unobtrusive methods in data collection (Kellehear, 1993; Webb, 2000).

Our primary focus will be on semiotic analysis and readers of this chapter should imagine that they have collected their data in the form of a sign or a series of signs. We use the example of a magazine cover (see below) in our discussion of semiotic analysis (after Barthes (1972 [1957])). Overall, we consider the focus on semiotic analysis appropriate because of the eclectic nature of data collection in social semiotics and because of the workings of a social constructivist epistemology within the approach. Epistemology refers to the theory of knowledge that informs how research is shaped in its broadest sense (see Chapter 1). Later in this chapter we will discuss some epistemological issues associated with the lack of methods *per se* in semiotics.

Semiotic analysis is an example of a case-centric approach. Case-centric approaches start with a case. They are an approach to research in which there are few cases and very many variables. As with other case-centric, case-first approaches, such as life history research (see Chapter 3), ethnographic research (see Chapter 4) and autoethnographic research (see Chapter 12), the core of this type of research is finding different sets of values (or measurable states) for the variables under investigation across a single or limited number of cases. In semiotics, the case(s) are signs or systems of signs, and the process of finding variables and values is decoding or deconstruction of the sign.

There are always multiple variables and values of meaning a researcher can decode or deconstruct from any sign(s). For example, the photographs someone posts on a social networking website are signs: they present messages (meanings/values) to others about who that person is, or at least how they would like to be seen. As a result, semiotics is one of a large number of qualitative approaches that focus on generating a data-matrix that is 'thick' or rich in its descriptive properties (Geertz, 1973: 6–30). This can be thought of in terms of analytical induction (Becker, 1993), the primary way of developing theory in case-centric research. In Chapter 1, we suggested that the best way of visualising this analytical process is as a spiral, the starting point of which is the naïve researcher, the outward curvilinear path the moments of research, and the end point is the researcher with greater knowledge or a new theory.

Analysing signs

Semiotic analysis is an approach that requires the researcher to have a sound grasp of some specific analytical tools before launching into study. Understanding and using this toolbox is probably the most challenging part of semiotic analysis. In this respect, semiotic analysis is similar to an otherwise very different approach, the survey (see Chapter 6). A researcher contemplating a survey should have confidence in the basics of statistical analysis, whereas one considering semiotics needs a similar appreciation of the basics of grammar. In semiotic analysis the use of grammar is the key mechanism by which variables are developed from signs and a host of meanings become values (or measurable states). In other words, using the analytical tools of semiotics, in the form of grammar, allows the researcher to decode or deconstruct a sign.

Grammar is the study of the rules of language. The use of grammar and a multitude of related terms reflects the origins of semiotics in linguistics. While semiotics has diversified enormously beyond linguistics to encompass the study of almost anything as a 'system of signs' (Jameson, 1972), the approach retains the notion that signs are rule-bound and that they are understandable through grammar. Regardless of their epistemological starting point (discussed below), semioticians agree that signs are not the product of chaos or chance but have to be understood in an orderly way.

Clearly, discovering the particularities of a relevant grammar is an important part of semiotic analysis, but at the same time emergent researchers must start the process with a grasp of some grammatical principles in order to develop the variables and values necessary for analysis. If a researcher does not have a grasp of the relevant grammar, he/she will not produce a good semiotic analysis. There are many grammars on offer (indeed every piece of semiotic analysis throws up its own version), but there are also some bedrock elements.

PRACTICE POINT 2

It is crucial for the researcher to have a familiarity with grammar, the study of the rules of language, in semiotics.

One very famous and widely used discussion of grammar and of the logic of its analysis is provided by Roland Barthes (1915–80) in his discussion of myth. Barthes was arguably the most important semiotician of the last century, especially in terms of transforming a linguistic approach into a social semiotics. His discussion of 'Myth today' in *Mythologies* is a foundational methodological work (Barthes, 1972 [1957]: 109–59) and his discussion of myth as a semiological chain is everywhere in introductions to the approach (Chandler, 2007: 138–41; Deacon et al., 2007: 141–50; Silverman, 1983: 25–32).

It is useful to understand the make-up of signs before opening the analytical toolbox. Barthes highlighted how a sign is meaningful and how it carries and conveys meaning to its readers or audience. Thus a sign is always interpreted by its readers as standing in for something else. Semioticians assume a sign carries meaning because it combines two elements: the signifier and the signified. A sign is a comprehensible combination of signifier and signified. This combination is also of form and content. The signifier is the physical form of the sign. It exists in a material way as spoken or written language, an image, or indeed as any object.

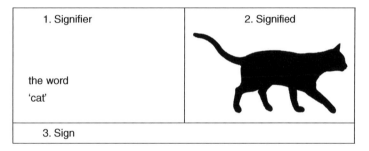

FIGURE 11.1 Example I of a signifier/signified pairing

The signified content exists within the sign in a non-material, psychological form, as a process of recognition and extrapolation on the part of the reader. There are an infinite number of examples of signifier/signified pairings. For example, Figure 11.1 uses the model of the sign developed by Ferdinand de Saussure. In this case, the word 'cat' is the signifier. It has physical form as written text on the page. The word 'cat' triggers a psychological process of recognition and extrapolation in the reader, which points to the concept and examples of 'cat'. This combination of form and content, of signifier and signified, results in the sign.

However, the same signifier can stand for different signifieds in different contexts. This diversity is called polysemy. A signifier can stand for a range of different signifieds and can therefore be a number of different signs. For example, the signifier 'fast' can be associated with concepts of moving quickly, adhering to something, standing true, fixing dye, not eating or being sexually promiscuous.

Conversely, any number of different signifiers can stand for the same signified within a sign. This diversity is called synonym. For example, the words 'Caledonian' and 'Scottish' are signifiers of the same signified (Figure 11.2).

Polysemy and synonym are mirror images: a signifier can stand for a range of different signifieds and a range of signifiers can stand for the same signified. Sorting this out is an important building block of semiotic analysis. This is crucial not just for classificatory purposes but because polysemy and synonym (and all other grammatical conventions) make language slippery and capable of multiple, hidden or coded messages. The basics of sorting and classifying the elements of a sign are absolutely necessary steps for making analysis of meaning.

This sorting process highlights how semiotic analysis is a true example of an inductive logic of research, sometimes referred to as a bottom-up logic. We have noted in earlier chapters how Bertaux and Bertaux-Wiam (1981) (see Chapter 3) talk of saturation in life histories, while Becker (1998) calls the process analytical induction when talking of solving puzzles in fieldwork. These descriptions outline the inductive research process as a constant movement between what the researcher knows from the existing literature or personal experience, and what the researcher learns from engaging with the data. In the case of semiotic analysis, the data – the case – is a sign. We suggested (in Chapter 1) that the best way of visualising this learning process is as a spiral: research spirals up and out from

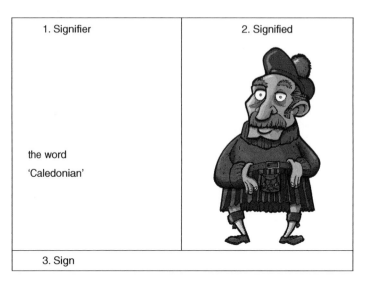

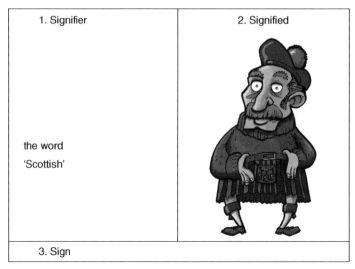

FIGURE 11.2   Example II of a signifier/signified pairing

an origin of knowing little to an end point of knowing a lot more. The most difficult component of inductive research in semiotic analysis is getting to know the grammar and its sometimes eye-watering terminology.

CONCEPTUAL CONCERN 2

Like most case-centric, case-first approaches, semiotic analysis enjoys an inductive approach to research.

For example, polysemy allows the use of double coded messages. Consider the situation where a couple are attending a party. As the party progresses one half of the couple is enjoying the night's events considerably more than the other. The happy partner, surrounded by a circle of friends, is unaware either of the passing of time or of his significant other's dissatisfaction and mind-numbing boredom. At some time, well past midnight, the dissatisfied partner whispers in the happy partner's ear 'It's late'. This semiological chain is a coded message and can be read in a variety of ways. At one level it is a statement about the time. At another it is a statement declaring that it is time for the happy-go-lucky partner to leave for home immediately.

CONCEPTUAL CONCERN 3

A sign is a comprehensible combination of signifier and signified. The signifier is the physical form of the sign. The signified is the psychological form of the sign, requiring recognition and extrapolation of the sign on the part of the reader.

Polysemy and synonym are fairly basic grammatical concepts. Clifford Geertz (1926–2006), who was perhaps the greatest social anthropologist of the twentieth century, suggests a far more complete and comprehensive grammar. There is not room here to provide definitions of all the grammatical terms mentioned by him (though we will discuss the more fundamental ones below). However, any social scientist contemplating semiotic analysis should have a competency with them. Geertz starts with metaphor and goes on to list several other conventions:

> Metaphor is, of course, not the only stylistic resource upon which ideology draws. Metonymy ('All I have to offer is blood, sweat and tears'), hyperbole ('The thousand-year Reich'), meiosis ('I shall return'), synechdoche ('Wall Street'), oxymoron ('Iron curtain'), personification ('The hand that held the dagger has plunged it into the back of its neighbor'), and all the other figures the classical rhetoricians so painstakingly collected and so carefully classified are utilized over and over again, as are such syntactical devices as antithesis, inversion, and repetition, such prosodic ones as rhyme, rhythm, and alliteration; such literary ones as irony, eulogy, and sarcasm … (Geertz, 1973: 213)

Barley (1983a, 1983b) posits three fundamentals of semiotic analysis: metaphor, metonymy and opposition. In metaphor and metonymy, the signifier and signified are associated in evocative ways, which could be thought of as particular examples of polysemy. (Remember, polysemy is when a signifier can stand for a range of different signifieds.) Metonymical signification occurs where the signifier and signified belong to similar semiotic domains or areas of speech. For example, the signifier 'the Crown' can substitute for signifieds including royalty, the state or government in Commonwealth countries. The signifier 'The White House' occupies a similar linguistic space in the USA.

Metaphor, in contrast, relies on the association of signifier and signified that are from otherwise different domains of language. For example, 'Love is a rose' (see Eco, 1976: 67–89, for an in-depth discussion of metaphor and metonymy). To further complicate things, metonymy is also associated with synecdoche – that is, the substitution of part of a thing for the whole. For example, 'Don't worry, the law will deal with him', in which case 'the law' stands as a substitute for the police and justice system. Both metaphor and metonymy are possible because sign systems are dynamic and the processes of signification allows for increasing complexity in meaning.

Barley suggests the opposition of signs as a third major tool of semiotic analysis. There are three dimensions to opposition:

1. **Antonym** (the opposite of synonym). This is where a signifier is associated with a logically opposite signified. An obvious example of this opposition is where the dead are dressed and made up by morticians, as if they were living people (Barley, 1983a). This (mis)representation of the dead as living can be understood as part of telling the story of the departed life – a core of all funerals. That is, it helps maintain the fiction for the bereaved that their dear departed are still with them.

2. **Comparison**. This is where signs can only be understood as elements in a ranking. For example, traffic lights as signs: green light = go, yellow light = get ready to stop, red light = stop.

3. **Absent signifier**. The most powerful form of opposition is the absent signifier (for example, a stop-sign encompasses the absent signifier 'go') in which missing signifiers shape the process of signification or the increasing complexity in meaning.

Polysemy and synonym; metaphor, metonymy and synecdoche; opposition – antonym, comparison and absent signifiers are introduced to make the point that a social researcher contemplating semiotic analysis needs an understanding of the relevant grammar (see the recommended readings at the end of this chapter). At the same time, the interconnectedness of all these terms – most can be understood as specific examples of each other – points to the interconnectedness of sign systems. Signs are always located within systems and semiological chains. The meaning of a sign is found not simply in and of itself, but in its relationships with other signs. Hence, the meaning of a sign – the meaning it conveys – must be explored by understanding the relationships between signs.

Barthes discusses the complexity of sign systems in terms of myth and the operation of denotation (the primary/obvious meaning of a sign) and connotation (all the other meanings of a sign) (Figure 11.3).

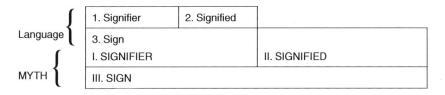

	1. Signifier	2. Signified	
Language	3. Sign		
	I. SIGNIFIER	II. SIGNIFIED	
MYTH	III. SIGN		

FIGURE 11.3 Language and myth (*Source*: Barthes, 1972 [1957]: 115)

Barthes' diagram illustrates the emergence of myth from language as an overlapping, two-stage process in which the association of signifier and signified in the sign, operating in the realm of language, is repeated in the realm of myth. The end point of denotative language (3. Sign) is the starting point of connotative myth (I. SIGNIFIER). This can be understood as a movement from a denotative semiological chain (1. Signifier, 2. Signified, 3. Sign) to a connotative chain (I. SIGNIFIER, II. SIGNIFIED, III. SIGN). One result is the growing complexity of communication. It is with these and other grammatical pointers that Barthes provides his wonderful semiotic analysis of a photograph on the cover of *Paris-Match*, a weekly glossy magazine. This is included as a sample or entrée to what semiotic analysis can achieve (Figure 11.4):

I am at the barber's, and a copy of *Paris-Match* is offered to me. On the cover, a young Negro[*sic*] in a French uniform is saluting, with his eyes uplifted, probably fixed on a fold of the tricolour. All this is the meaning of the picture. But, whether naïvely or not, I see very well what it signifies to me: that France is a great Empire, that all her sons, without any colour discrimination, faithfully serve under her flag, and that there is no better answer to the detractors of an alleged colonialism than the zeal shown by this Negro in serving his so-called oppressors. I am therefore again faced with a greater semiological system: there is a signifier, itself already formed with a previous system (a black soldier is giving the French salute); there is a signified (it is here a purposeful mixture of Frenchness and militariness); finally, there is a presence of the signified through the signifier. ... In myth (and this is the chief peculiarity of the latter), the signifier is already formed by the signs of the language. ... Myth has in fact a double function: it points out and it notifies, it makes us understand something and it imposes it on us ... (Barthes, 1972 [1957]: 116)

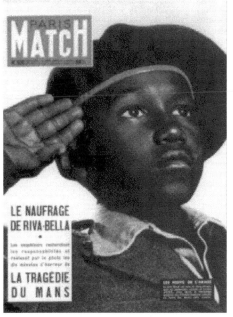

FIGURE 11.4 Front Cover of *Paris Match*, No. 326, June 1955

Reprinted with permission from Paris Match

PRACTICE POINT 3

The grammatical elements used by researchers in semiotic analysis include: polysemy and synonym; metaphor, metonymy and synecdoche; opposition – antonym, comparison and absent signifiers.

SOME ISSUES IN RESEARCH

Unfortunately for textbook writers and their readers, Barthes, Eco and other important proponents of semiotics and semiotic analysis provide very little in the discussion of methods. Even Daniel Chandler's wonderful *Semiotics: The basics* (2007) doesn't read like a procedural methods textbook, and similarly Judith Williamson's influential primer *Decoding advertisements: Ideology and meaning in advertising* (1978) is far removed from any how-to-do book in the social sciences. Further, when the methods component of semiotic analysis is discussed, the emphasis is on aspects of linguistic techniques (e.g., on illuminating the material about grammar touched on above) rather than the logical and contextual sequencing of procedures. In the opening section of this chapter it was suggested that semiotics cross-cuts and overlaps the social sciences. This in part explains what to social scientists looks like deficiency in the approach. We might ask: 'Where is the method?' One answer is that semiotics, and even our narrower formulations of social semiotics and semiotic analysis, are unable to support a standardised approach. This apparent lack has an epistemological or philosophical justification.

PRACTICE POINT 4

The leading practitioners of semiotic analysis have little to say about methods. This reflects their greater interest in the unique properties of deconstruction.

Jacques Derrida (1930–2004), until his death the leading advocate of discourse analysis, provides the rationale for the absence of methods in discussions of semiotics.[3] He argued that semiotics suggests a methodology but cannot sustain a

---

[3]In the balance of this chapter, the term 'text' is used interchangeably for signs as semiological chains. This is, a text is considered to be a series of linked signs, a semiological chain, which is the basis for the movement of language beyond the denotative to the connotative. From this perspective, discourse analysis or deconstruction are understood as stands of a social semiotics. Many scholars would disagree with this formulation. For example, Lee and Poyton (2000) discuss discourse analysis with no mention of semiotics.

method. Methodology is understood as a logic of the processes shaping research, while methods refers to a repeatable set of procedures:

> Every discourse, even a poetic or oracular sentence, carries with it a system of rules for producing analogous things and thus an outline of methodology. That said, at the same time I have tried to mark the ways in which, for example, deconstructive questions cannot give rise to methods, that is to technical procedures that can be transposed by analogy – this is what is called a teaching, a knowledge, applications – but these rules are taken up in a text which is in each time a unique element and which does not let itself be turned totally into a method. (Derrida, 1995: 200)

Derrida is highlighting an issue of epistemology. Let's break this down. By epistemology we mean the theory of knowledge that informs how research is shaped in its broadest sense (see Chapter 1). As we noted in Chapter 1, there are three main epistemological positions: positivist, social realist and social constructivist.

To recap: Positivists accept as true a social reality that exists independently of our perceptions of it. They emphasise the techniques of observation and measurement and the potential for scientists to form objective understandings. This assurance informs their practice and is the justification for doing science.

Social realists also accept an external and measurable social reality, but one that exists through the mediation of our perceptions and actions. Where positivists strive for objectivity, social realists insist on forms of subjectivity and the appreciation of factors like power, meaning and researcher reflexivity. For social realists, the scientific endeavour is still a legitimate goal but it is understood as a limited and somewhat contextual project. This social realism is the mainstream position within the social sciences today and is the one underlying this textbook – although it is probably not the epistemology underlying most semiotics (see Chandler, 2007: xiii–xvi).

Social constructivists have little faith in science as a project that generates anything resembling universal rules, laws or theorems. In this epistemology, it is impossible to differentiate truth-claims based in science, or folklore, or commonsense, or metaphysics because individuals or actors actively create the social world and all potential measures of that social world.

In the extract Derrida plays out a social constructivist logic in two ways. First, he argues that every text, every sign, is so exceptional that it has to be treated differently from every other text or sign. That is: 'rules are taken up in a text which is in each time a unique element and which does not let itself be turned totally into a method'. In other words, what works in understanding one sign will not work in understanding another. Second, by emphasising the exceptionality of signs Derrida is also asserting social constructivism. He assumes no commonality of interpretation (reading) and as a result no potential for science or the assessment of truth-claims. Instead, every text can be deconstructed in multiple ways as there are no universal rules or truths that can be revealed through the appropriate application of a method. In effect, the concerns of social scientists regarding validity and reliability are left far behind (see Chapter 1).

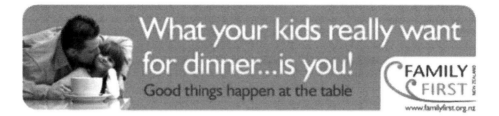

FIGURE 11.5 Example of a billboard campaign

Reprinted with permission, www.familyfirst.org.nz

CONCEPTUAL CONCERN 4

Semiotics, primarily deconstruction, provides a way for social constructivists to comment on society in general while eschewing (what they consider to be) the pitfall of social realism and positivism.

Scott (2006: 39) provides an encapsulation of the exceptionality of texts, and hence lack of method for social constructivists. He focuses in the 'internal' meaning or multiple potential meanings of any text:

> But this internal meaning cannot be known independently of its reception by an audience. As soon as a researcher approaches a text to interpret its meaning, he or she becomes a part of its audience. The most that can be achieved by a researcher is an analysis which shows how the inferred internal meaning of the text opens up some possibilities for interpretation by its audience and closes off others. (Scott, 2006: 39)

Providing a bullet point list of how to do a semiotic analysis flies in the face of the social constructivists who have championed the approach. That said, here are some ideas an emergent researcher should think about when considering semiotics. It might be useful to think about these questions while considering the image in Figure 11.5. The image is from a billboard campaign by an organisation called Family First (http://www.familyfirst.org.nz).

- What are the two elements that make up the sign? What is the signifier and what is signified? What is the physical form of the sign? What is its psychological form? For example, why a billboard campaign (facing traffic heading into the Central Business District)?

- What aspects of the grammar of semiotics captures your imagination?

- Does the sign use metaphor? Are the signifier and signified associated evocatively through the use of different domains of language (including imagery)? For example, what is the purpose of the big white bowl? Does this look like dinner, an evening meal?

- Does the sign use the more prosaic practices of metonymy, using similar domains of language to make an association? For example, what is the purpose of the kiss?

- Does the sign use opposition? Antonym, comparison, absent signifier? Often the absent signifier is a rewarding starting point for analysis. For example, why is there no mother in this particular image?

- How is the sign located within a sign system? How does the end point of denotative language become the starting point for connotative language or myth? For example, what myth or stereotypes are being supported or challenged in the sign?

An aside on rigour

In Chapter 6 we discussed survey research which in many respects is the antithesis of semiotic analysis. On the one hand, semiotics is case-centred and strongly social constructivist in its epistemology. Derrida argues that the one-off cases that are its focus are unique to the extent their investigation cannot support a method. On the other hand, survey research is variable-centred and its practitioners are often old school positivists. Further, semiotics is radical; survey research is intrinsically conservative or modest in its claims-making. But there are two strong similarities between the approaches. First, (as noted above) semiotic analysis and survey research both require the researcher to have a sound grasp of a specialist knowledge: grammar and statistics respectively. Second, semiotic analysis shares with survey research the need for rigour. Statistical analysis, which is the lodestone of survey research, depends on proper sampling strategies and precision in developing variables. Similarly, the decoding or deconstruction of a sign through semiotic analysis requires as much rigour in the development and use of variables. Derrida's argument about the impossibility of a method in semiotic analysis must not be confused for 'any old application of grammatical concepts will do'. There are good and bad examples of semiotic analysis and the best adhere to the principles around independent, dependent and intervening variables and mutually exclusive and collectively exhaustive values every bit as much as do survey researchers (see Chapter 6). These components of research operate at the level of logic and plausibility. The dilemma for emergent researchers in this respect is that semioticians never seem to discuss this in their publications.

Structuralism and post-structuralism

Derrida's position exemplifies one far removed from the epistemology of the founders of semiotics. Ferdinand de Saussure (1857–1913) and Charles Peirce (1839–1914) were positivists and structuralists. They saw semiotics as a science (positivism) that would enable the study of languages, meta-languages and other sign systems in ways that would transcend day-to-day contexts of human interaction.

Semiotics was intended as the first truly comparative study of humanity as, they reasoned, all cultures had language and all languages were ordered by underlying rules (structures).

Structuralism can also be described as being 'decentred', meaning semioticians did not study what individuals or groups thought of the world but how their use of signs/language was structured by rules that they may well be unaware of. Much of early semiotics was linked to the growth of anthropology and its efforts at cross-cultural comparisons dating from the late nineteenth century. In contrast, in the late twentieth century, Derrida and, perhaps even more famously, Jean Baudrillard (1929–2007) were social constructivists and post-structuralists. Where the founders of semiotics saw *commonality* in sign systems and an imperative for science, the more recent champions of the approach saw *exceptionality* and understood science as only one of many truth-claims.

The differences are between social constructivism and positivism and can be understood as a break, as a discontinuity. However, the differences between structuralism and post-structuralism are more about continuity. Structuralism was decentred in its theory and practice. Post-structuralism is a form of hyper-decentring (see Seidman, 1994: 194–233, for an interesting discussion of the 'French post-structuralists'). In both cases research is not centred on individuals or actors or agents (as with almost all other approaches), but on the ways rules of language or discourses (Derrida, 1995) or simulacra (Baudrillard, 1995) play across different sites, of which humans are but one example. In essence, the difference between structuralism and post-structuralism is about truth-claims. For the founders of semiotics, decentring the focus of research provided the basis for science. However, for the post-structuralists the logic of decentring, of subordinating the individual, provides a further rationale for the abandonment of science as a privileged truth-claim.

The above discussion of epistemology borders on the esoteric or obscure. More practically, the decentred epistemological starting point of both structuralist and post-structuralist semiotics suggests one explanation for the overwhelming discussion on analysing data rather than on collecting it. At the same time, a more concrete way of highlighting the differences within semiotics is to contrast decoding and deconstruction. Decoding can be thought of as a process, a repeatable set of procedures that can be applied to a sign in order to better reveal its character. We consider the long extract from Barthes (on p. 251) to be an example of decoding: a photograph is analysed to reveal its role in perpetuating certain myths and ultimately the dominant nationalistic ideology of France. When a researcher engages in decoding, the result of this analysis is intended to better reveal the workings of the social world. What is revealed by decoding are hidden meanings, sub-texts and linguistic subterfuges. The researcher is either explicitly or implicitly making a truth-claim. But post-structuralists argue that signs cannot be straightforwardly decoded to reveal their meaning. Instead, signs or texts can be subjected to deconstruction. Deconstruction is technically similar to decoding in so far as it uses linguistic techniques – an appreciation of grammar – to reveal how signifiers and signifieds might relate. However, deconstruction is epistemologically distinct from decoding. Most importantly, any deconstruction provides only one reading of the sign (of many possible readings) and can itself be further and endlessly deconstructed.

CONCEPTUAL CONCERN 5

Semiotic analysis has structural and post-structural variants. Structuralism 'decentres' research and emphasises universalistic factors, including the rules of human language. Post-structuralism extends the decentred research focus of structuralism to produce a hyper-decentring that challenges the privileged position of science in making truth-claims.

PUTTING THE APPROACH IN CONTEXT

Semioticians enjoy a fluid framing of research (see Chapter 1) and this is apparent in the moment of research we have designated as semiotic analysis. The researcher using semiotics is able to engage with data and the tools of analysis in a highly iterative process, largely unfettered from the resource constraints, other than time and deadlines, that impact on more fixed and sequential approaches (see Chapter 6 on survey research and Chapter 9 on content research for a more focused discussion of fixed framings). This fluidity means that partial answers, suppositions and guesses can be firmed up by the researcher through the inclusion of more data either by conducting more fieldwork or, as is often the case with media research, selecting from the data broadcast to them. Fluidity in research practice no doubt makes the approach more attractive to emergent researchers. Similarly, the focus on signs, the ease with which these signs can be 'collected' and the authoritative voice of many practitioners are all likely attractors.

CONCEPTUAL CONCERN 6

Like most case-centric, case-first approaches, semiotic analysis enjoys a fluid framing of research. The researcher is free to conduct research as an iterative process, moving between data and analysis as she or he sees fit.

The popularity of semiotics reflects dynamics in contemporary society, in particular the increasing media saturation of the social world. The rise of new information and communication technologies (ICTs), such as Web 2.0 internet, wireless communication, digital technologies, narrowcasting and so on, has dramatically expanded what Eco (1976) called the semiotic field and the potential for what Hodge (2008) called social semiotics. The new ICTs have opened up new realms of research. For example, the practice of 'happy slapping', where young people use mobile phones and social networking sites to record their assaults on friends and strangers (Haddon, 2007), was unimagined ten years ago and is passé now. Researchers are enmeshed with new media, new technologies and new channels in their everyday life and these are also mechanisms for accessing and constituting signs and sign systems for study. The new technologies are important and engaging. Also, a significant part of the initial studies by social scientists on any 'new technology' is undertaken by researchers who are also enthusiastic users. The ICTs that provide the infrastructure for the increasing media saturation of the social world are no exception in this respect. Researchers who engage in semiotic analysis also tend to be technologically savvy and fans of what they study (Jenkins, 2004).

Nevertheless, practitioners of semiotics and semiotic analysis seem resistant to new technologies as tools of analysis. Here we are referring not to the technologies such as the internet, social networks, user-generated content or wireless telephony that mediate the broadcasting (and narrowcasting) of semiotic 'data', but to the host of software packages that purport to help in data analysis. Specifically, the tendency in content research (see Chapter 9) and in in-depth interviewing (see Chapter 2) to use specialised software (see Bryman, 2008: 264–84 on NVivo; Lowe, n.d.) to collect and analyse data is not apparent in semiotics. The benefits of a fluid framing of research, in particular the flexibility in the ordering of research and resources, is most likely the telling factor. That, and the relatively small-scale nature of much semiotic analysis undertaken by emergent researchers, makes the set-up costs of most analytical software – including the time it takes to program pre-coded variables and values – somewhat unattractive.

CONCLUSION

As noted in the introduction (see Chapter 1), the social sciences are subjected to waves of criticism, and the integration of this critique. This process inevitably involves putting methodological orthodoxies that have been inherited from various founding fathers (for example, Durkheim, James, Levi-Strauss, Malinowski, Radcliffe-Brown, Weber, Wundt) under intense scrutiny. The collective results of these challenges can be in part captured by the diversity of research approaches sampled in this textbook. These waves of criticism tend to be played out in disciplinary contexts and with different results. Since the Second World War, sociology has proven most amenable to change and has fully integrated the critique of positivism, forms of qualitative research and social constructivism. The subdisciplines of cultural anthropology and social anthropology are in many respects the results of epistemological and methodological criticism of what, in the 1940s and 1950s, was a thoroughly positivistic anthropology and psychology.

Without a doubt the increased popularity and application of semiotics formed part of this ongoing and multi-pronged challenge to prevailing norms in the social sciences. Specifically, semiotics and post-structuralism constituted part of a 'linguistic turn' (Rorty, 1967) which pushed a critique of positivist and social realist epistemologies that underpinned the social sciences – the core of this challenge is covered in our discussion of post-structuralism and decentring research, above.

At the same time, social scientists – anthropologists, social psychologists, sociologists – are highly critical of semiotics. For example, Jameson (1972) provided an early and sustained critique of structuralism and semiotics in terms of their formalism and detachment from the material world. This social realist critique of semiotics is an enduring one. Further, the criticism of semiotics tends to be most damning from researchers who are most interested in transforming aspects of the social world. For many such researchers, semiotics is not an appropriate approach because its focus on signs and sign systems makes it detached from the social world.

It is argued that the social constructivism that underpins semiotics prejudices it towards asocial agnosticism. 'Social agnosticism' refers to efforts to put aside issues of injustice and inequalities. This scepticism about all facets of society may have been ethically problematic for Derrida but straightforwardly informed the later Baudrillard. Baudrillard's approach was logical but socially agnostic, in that he argued that the social world is so saturated with signs, especially those generated by the media, that it is impossible to distinguish between real and unreal. In this context, social science is an outright impossibility because we are surrounded by the hyper-real, the verisimilitude of which cannot be proven. Deconstructed readings – themselves open to further endless deconstruction – is all that is on offer (see Baudrillard, 1995).

More concretely, Leiss, Kline and Jhally (1990) detail drawbacks that are worth quoting. Their focus is on advertising, but their comments can be generalised. They argue that semiotics:

> ... suffers from a number of related weaknesses. First, it is heavily dependent upon the skill of the individual analyst. In the hands of someone like Roland Barthes or Judith Williamson, it is a creative tool that allows one to reach the deeper levels of meaning-construction in ads. A less skilful practitioner, however, can do little more than state the obvious in a complex and often pretentious manner. As a result, in these types of studies there is little chance to establish consistency or reliability – that is, a sufficient level of agreement among analysts on what is found in the message. ... Second, because the semiological approach stresses individual readings of messages, it does not lend itself to the quantification of results; it is impossible to base an overall sense of constructed meanings on the examination of a large number of messages. What insights may be extracted from the approach must remain impressionistic. Third, ... [the] procedure courts the danger of self-confirming results, the conclusions should, strictly speaking, be confined to those instances alone and not generalized to the entire range of advertising. (Leiss et al., 1990: 214)

Leiss, Kline and Jhally (1990) are perhaps too harsh in so far as their comments can really be applied to all research approaches and there is more than a whiff of old-fashioned positivism in what they say. More often than not, unskilful researchers produce poor results, research doesn't need to be validated through quantification to be plausible, all research can be self-confirming if poorly designed. Plainly, skilful researchers can produce plausible results from semiotic analysis of quite unexpected sets of social relations. For example, Anderson, Standen and Noon (2005) conducted a semiotic analysis of suicidal behaviour. Their focus was on nurses' and doctors' perceptions. After extensive interviewing and observation, Anderson, Standen and Noon conceptualised suicidal behaviour as a sign, comprising both signifier and signified. Suicidal behaviour was foregrounded as an example of an absent signifier, the absence being the inability of young people to verbally express negative emotions. The conclusions they drew from this were intentionally practical and focused on the training of health professionals to better read (we might say decode) suicidal behaviour and its precursors as a semiological chain.

PRACTICE POINT 5

While semiotic analysis has the promise of allowing the researcher to speculate on very significant issues at relatively low cost, emergent researchers are urged to be cautious with the approach and to ensure that they have a sound grasp of the grammatical requirements.

Nevertheless Leiss, Kline and Jhally (1990) rightly underline that semiotics or semiotic analysis – like all approaches – has its particular weaknesses. In this case emergent researchers are cautioned to be modest in their initial expectations and plans for research. Semiotic analysis has the promise of allowing the researcher to speculate on very significant issues. But while Barthes, Derrida and Baudrillard were public intellectuals of the highest order, their books and articles cannot be considered as models for emergent researchers. These writers, like most public intellectuals, were excused from 'showing their workings' or justifying their claims-making in ways that most academics and emergent researchers are not.

FURTHER READINGS

Daniel Chandler's (2007) *Semiotics: The basics* is the most comprehensive reader on semiotics. His approach is detailed and accessible. He has also maintained the best site on the internet dealing with semiotics. This is called 'Semiotics for Beginners' and is freely available on the Aberystwyth University webpage at: http://www.aber.ac.uk/media/Documents/S4B/semiotic.html.

Roland Barthes' (1972 [1957]) *Mythologies* remains the best formulation of semiotics for researchers interested in social semiotics. His chapter on 'Myth today' is an inspirational discussion about revealing the construction of meaning and its consequences.

Judith Williamson's (1978) *Decoding advertisements: Ideology and meaning in advertising* is somewhat dated in terms of its content (1970s TV advertisements) but is still an excellent example of sustained semiotic analysis. Williamson cites a number of structuralists in her select bibliography from both the semiotic tradition (Saussure, Barthes, Lacan, Lévi-Strauss) as well as Louis Althusser, the champion of structural Marxism. However, this selection is leavened with the inclusion of Benjamin, Brecht, Freud and Gramsci. As a result, her primer has none of the social agnosticism associated with Baudrillard et al., but represents a now sadly old-fashioned attempt at consciousness-raising.

The following are also highly recommended: Derrida (1976), Haddon (2007) and Lee and Poynton (2000).

REFERENCES

Anderson, M., Standen, P. J. & Noon, J. P. 2005. A social semiotic interpretation of suicidal behaviour in young people. *Journal of Health Psychology*, 10, 317–331.

Barley, S. 1983a. The codes of the dead: The semiotics of funeral work. *Journal of Contemporary Ethnography*, 12, 3–31.

Barley, S. 1983b. Semiotics and the study of occupational and organizational culture. *Administrative Science Quarterly*, 28, 393–413.

Barthes, R. 1972 [1957]. *Mythologies*. New York: Hill & Wang.

Baudrillard, J. 1995. *The Gulf War did not take place*. Bloomington, IN: Indiana University Press.

Becker, H. S. 1993. How I learned what a crock was. *Journal of Contemporary Ethnography*, 22, 28–35.

Becker, H. S. 1998. *Tricks of the trade: How to think about your research while you're doing it*. Chicago: University of Chicago Press.

Bertaux, D. & Bertaux-Wiam, I. 1981. Life stories in the bakers' trade. In: Bertaux, D. (ed.), *Biography and society: The life history approach in social sciences*. London: Sage.

Bryman, A. 2008. *Social research methods*. Oxford: Oxford University Press.

Chandler, D. 2007. *Semiotics: The basics*. London: Routledge.

Deacon, D., Pickering, M. & Golding, P. 2007. *Researching communications: A practical guide to methods in media and cultural analysis*. London: Hodder Arnold.

Derrida, J. 1976. *Of grammatology*. Trans. Gayatri C. Spivak. Baltimore, MD: Johns Hopkins University Press.

Derrida, J. 1995. *Points … : Interviews, 1974–1994*. Stanford, CA: Stanford University Press.

Eco, U. 1976. *A theory of semiotics*. Bloomington, IN: Indiana University Press.

Geertz, C. 1973. *The interpretation of cultures*. New York: Basic Books.

Haddon, L. 2007. *More than a phone: Emerging practices in mobile phone use amongst children* [Online]. Budapest: Towards a Philosophy of Telecommunication Convergence, T-Mobile Hungary/Hungarian Academy of Sciences. Available at: www.socialscience.t-mobile.hu/2007/prepro2007_szin.pdf#page=123 [Accessed 12 September 2009].

Hodge, B. 2008. Social semiotics [Online]. *Semiotics Encyclopedia Online*. Available at: www.semioticon.com/seo/S/social_semiotics.html# [Accessed 20 May 2011].

Jameson, F. 1972. *The prison-house of language: A critical account of structuralism and Russian formalism*. Princeton, NJ: Princeton University Press.

Jenkins, H. 2004. The cultural logic of media convergence. *International Journal of Cultural Studies*, 7, 33–43.

Kellehear, A. 1993. *The unobtrusive researcher: A guide to methods*. St Leonards, NSW: Allen & Unwin.

Lee, A. & Poynton, C. 2000. *Culture and text: Discourse and methodology in social research and cultural studies*. St Leonards, NSW: Allen & Unwin.

Leiss, W., Kline, S. & Jhally, S. 1990. *Social communication in advertising: Persons, products and images of well-being*. London: Routledge.

Lowe, W. 2003. *Software for content analysis: A review* [Online]. Available at: http://kb.ucla.edu/system/datas/5/original/content_analysis.pdf [Accessed 20 May 2011].

Manning, P. K. & Cullum-Swan, B. 1994. Narrative, content, and semiotic analysis. In: Denzin, N. K. & Lincoln, Y. S. (eds.), *Handbook of qualitative research*. Thousand Oaks, CA: Sage.

Rorty, R. 1967. *The linguistic turn: Recent essays in philosophical method*. Chicago: University of Chicago Press.

Scott, J. 2006. Assessing documentary sources. In: Scott, J. (ed.), *Documentary research*. London: Sage.

Seidman, S. 1994. *Contested knowledge: Social theory in the postmodern era*. Oxford: Blackwell.

Silverman, K. 1983. *The subject of semiotics*. New York: Oxford University Press.

Webb, E. J. 2000. *Unobtrusive measures*. Thousand Oaks, CA: Sage.

Williamson, J. 1978. *Decoding advertisements: Ideology and meaning in advertising*. London: Marion Boyars.

TWELVE

AUTOETHNOGRAPHIC RESEARCH – WRITING AND READING THE SELF

CONTENTS LIST

Key words: autoethnography – autobiography – reflexivity – analytical autoethnography – evocative autoethnography

---

SUMMARY

An overview of autoethnography, covering the role of autobiography and reflexivity in autoethnography, links to assumptions about epistemology, practical considerations including multiple-perspective and multiple-voicing practices and guidelines for writers, and the evaluation of autoethnographic as well as conceptual issues including distinctions between analytical and evocative autoethnography.

In Chapter 4 we discussed ethnographic approaches to research: the studying of *groups* in their natural settings. In this chapter we turn to autoethnography: the study of the *self*. In autoethnography, which (like ethnography) has its origins in anthropology, data is collected and analysed as part of the researcher's own autobiographical writing.

Key topics in this chapter include the role of autobiography and reflexivity in autoethnography. We argue that reflexivity should be pursued by autoethnographers as an integral part of data collection and analysis. We discuss the ways in which this is linked with assumptions about epistemology. We examine multiple-perspective and multiple-voicing practices and guidelines for writers in this genre and we evaluate autoethnographic research. Conceptual issues include distinctions between analytical autoethnography and evocative autoethnography.

DOING DATA COLLECTION AND ANALYSIS

Autoethnography is an autobiographical genre of writing and research that displays multiple layers of consciousness. Back and forth autoethnographers gaze, first through an ethnographic wide angle lens, focusing outward on social and cultural aspects of their personal experience; then, they look inward, exposing a vulnerable self that is moved by and may move through, refract, and resist cultural interpretations. As they zoom backward and forward, inward and outward, distinctions between the personal and cultural become blurred, sometimes beyond distinct recognition. Usually written in first-person voice, autoethnographic texts appear in a variety of forms – short stories, poetry, fiction, novels, photographic essays, personal essays, journals, fragmented and layered writing, and social science prose. In these texts, concrete action, dialogue, emotion, embodiment, spirituality, and self-consciousness are featured, appearing as relational and institutional stories impacted by history and social structure, which themselves are dialectically revealed through actions, feelings, thoughts, and language. (Ellis, 1999: 673)

Carolyn Ellis (1999) notes that autoethnography is an 'autobiographical genre of writing and research'. Ellis also comments that autoethnographers alternate between outward and inward focuses in their writing. These personal narratives can take many forms, including fiction. Indeed, autoethnographic research lies at the boundary of social science and literary endeavours, and one strand involves poetic takes on autobiography (Freeman, 1993).

PRACTICE POINT 1

In autoethnography data is collected and analysed as part of the researcher's own autobiographical writing.

The unifying theme of the approach is twofold: autobiography and reflexivity. The researcher's autobiography or, more often, a fragment of personal narrative provides both data collection and data analysis in the research process. This process is reflexive in that it requires an interrogation of the self. Reflexivity is the process of being self-reflective.

CONCEPTUAL CONCERN 1

Autoethnographic texts take a variety of forms. They have in common: (1) the autobiographical genre and (2) an explicit commitment to reflexivity. Reflexivity is the process of being self-reflective.

More recently, Ellis said:

> As an autoethnographer, I am both the author and the focus of the story, the one who tells and the one who experiences, the observer and the observed, the creator and the created. I am the person at the intersection of the personal and the cultural, thinking and observing as an ethnographer and writing and describing as a storyteller. (Ellis, 2009: 13)

She identifies an imperative in autoethnography which transcends narcissism or mere self-interest. This is the modest belief that autoethnographic writing 'might be of value to someone besides ourselves' (Freeman, 1993: 229).

An autoethnographic aside

Autoethnographic research is the most recently developed of the approaches covered in this textbook. Autoethnography has its distant origins in anthropology and ethnographic research but has emerged as a distinct approach only since the 1980s. Perhaps unsurprisingly this newness is accompanied by considerable flux among its proponents and practitioners – about epistemology, on the one hand, and method on the other. The approach is most closely associated with a strong social constructivist epistemology, and social constructivists have severe doubts about the possibility for a standard social science. In recent years, however, the social constructivist take on autoethnography has been challenged by champions of a social realist epistemology, who do have hopes for the research approach as a radical variant of social science (Anderson, 2006).

This newness and flux are joined with a paucity of textbooks, a fascination for methodology rather than method, and the commitment of autoethnographers to witness through reflexivity. Together, these make this, the final chapter in our textbook, somewhat different from those that precede it. The reader will therefore notice several things. First, most obviously, we include autoethnographic research, surely the most singular of the single-case, case-centric approaches, as part of the cache of research approaches available to emergent researchers. Second, we have taken the narrative contention of autoethnographers seriously and, where possible, we use their words directly, so this chapter, unlike earlier ones, has many longish quotes. Third, the 'debate' between social constructivists and social realists – or what Anderson (2006) calls evocative and analytical autoethnographers – is unresolved. Where possible we have paid attention to both perspectives, but there is an element of each side talking past the other that we have not necessarily resolved.

Origins of the approach

> The concept of autoethnography … reflects a changing conception of both self and society. … It synthesizes both a postmodern ethnography, in which realist conventions and objective observer position of standard ethnography have been called into question, and a postmodern autobiography, in which the notion of the coherent, individual self has been similarly called into question. The term has a double sense – referring either to the ethnography of one's own group or to autobiographical writing that has ethnographic interest. (Reed-Danahay, 1997: 2)

Autoethnography has its origins in anthropology. Deborah Reed-Danahay (1997) points to the origins of autoethnography in both postmodernism and an 'anthropological angst' in which the certainties of standard ethnography and of the role of anthropologists in reporting back to metropolitan audiences about exotic peoples and locales became problematic (see Geertz, 1995). Our interest in this chapter is with the autobiographical genre rather than the phobias of anthropology (see also Chapter 3 on life history research). This also reflects changes to autoethnography; as it has moved beyond its home discipline, it has become more focused on autobiographical writing rather than 'the ethnography of one's own group' (see Ellis, 2009). In fact, autoethnography is now most popular among the vocational disciplines: training nurses, social workers and teachers (see Foster et al., 2006; Nash, 2004; Riessman and Kohler, 2005; Roth, 2005). These somewhat marginalised disciplines were most attracted to postmodern arguments about the shifting character of society, science and the self.

Autoethnographic research is one of the legacies of postmodernism. It is arguably the exemplar of postmodern research, combining a focus on the self with a commentary on the social world. While postmodernity is increasingly dismissed or simply forgotten, Matthewman and Hoey (2006) are generous in their assessment:

> 'Critics on the Left concede that postmodern theorizing forced a greater attention to context, geography, historical specificity, gender, ethnicity, and sexuality. While supporters championed postmodernism for 'refocusing the sociological narrative on experience, emotion, "the sensual", "identification" and other events and processes all anchored in the subject.' (2006: 530)

CONCEPTUAL CONCERN 2

Autoethnographic research is one of the legacies of postmodernism. It is centrally concerned with the shifting character of society, science and the self.

Autobiography and reflexivity as a case

While life history research may explore the biography of an individual (see Chapter 3), ethnographic research a group bounded by space, time or social relations (see Chapter 4), and semiotic analysis a sign (see Chapter 11), and can all be labelled single-case approaches, autoethnographic research combines the single-case with autobiography and reflexivity. As a result, autoethnography is a particular form of research. More than any other it represents the single-case approach. One life, that of the writer, or a fragment of it, is explored through many variables and values. These variables and values are discovered through a reflexive process of writing. This, then, is a voyage of self-discovery, at least in part. In this respect, 'reflexive' can be thought of as a variant of analytical induction, the primary way of developing theory in case-centric research. The researcher starts knowing little and reaches an end point of knowing more (see Chapter 1).

CONCEPTUAL CONCERN 3

Autoethnographic research is a case-centric, single-case approach. One life, that of the writer, or a fragment of it, is explored through many variables and values. These variables and values are discovered through a reflexive process of writing. In this respect, 'reflexive' can be thought of as a variant of analytical induction.

Below we will discuss reflexivity as a practice that should be pursued by autoethnographers as part of data collection and analysis. Much of this material is linked with assumptions about epistemology. It is useful to start thinking about reflexivity in terms of the slightly less intimidating notion of being self-reflective. We borrowed the following bullet points from the Open University (2010) *Skills for OU study*. They are a ubiquitous set of points for coming to grips with reflexivity:

Thinking about your own skills and being aware of those you tend to use may help you to:

- see how you might make changes
- develop new ways of working
- become more aware of the different techniques you could devise.

Reflection has an important role to play in learning and self-development. There are some key elements of reflection, and you'll need to decide on your preferred ways.

Reflection could be described as:

- thinking with a purpose
- being critical, but not negative
- analysing how effective your learning is
- questioning and probing
- making judgements and drawing conclusions.

Get used to reflecting on your experiences as part of your everyday learning. In this way, each experience – whether positive or negative – will contribute to your development and personal growth. An experience that is repeated without reflection is just a repetition, which does not help you to learn. Record your reflections in a learning journal or on audio.

PRACTICE POINT 2

Reflexivity begins with an awareness of your skills and assumptions. It should move on to challenging those assumptions.

Data collection and analysis and reflexivity

Data collection and analysis in autoethnographic research centres on reflexive writing. Alvesson, Hardy and Harley (2008) provide four dimension or practices for reflexivity. We have modified these slightly:

1. **Reflexivity as multiple-perspective practices**: All writers are confronted with a multitude of paradigms, theories and perspectives that claim explanation. The reflexive writer uses this contestation or tension between perspectives as a resource. Specifically, the reflexive writer may look for what is shared and overlooked by the perspectives, what is stated or left unstated. The aim is to

expose assumptions and open up new ways of thinking (see Chapter 10 on secondary research for another discussion of these issues). Alvesson, Hardy and Harley argue that the key questions here are: 'What are the different ways in which a phenomenon can be understood? How do they produce different knowledge(s)?'

2. **Reflexivity as multiple-voicing practices**: Obviously, author and authority are words with a common origin. Unreflexive writing accepts the voice of the author as having authority. However, the reflexive writer, the autoethnographer, has to challenge the authority and authenticity of his or her *own* voice. This can be attempted by the autoethnographer treating his/her voice like all others used in the personal narrative. The motivations and assumptions of the author have to be exposed, explained and their limitations assessed. Only at this moment does the autobiographical voice become authentic.

3. **Reflexivity as positioning practices**: Alvesson, Hardy and Harley (2008) are particularly excited by social constructivist writings that examine the broader network or field that situates the autoethnographer. The above practices focus on the relationships between the writer and existing claims, and the writer and their own claims to authority. Positioning practices try to situate all of these relationships within a nexus. Alvesson, Hardy and Harley quote Collins (1998: 297): 'The networks of beliefs, practices, and interests that favour one interpretation over another; and, ideally, the way that one interpretation rather than another comes to predominate.' Alvesson, Hardy and Harley (2008: 485) restate the key question as: 'What is the network of practices and interests that produces particular interpretations of knowledge?'

4. **Reflexivity as destabilising practices**: This is the most political of the four practices and sees reflexivity as a component of the postmodern critique. Alvesson, Hardy and Harley claim the key question here is: 'What are the conditions and consequences of the construction of a theory or a "fact"?' The aim of destabilising practices is to question and challenge epistemological and theoretical assumptions, precisely because they lack a reflexive, overly authoritarian voice.

Taken collectively, the practices advanced by Alvesson, Hardy and Harley are an explicit challenge to social science. They champion a social constructivist epistemology. They also echo the criticisms of radical feminists in the 1960s and 1970s and of postmodernists in the 1990s (see Chapter 11 on semiotic analysis).

Guidelines for writers

Nash (2004: 56–70), an enthusiast of autoethnography in the form of the 'scholarly personal narrative', provides ten guidelines for writers. These are reflexive insights as well as a scholarly call-to-arms. Nash clearly agrees with 'reflexivity as destabilising practices', suggested by Alvesson, Hardy and

Harley (2008). Nash encourages the researcher as writer to produce a narrative, an exemplar, that allows others to learn from their life:

1. **Establish clear constructs, hooks and questions**: Nash identifies the importance of integrating the narrative around a theme or construct. The construct is a conceptual guide. The hook is needed to make the narrative compelling. Writers are urged to question themselves about the purpose of their writing. A pertinent question is 'What message do you think your life sends to others?'

2. **Move from the particular to the general and back again ... often**: An effective personal narrative combines general and particular elements, moving from what Mills (1959) would have called private troubles into public issues. This movement is necessary for both narrative (storytelling) and substantive reasons. A narrative that focuses solely on the particulars of a life story is likely to be both boring and of little impact. On the other hand, a narrative in which the life story disappears into an account of general patterns is also of questionable worth.

3. **Try to draw larger implications from your life story**: In many respects this is a restatement of the *raison d'être* for autoethnography. In order to be anything more than an exercise in narcissism the personal narrative has to be written with the reader in mind. Mostly, the reader is seeking the implications that can be drawn from a life story, looking for commonalities and differences between the autoethnographer's and his/her own life experiences.

4. **Draw from your vast store of formal background knowledge**: Writing personal narratives may appear as an informal, even iconoclastic, project. It is also a scholarly project which will be subjected to peer review prior to publication. This background knowledge, including academic expertise, should be made clear in the text.

5. **Always try to tell a good story**: An interesting and engaging story provides the best vehicle for personal narratives. Nash points to the key elements of good storytelling: plot, colourful characters, suspense, a climax, a denouement, and significant lessons to be learnt.

6. **Show some passion**: Nash urges writers to 'stand for something'. He says: 'Resist the conventional academic temptation to be "objective" – stoical, qualified, subdued and distant' (2004: 63).

7. **Tell your story in an open-ended way**: By this Nash means that a personal narrative should help the reader to see the world a little differently. He argues that the aim of the personal narrative should be to encourage the reader to accept that there is a range of viewpoints rather than accept any one viewpoint. The trick is to write 'softly and subtly'.

8. **Remember that writing is both a craft and an art**: Personal narratives are undermined by poor presentation, writing and editing. In this respect, they are the same as all academic writing.

9. **Use citations whenever appropriate**: More generally, Nash claims: 'To some extent, writing is about recirculating others' ideas within the framework of the personal narrative that only you are living and narrating. If you are truly honest with yourself, you know that, at most, you will be able to circulate and describe no more than one or two original ideas in all the writing that you will do for all your days' (2004: 66).

10. **Love and respect clear language**: Nash calls this eloquence.

PRACTICE POINT 3

Autoethnographic research has to succeed as both an example of social science and as a literary work. An important aim is to make the personal narrative an exemplar from which others may learn.

Analytical autoethnography

Alvesson, Hardy and Harley (2008) make an appeal for reflexivity, the constant questioning of authorial voice, and a challenging political agenda. Autoethnographic research appears as the perfect vehicle for the reflexive practices they champion. Similarly, Nash (2004) provides guidelines that seek to inspire researchers as well as guide them. Both sets of exemplars stress the autobiographical and at times poetic character of autoethnography. Hopefully, readers will be unsurprised that Alvesson, Hardy and Harley (2008) and Nash (2004) are writing from a social constructivist epistemology. But this is not the whole story in autoethnography. Some autoethnographers argue for an incorporation of social realist scholarship. For example, Duncan (2004: 5) argues:

> Although ethnographic and autoethnographic reports are presented in the form of personal narratives, this research tradition does more than just tell stories. It provides reports that are scholarly and justifiable interpretations based on multiple sources of evidence. This means autoethnographic accounts do not consist solely of the researcher's opinions but are also supported by other data that can confirm or triangulate those opinions. Methods of collecting data include participant observation, reflective writing, interviewing, and gathering documents and artefacts. ... Of these various methods, participant observation is by far the most characteristic of ethnographic work and the most important for autoethnographers. ... The challenge of participant observation in an autoethnography lies in mastering the art of self-reflection. A system of keeping reflections must be found that suits the nature of the research setting.

Duncan represents a minority position among autoethnographers, one that Anderson (2006) also supports. Anderson categorises the variants of autoethnography discussed in this chapter thus far as 'evocative autoethnography'. His preference is for an 'analytical autoethnography'. Its main features are:

1. **Complete member researcher (CMR) status**: The autoethnographer/researcher must be a complete member in the social world under study. It is interesting to note that Anderson uses the term researcher. This term is largely eschewed by the proponents of evocative autoethnography and is not really a part of the social constructivist epistemology. Anderson very clearly seeks to return autoethnography to the ethnographic fold: 'While most members are concerned only with participating in setting activities, the autoethnographer (like all participant observers) must also record events and conversations, at times making fieldwork 'near[ly] schizophrenic in its frenzied multiple focus (Adler and Adler, 1987: 70)' (Anderson, 2006: 380).

2. **Analytic reflexivity**: Anderson (2006: 382) argues that: 'reflexivity involves an awareness of reciprocal influence between ethnographers and their settings and informants. It entails self-conscious introspection guided by a desire to better understand both self and others through examining one's actions and perceptions in reference to and dialogue with those of others.'

3. **Narrative visibility of the researcher's self**: His next point is the importance of making the writer visible (Anderson, 2006: 384): 'By virtue of the autoethnographer's dual role as a member in the social world under study and as a researcher of that world, autoethnography demands enhanced textual visibility of the researcher's self. Such visibility demonstrates the researcher's personal engagement in the social world under study. Autoethnographers should illustrate analytic insights through recounting their own experiences and thoughts as well as those of others. Furthermore, they should openly discuss changes in their beliefs and relationships over the course of fieldwork, thus vividly revealing themselves as people grappling with issues relevant to membership and participation in fluid rather than static social worlds.'

4. **Dialogue with informants beyond the self**: Anderson also picks up on Duncan's (2004) point, that autoethnography should use multiple sources of evidence. Thus: 'Given that the researcher is confronted with self-related issues at every turn, the potential for self-absorption can loom large … solipsism and author saturation in autoethnographic texts are symptoms rather than the underlying problem. They stem from failure to adequately engage with others in the field. No ethnographic work – not even autoethnography – is a warrant to generalize from an "N of one"'(Anderson, 2006: 385). Certainly, narcissism is a major drawback of autoethnography – we will discuss this later.

5. **Commitment to theoretical analysis**: Anderson's final point is that there is more to autoethnography than representing the social world. Anderson asserts there is an imperative to analyse it and to develop theory.

Aims of autoethnography

Finding a definition of autoethnography is no easy task. This reflects the mutable character of the approach and a focus among the edited collections on the use of exemplars rather than how-to-do textbooks. For example, Stacey Holman Jones offers this gem: 'Autoethnography is … a balancing act', while '[w]riting about autoethnography is also a balancing act. In a handbook chapter that wants to move theory and method to action, what do I leave in and leave out?' (Holman Jones, 2005: 764). As it turns out, Holman Jones spends a considerable portion of her short-ish chapter asking these sorts of questions. The best definition she strikes is drawn from Ellis (1999), which we use as an introduction to the chapter.

Holman Jones is both frustrating and accurate. Autoethnography is slippery to define because a majority of its practitioners are committed to a social constructivist epistemology. One way to get a handle on autoethnography is to examine its aims. These vary between authors but provide a way into the approach:

- **Autoethnography as self-examination**: This is the most personal and inward-looking aim of the approach. Autoethnography is an autobiographical genre and the voice that is heard is primarily that of the author. Indeed, Carolyn Ellis argues in the introduction to her *Revision: Autoethnographic reflections on life and work* (2009) that autoethnography is part of her life work. This is a daunting but significant personal project. It highlights how autoethnography faces in two directions: one towards an engagement with the arts, humanities and social sciences; the other towards the existentialist concerns of living a conscious and thoughtful life. Plato records Socrates as giving the existentialist credo: 'The unexamined life is not worth living.' This means that the meaning in life is found in its examination and reflection. We will discuss this philosophical (non-social science) aspect of the approach in the conclusion (below).

- **Autoethnography as post-structural ethnography**: Roth (2005) argues that autoethnography remains a form of ethnography regardless of its autobiographical nature. At first sight autoethnography generates idiographic material which cannot be generalised. Roth disputes this in a somewhat convoluted manner. He argues two ways, applying social constructivist and post-structuralist principles (see Chapter 11 on semiotic analysis). On the one hand, he (after Jacques Derrida) argues for no commonality of interpretation or reading texts (or series of linked signs). In this respect, autoethnographic texts are no different from ethnographic texts. Each text is unique. On the other, all texts are linked by deep, structural commonalities in language. This means that autoethnographies are available as resources for people to deconstruct and use.

- **Autoethnography as witnessing trauma, loss and marginalisation**: Ellis (2009) and Roth (2005) point to fairly abstract and philosophical aims of autoethnography, but also engage in the more concrete, and at times explicitly political activity of witnessing. Sparkes (2002: 221, original italics) argues that autoethnographies 'become a call to *witness* for both the author and the reader. The witness offers testimony to a truth that is generally unrecognised or suppressed.' Autoethnographic research has been used most widely to give witness to trauma, loss and marginalisation. The edited collections of autoethnography focus almost exclusively on this sort of autobiography. For example, the early collection by Reed-Danahay (1997) has chapters on: Pan-Mayan writers, political resistance in socialist Romania, Swedish prisoners, ethnic Kabyle singers in Algeria, homeschooling in rural France, personal narrative in Corsica, reflections in fieldwork in Crete, and a feminist account of three women's lives in Portugal. We noted above that the Reed-Danahay collection is closely linked with an anthropological take on ethnography and the approach has since become more autobiographical. If anything, personal narratives have intensified the focus on witnessing (see Bochner and Ellis, 2002).

- **Autoethnography as praxis**: Autoethnography is most accepted among vocational disciplines: training nurses, social workers and teachers (see Foster et al., 2006; Nash, 2004; Riessman and Kohler, 2005; Roth, 2005). In these contexts, autoethnography is a self-centred approach used to examine the praxis (that is, the theory and practice) of teaching, nursing, social work. Praxis can be thought of as a special kind of witnessing: expert practitioners reflect on and share their insights with others. Autoethnography provides an insight into praxis because the account is produced in a reflexive manner (see both quotes from Ellis, above) and can be used as an exemplar. An exemplar is used in the physical sciences to refer to an unproblematic, tried-and-true building block of scientific theory. As many autoethnographers are at best agnostic about the possibility for science, an exemplar is somewhat looser and more political:

  > But surely it is not outside the bounds of possibility to suppose that some of the work we do, even if its primary role is but an exemplary one – i.e. 'This is what a life can be like', 'This is how someone can be defeated or rendered unconscious', 'This is how someone can reclaim his or her history', and so on – might be of value to someone besides ourselves. As an aside, it should be noted that, whether we intend it so or not, the work we do does indeed have an impact on people, even if only in what might appear to be relatively insignificant ways; for better or worse, it often steps outside the offices, labs, and so forth we inhabit. To the extent that this is so, we had better be cognizant both of what it is we are doing and what sort of impact we would like it to have. (Freeman, 1993: 229)

- **Autoethnography as postmodern 'social science'**: Freeman's (1993) notion of exemplars being of use to others, Sparkes' (2002) use of witnessing, and Roth's (2005) nod to post-structural linguists all point to the possibility at least for a postmodern form of social science. Each of those mentioned above provide ways of moving from autoethnography as idiographic research (that cannot be generalised) to nomothetic research that can. Of course the search for a postmodern variant of social science is not new. Bauman (1988) covered this ground with mixed success. Further, while autoethnographic research is dominated by social constructivist voices, there are also social realists who attempt to deal with more mainstream arguments about validity and reliability (see below).

SOME ISSUES IN RESEARCH

We have discussed issues of epistemology and the scientific concepts of validity and reliability. At first consideration it would appear that nowhere are these claims more difficult to uphold than with autoethnographic research. How, for example, can another researcher possibly attempt to replicate the findings of an autoethnographic researcher? However, in this section we discuss how these challenges may be faced and how autoethnographic research may be evaluated.

Epistemology and claims for validity and reliability

Reliability and validity are the core claims of research approaches that aim to be scientific. Reliability measures the extent to which the analysis of data yields results that can be repeated or reproduced at different times or by different researchers. Validity measures the extent to which the research is accurate and the extent to which claims can be made based on the research.

In the above section we referred to a split in autoethnographic research between social constructivist and social realist writers. To recap: Social constructivists have little faith in science as a project that generates anything resembling universal rules, laws or theorems. In this epistemology it is impossible to differentiate truth-claims based in science, or folklore, or common sense, or metaphysics because individuals or actors actively create the social world and all potential measures of that social world (see Chapters 10 and 11 on secondary research and semiotic analysis for a comparison). In contrast, for social realists, doing science is a legitimate goal, but it is understood as a project that is limited by factors that social scientists have great difficulty in controlling for or being objective about. Social realists emphasise subjectivity and the appreciation of factors like power, meaning and the need for researcher reflexivity (or self-awareness). As a result, any search for truth is always clouded by, among other things, the ways in which researchers and institutions impose bias.

The debate between evocative autoethnography and analytical autoethnography (Anderson, 2006) is most obvious in the discussion of reliability and validity. In effect, only the latter, the social realists, contribute to this debate. For example, in a discussion with Anderson (2006) about the future of autoethnography Norman Denzin describes his work thus:

It enacts a critical cultural politics concerning Native Americans and the representations of their historical presence in Yellowstone Park and elsewhere (Denzin, 2006). With Pelias (2004), I seek a writing form that enacts a methodology of the heart, a form that listens to the heart, knowing that 'stories are the truths that won't stand still' (Pelias, 2004, 171). In writing from the heart, we learn how to love, to forgive, to heal, and to move forward. (Denzin, 2006: 422–3)

He then offers a sample which talks of his watching cowboy and Indian movies as a child. His approach to autoethnography seems to have left social science research and has embraced literary forms. In this perspective, issues of reliability and validity are of secondary importance at best. The key driver is to be evocative, even poetic. Similarly, Carolyn Ellis and co-author Arthur Bochner (Bochner and Ellis, 2002) stage the following at a seminar:

Art (Stands and raises his hand; Carolyn nods.): Dr Ellis, I really appreciated your talk. Social science does indeed need more heart and emotion. I have only one small point to raise. You seem to accept the terms that orthodox social scientists use to describe their work – objectivity, validity, reliability. This ends up making you sound very defensive. Why not drop all the science talk? Just take for granted that what you are doing is important. It only distracts you and your readers from the very human sense of suffering and loss you communicate so beautifully... (Ellis, 2009: 111–12)

Clearly, there is an element of misrepresentation in this portrayal of analytical autoethnographers as positivists interested in objectivity rather than the more nuanced social realist position. But it does underscore that only the social realists are intrinsically interested in reliability and validity.

CONCEPTUAL CONCERN 4

Autoethnography has evocative and analytical variants (Anderson, 2006). Analytical autoethnography is social realist in terms of reliability and validity. By and large it views the approach as part of a broader 'reflexive ethnography'. Evocative autoethnography is social constructivist and literary in its orientation. In this perspective, issues of reliability and validity are of secondary importance at best. The key driver is to be emotive rather than analytical, poetic rather than scientific.

At the same time, reliability and validity are important for champions of evocative and analytical autoethnography alike. This is because autoethnographic researchers are challenging norms of science, but at the same time are seeking publication in academic journals and monographs. As a result, the issues around doing good or credible social science, including peer review, can become acute, especially when autoethnographers have their writing rejected (see Holt, 2003).

- **Reliability with a single-case**: The main tenet of reliability is reproducibility. To be reliable the data generated by a piece of research should be able to be reproduced by other researchers. This is an extremely problematic notion for autoethnography, where data is collected and analysed as part of the researcher's autobiographical writing. Autoethnography is a single-case variant of case-centric, case-first research. What passes for analytical induction in this is a reflexive process involving the author. Yin suggests that a case protocol can assist reliability in single-case research. He argues that a case study protocol 'is a major way of increasing the *reliability* of case study and is intended to guide the investigator in carrying out data collection from a single-case study' (Yin, 2003: 67). The protocol provides at least a hypothetical basis for other researchers to repeat the study. The protocol requires researchers to spell out: (1) an overview of the case study project; (2) field procedures – accessing the participants, etc.; (3) the schedule of questions; and (4) the guide for data analysis and reporting. Duncan (2004: 11) modifies the protocol developed by Yin:

This basic protocol required that:

1. the study be located in the practitioner's work setting;
2. extra time be allowed for the job of making tacit knowledge explicit, recording and developing reflections, and conducting a literature review; in the first instance, a retrospective account be developed to sensitize the researcher to important themes and issues already present in the research setting;
3. a reflective journal be kept systematically;
4. files for documentary evidence be kept based on significant events or project stages;
5. multiple sources of data be collected and categorized;
6. data collection and analysis be ongoing and used to inform practice;
7. a narrative account be constructed based on the data and conclusions drawn from that account; and
8. the account be reviewed by others involved in the research setting.

Duncan also provides an assessment of validity that is close to some of the categories we use in our discussion in Chapter 9 on content research. The variants of validity associated with autoethnography are somewhat truncated because of the single-case and reflexive character of the writing. They seek affirmation of the variants of validity that have little or nothing by way of a quantifiable component.

- **Content or construct validity**: Content or construct validity focuses on the comprehensiveness of the variables used. Duncan (2004) again refers to Yin (2003). She argues that her writing attained construct validity because the autobiographical/autoethnographic text was the primary source of evidence, but this account was also substantiated in three main ways:

1. 'Multiple sources of evidence were used along with the researcher's personal account. These additional sources of evidence included letters, memos, meeting minutes, computer interactions stored on disk, prints of screen designs, preparatory sketches, visitors comments, e-mails, and other related items' (Duncan, 2004: 10).

2. 'A chain of evidence was established in which data were catalogued and indexed, and recurring or developing themes recorded in a way that facilitates retracing' (Duncan, 2004: 10).

3. 'Drafts of the narrative account were reviewed by three other key members of the design team' (Duncān, 2004: 10). This reading of drafts of the autoethnography was used by Duncan to verify her interpretation of events, and is clearly an effort to move autoethnography beyond idiographic material, which cannot be generalised.

- **Face or instrumental validity**: Autoethnographers are acutely aware that their accounts can be called self-serving (see Freeman, 1993). Duncan uses the notion of autoethnography being helpful to others as both a rejoinder to this criticism and a version of the common-sense measure of validity. She asks a version of the question 'Does the research seem to work? Is it instrumental or helpful to other researchers?' Unfortunately, this measure of validity has little empirical content, although perhaps a measure of impact factors – how widely an article is read or cited – might be useful.

- **Peer validity**: This assessment of validity is made by peer review. Whereas face validity relies on the opinion of the researcher, peer review relies on the opinions of a community of academics and other researchers. Peer validity carries with it the notion that an autoethnography will be judged in comparison with others both in terms of process and results. Duncan believes that this aspect of peer review will ensure a scholarly account. It should be noted that evocative autoethnographers seem more likely to bemoan peer review (Holt, 2003).

Evaluating autoethnographies

Arguably a holistic evaluation of autoethnographic research is a more sensitive and appropriate measure than standard reliability and validity. Richardson (2000: 254) described five factors she uses when reviewing ethnographic articles – including autoethnographies – that combines scientific and literary approaches. Richardson's work is very useful because she straddles the social constructivist/social realist divide or the distinction between evocative and analytical autoethnography (Anderson, 2006). Her focus is on what makes a good and useful autoethnography rather than the more abstracted issues of epistemology. Her criteria are posed as questions:

1. **Is there a substantive contribution?** This criteria is located squarely within the social sciences. Does the article add to the understanding of social life? Richardson is particularly interested in the extent to which autoethnographers show how their experiences are of relevance to others.

2. **Is there aesthetic merit?** Does this piece succeed aesthetically? With this criteria Richardson focuses on the literary aspects of autoethnography rather than the social sciences. This is a key dimension to remember if contemplating the approach. She asks: 'Is the text artistically shaped, satisfying, complex, and not boring?'

3. **Is the text reflexive?** Here we will just list the questions she asks: 'How did the author come to write this text? How was the information gathered? Ethical issues? How has the author's subjectivity been both a producer and a product of this text? Is there adequate self-awareness and self-exposure for the reader to make judgements about the point of view? Do authors hold themselves accountable to the standards of knowing and telling of the people they have studied?' (Richardson, 2000: 254). The last question touches on the problem of validity and reliability, which we have discussed above.

4. **Does it have impact?** Here Richardson combines scientific and literary concerns. For her, impact is not simply a measure of how widely an account is read, but includes its emotional force. Indeed, she frames the emotional impact as key in opening up new questions and areas of research for readers.

5. **Does it express a reality?** Again, Richardson combines scientific and literary concerns. She questions whether the account provides a credible interpredation of 'a cultural, social, individual, or communal sense of the "real"?'. She is less clear, a lot less clear, on how reality might be assessed.

PUTTING THE APPROACH IN CONTEXT

Autoethnographic research is a case-centric, case-first approach that is based on the reflexivity of the writer dealing with her/his autobiography. It is a single-case approach. While Duncan (2004) and other analytical autoethnographers might seek to fold in forms of triangulation – using multiple methods to double and triple check results – the majority of social constructivist writers would see this as an unnecessary and inelegant burden. As a result, autoethnographic research is highly individualistic and very fluid in the way it is undertaken. Indeed, the reflexive imperative of the approach demands that writing be reviewed, reworked and rewritten. Ellis (2009) seems to suggest that this fluid engagement with data and analysis is a life's work.

CONCEPTUAL CONCERN 5

Like most case-centric, case-first approaches, autoethnography has a fluid framing of research. The researcher is free to conduct research as an iterative process, moving between data and analysis as he or she sees fit. Indeed, the reflexive imperative of the approach demands that writing be reviewed, reworked and rewritten.

Motivations: the forms of personal documents

Given the long-term commitment that the main protagonists of autoethnography have to writing and reflection and their aversion to standard social sciences procedures, it is useful to explore some possible motivations.

PRACTICE POINT 4

Anyone contemplating autoethnography should keep a diary and revisit it often as part of the process of being reflexive.

Gordon Allport (1897–1967) was an American psychologist. Writing in 1942, long before autoethnography, he proposed thirteen reasons for the authoring of personal documents. He points to the psychological underpinnings and interpretations of personal narratives. These can all be restated for the social sciences.

1. **Special pleading:** Writers may be interested in self-justification, particularly in blaming others for the faults that are assigned to them. Allport concludes that no autobiography is free from self-justification and, indeed, the more extreme the self-justification is, the more use it may be for analysing motivation.

2. **Exhibitionism:** 'Closely related is the document in which egotism runs riot' (Allport, 1942: 5). Authors portray themselves in the best possible light. This is a form of narcissism or self-absorption.

3. **Desire for order:** This is a compulsive need to record the events of the day.

4. **Literary delight:** Allport argues that the personal narrative can be the mechanism for aesthetic or artistic motives.

5. **Securing personal perspective:** The personal narrative can, and should, be used to take stock of a life, especially after a period of change or transition.

6. **Relief from tension**: Writing a diary or personal narrative can be cathartic or therapeutic. This is especially so if there is no other obvious mechanism for securing relief.

7. **Monetary gain**: In the context of autoethnography and what Nash (2004) calls scholarly personal narrative, advancing an academic career is probably a better term than simple monetary gain. Allport made the point that monetary/professional gain does not necessarily undermine the autobiography.

8. **Assignment**: Nash (2004) would be delighted with Allport's comment: 'In college courses students can be required to write autobiographies. ... In writing under such conditions, the student at first is merely carrying out an assigned task, but in the process of writing, his interest becomes deeper and personal motives are brought into play' (Allport, 1942: 7).

9. **Assisting in therapy**: Some personal narratives are written explicitly as part of a therapeutic process.

10. **Redemption and reintegration**: Autobiography often has a confessional element. Confessions, whether religious or secular, are normally offered by writers seeking forgiveness and reintegration.

11. **Scientific interest**: Allport argues that 'candid' or 'cultivated' students can offer their personal narratives in the belief that their unique experiences will be of benefit to scientists. Allport talks here of psychologists' interests in issues of personality. It seem only a small leap to include the social sciences more broadly and the autoethnography.

12. **Public service and example**: This approach is favoured by social reformers who use their life struggles and insights to advance a cause.

13. **Desire for immortality**: More generally, this notion can be thought of as a desire to be heard and acknowledged.

Allport's review is somewhat cynical and world-weary. It is a long way from the enthusiasm of Carolyn Ellis and Norman Denzin. We feel that Allport would be somewhat shocked by the confessional and narcissistic elements of autoethnography. Its self-contained, self-referential, if not self-serving, elements are a little hard to take at times. But the world has moved on since Allport, most notably with the rise of the internet, and a host of digital and wireless technologies.

Autoethnography where '... I am both the author and the focus of the story, the one who tells and the one who experiences, the observer and the observed, the creator and the created' (Ellis, 2009: 13) dominates the internet and new media. These sorts of postings are central to social networking (e.g., blogs, tweets, daily posting about 'what's on your mind?'). Arguably, the perspective of evocative autoethnographers, i.e., that emotion should trump analysis, has won out in cyberspace, if not yet in peer-reviewed journals. Such variants of autoethnography seem to capture the *Zeitgeist* or spirit of the age.

CONCEPTUAL CONCERN 6

Autoethnography is an increasingly popular form of self-expression, and is aligned with the most rapidly developing, contemporary technologies and media. Variants of autoethnography seem to capture the *Zeitgeist* or spirit of the age. It is hard to believe that autoethnography will not grow as a legitimate research approach.

Marshall McLuhan (1911–80) used the phrase 'the medium is the message' to suggest that new technologies themselves play a powerful role in shaping the content of media and the attitudes of the public (McLuhan, 1967). From this perspective, if social networking is the medium, what is the message? The new technologies allow us to stay in contact almost continuously with friends, families, employers and employees, news and entertainment sources, etc. But do they also encourage narcissism? Narcissism is a synonym of vanity, conceit and self-absorption. Often, such networking isn't very social at all: there are literally millions of posts to hundreds of online and wireless fora that are unread by anyone except the poster and their closest friends.

CONCLUSION

Autoethnographic research is a particular form of case-centric research, representing the single-case approach. It is highly individualistic and very fluid in the way it is undertaken. Autoethnographic texts have a variety of forms. They have in common the autobiographical genre and an explicit commitment to reflexivity as a means of generating and analysing data.

Due to the mutable character of the approach, defining autoethnography is a challenging task. One way of developing an understanding of autoethnographic research is to examine its aims. These vary between authors but include autoethnography as self-examination, as post-structural ethnography, as witnessing trauma, loss and marginalisation, and as a self-centred approach used to examine praxis (i.e., the theory and practice) of vocational work in particular.

Issues of reliability and validity are particularly problematic for autoethnographers. Arguably, a holistic evaluation of autoethnographic research is a more sensitive and appropriate measure than standard reliability and validity. Richardson (2000) combines scientific and literary concerns in her discussion of aspects of 'good' autoethnography, considering the substantive contribution to knowledge, aesthetic merit, reflexivity, impact and expression of 'reality'.

Overall, it is helpful to view autoethnography in terms of the *Zeitgeist* discussed in the previous section, when making an assessment of the approach. On the negative side are all the shortcomings of the approach in terms of reliability and validity, and just outright clarity of method. One problem with facilitating multiple voices is that you end up with multiple voices on what to do and not to do! Further, the approach, especially evocative autoethnography, can collapse to narcissism and smugness. Your authors confess to experiencing a degree of eye-rolling when collating the quotes used in this chapter. On the positive side, autoethnography is an increasingly popular form of self-expression and is aligned with the most rapidly developing, contemporary technologies. We believe its popularity creates an imperative to harness and use autoethnography as research.

FURTHER READINGS

More than any other approach covered in this textbook, autoethnography is the product of postmodernity. The classic discussion of postmodernity is by Frederick Jameson (1990) and there is a sustained critique by Alex Callinicos (1991). Zygmunt Bauman's 'Is there a postmodern sociology?' (1988) is a brave attempt to turn the postmodern critique into a contemporary discipline. The article by Steve Matthewman and Doug Hoey 'What happened to postmodernism?' (2006) is a generous retrospect of the moment. Steven Seidman (1994) wrote an introduction to social theory that brilliantly captures the highwater mark of postmodernism.

REFERENCES

Adler, P. A. & Adler, P. 1987. *Membership roles in field research*. Thousand Oaks, CA: Sage.

Allport, G. W. 1942. *The use of personal documents in psychological science*. New York: The Committee on Appraisal of Research.

Alvesson, M., Hardy, C. & Harley, B. 2008. Reflecting on reflexivity: Reflexive textual practices in organization and management theory. *Journal of Management Studies*, 45 (3), 480–501.

Anderson, L. 2006. Analytic autoethnography. *Journal of Contemporary Ethnography*, 35 (4), 373–395.

Bauman, Z. 1988. Is there a postmodern sociology? *The Journal of Theory, Culture & Society*, 5 (2), 217–237.

Bochner, A. P. & Ellis, C. 2002. *Ethnographically speaking: Autoethnography, literature and aesthetics*. Walnut Creek, CA: Altamira Press.

Callinicos, A. 1991. *Against postmodernism: A Marxist critique*. Cambridge: Polity Press.

Collins, W. H. 1998. The meaning of data: open and closed evidential cultures in the search for gravitational waves. *American Journal of Sociology*, 1042, 293–338.

Denzin, N. 2006. *Searching for Yellowstone: Performing race, nature and nation in the New West*. Walnut Creek, CA: Left Coast Press.

Denzin, N. K. 2006. Analytic autoethnography, or *déjà vu* all over again. *Journal of Contemporary Ethnography*, 35, 419–428.

Duncan, M. 2004. Autoethnography: Critical appreciation of an emerging art. *International Journal of Qualitative Methods*, 3, 1–24.

Ellis, C. 1999. Heartful Autoethnography. *Qualitative Health Research*, 9, 669–683.

Ellis, C. 2009. *Revision: Autoethnographic reflections on life and work*. Walnut Creek, CA: Left Coast Press.

Foster, K., MCallister, M. & O'Brien, L. 2006. Extending the boundaries: Autoethnography as an emergent method in mental health nursing research. *International Journal of Mental Health Nursing*, 15, 44–53.

Freeman, M. 1993. *Rewriting the self: History, memory, narrative*. London: Routledge.

Geertz, C. 1995. *After the fact: Two countries, four decades, one anthropologist*. Cambridge, MA: Harvard University Press.

Holman Jones, S. 2005. Autoethnography: Making the personal political. In: Denzin, N. K. & Lincoln, Y. S. (eds.), *Handbook of qualitative research*. Thousand Oaks, CA: Sage.

Holt, N. L. 2003. Representation, legitimation, and autoethnography: An autoethnographic writing story. *International Journal of Qualitative Methods*, 2(1) 18–28.

Jameson, F. 1990. *Postmodernism, or, The cultural logic of late capitalism*. London: Verso.

Matthewman, S. & Hoey, D. 2006. What happened to postmodernism? *Sociology*, 40, 529–547.

McLuhan, M. 1967. *Understanding media: The extensions of man*. London: Sphere Books.

Mills, C. W. 1959. *The sociological imagination*. New York: Oxford University Press.

Nash, N. 2004. *Liberating scholarly writing: The power of personal narrative*. New York: Teachers College Press.

Open University. 2010. *Skills for OU study*. Available at: www.open.ac.uk/skillsforstudy/being-reflective.php [Accessed 10 May 2011].

Pelais, R. A. 2004. *Methodology of the heart*. Walnut Creek CA: Altamira Press.

Reed-Danahay, D. E. 1997. *Auto/ethnography: Rewriting the self and the social*. Oxford: Berg.

Richardson, L. 2000. Evaluating ethnography. *Qualitative Inquiry*, 6, 253–254.

Riessman, C. & Kohler, C. 2005. Narrative in social work: A critical review. *Qualitative Social Work*, 4, 391–412.

Roth, W. 2005. *Auto/biography and Auto/ethnography: Praxis of research method*. Rotterdam: Sense Publishers.

Seidman, S. 1994. *Contested knowledge: Social theory in the postmodern era*. Oxford: Blackwell.

Sparkes, A. C. 2002. Autoethnography: Self-indulgence or something more. In: Bochner, A. P. & Ellis, C. (eds.), *Ethnographically speaking: Autoethnography, literature and aesthetics*. Walnut Creek, CA: Altamira Press.

Yin, R. K. 2003. *Case study research: Design and methods*. London: Sage.

GLOSSARY

Analytical induction: Analytical induction is associated with case-centric research. This means that researchers who start with exploring a case do so with something of a blank slate. This is not to say that they have forgotten all that they know of anthropology, or psychology, or sociology, etc., but it does mean that they enter the field with a lot to learn. This is called an analytical inductive approach. Inductive means reaching a conclusion based on observation. Some textbooks describe inductive research as a bottom-up approach. The researcher builds up a new theory from observations, and then developing propositions and hypotheses about them. In other words, when beginning with a case (or a limited number of cases), the researcher has to determine what the key variables and associated values are, and the significant relationships between them. Associated techniques include grounded theory and thematic analysis (see Chapter 2 – In-Depth Interviewing).

Case: The closest synonym to 'case' is 'example'. A case or a set of cases is the thing that a researcher is interested in studying. A case, or cases, is ultimately defined by the researcher. Common cases include people, groups of people, places, texts, objects, writing, images, audio-visual material. All of these things, and many more, can be constituted as cases suitable for social scientific research.

Case-centric, or case-first research: The researcher begins with the exploration of a case (a place, a person, a body of writing, and image, etc.). This learning – we use the term analytical induction – centres on finding which variables and associated values best describe the interesting aspects of the case. Case-centric research is associated with a single or a few cases and many variables. The classic example of case-centric research is traditional ethnography in which the researcher (i.e., a western anthropologist) lives among a group of indigenous peoples – the case – for a sustained period, and in doing so details their daily lives, rituals and customs – the variables (see Chapter 4, Ethnographic Research).

Closed questions: Closed questions can be answered with a 'yes' or 'no' of statement of fact, or through a predetermined selection. For example: How strongly do you agree or disagree with the following statement: 'I enjoy being a university student?' Example survey answer options: (1) Strongly agree, (2) Agree, (3) Neither agree nor disagree, (4) Disagree, (5) Strongly disagree.

Coding: Coding is a process of sorting and categorising data for further analysis. It can be undertaken with case-centric and variable-centric data. In its most narrow terms, coding refers to making data readable by software packages – either numeric or non-numeric. Coding tends to make data more amenable for forms of statistical analysis and for making case-centric data countable. However, grounded theorists (see Chapter 2) use coding as the basis of building theory from interview material.

Data collection and analysis: Data collection is the phase of research in which the needed material is sourced. The methods used to collect data differ markedly according to the research process. Data analysis involves the checking of the material against what is expected (as in the case of hypothesis-testing), or the use of the technique of analytical induction.

Epistemology: Epistemology refers to the theory of knowledge that informs how research is shaped in its broadest sense. Epistemology generates differing attitudes to making and understanding observations of the social world, and the possibilities for science. We discuss three epistemological positions in this textbook: (1) positivism, (2) social realism and (3) social constructivism (see below).

Fixed analytical framing: A fixed analytical framing means that the researcher must adhere to a sequence of procedures. There is very little scope for the researcher to revisit earlier phases of the research, especially data collection. Fixed framing is associated with variable-centric research and hypothesis-testing.

Fluid analytical framing: A fluid analytical framing means that the researcher is free to revisit and significantly modify earlier stages of research. This can include the overall focus of the research. Fluid framing is associated with case-centric research and analytical induction.

Giving voice: Giving voice is a research goal that is sometimes at odds with the demands of reliability and validity. Giving voice means using a research project as a mechanism for the research participants to speak to a broader academic or mainstream audience.

Grounded theory: This is a key form of data analysis associated with case-centric data. It was developed by Anselm Strauss, Barney Glaser and Juliet Corbin (see Chapter 2).

Hypothesis: An hypothesis is a proposition about the relationship between at least two variables. For example, an increase in the variable 'Price of Petrol' will generate increases in the variable 'Use of Public Transport'.

Hypothesis-testing: Hypothesis-testing is a top-down approach to theory and research. It is a deductive way of doing research. Deductive means finding the solution to a problem based on evidence. A more formal name for this approach to research is 'hypothetico-deductive reasoning'. The researcher begins with a developed problem, in the form of a hypothesis about the relationship between some variables, and seeks a solution by testing this theory across a number of cases.

Interactive and non-interactive research: Interactive research involves the creation of data at the point or moment of its collection. Common forms of interactive research include interviewing, participant observation and experiments. Almost all forms of research involving participants is interactive. Non-interactive research is either unobtrusive, involving covert surveillance or relies on the collection and analysis of inanimate data: texts, audio-visual materials, secondary research, etc.

Interviewing: There are three main variants of interviewing: (1) structured interviewing, in which the interviewer follows, and does not deviate from, an interview schedule; (2) semi-structured interviewing, where the schedule can be augmented with questions developed in response to the interview situation. In some examples, the interview schedule is a list of topics that does not include the wording of questions; (3) unstructured interviewing, in which the interviewer begins with only a topic of conversation in mind.

Methodology: Methodology is the logic of methods or of research. In this textbook we have tended to use the term 'research approach' rather than methodology. Methodology occupies a conceptual 'space' that is more abstract than 'methods' and less abstract than 'epistemology' (see above). It refers to how and why different sets of methods are bundled together.

Methods: Methods are a repeatable set of procedures or techniques undertaken in research.

Non-interactive research: *See* **Interactive research**

Open questions: Open questions are those that cannot be answered with a simple 'yes' or 'no' or by stating a fact. Open questions are more probing. They are commonly used in in-depth interviewing. For example: 'Tell me how you got on with your brother?' and 'What stands out most clearly for you when you recall that first day in prison?'

Participant observation: In participant observation research the researcher immerses him/herself in a social group. Such immersion can be to a greater or lesser degree. Covert participation observation involves the participation of the researcher without informing members of the social group. Overt participant observation involves the researcher notifying the group of his/her intentions. Participant observation usually requires the help of a gatekeeper to the group or a sponsor.

Positivism: Positivism is an epistemological position. Positivists stress the techniques of observation and measurement and the potential for scientists to form objective, unbiased understandings of the social world. For them, good science is objective science, and the methods of doing research are largely about eliminating a subjective stance or bias on the part of the researcher and the research participants. This is an important – but tacit – 'political' agenda and as a result positivism is commonly accused of ignoring issues like power, subjectivity (meaning) and cultural relativism.

Post-structuralism: *See* **Structuralism**

Reflexivity: Reflexivity is the process of researchers being self-reflexive or self-aware in the research process. Reflection could be described as: (1) thinking with a purpose; (2) being critical, but not negative; (3) analysing how effective your learning is; (4) questioning and probing; (5) making judgements and drawing conclusions.

Reliability: Is a way of discussing and assessing the rigour of research. Reliability measures the extent to which the analysis of data yields reliable results that can be repeated or reproduced at different times or by different researchers.

Sampling: Sampling is the process of making a selection of cases to be studied (e.g., people, texts, objects, films, etc.) from the entire population of such cases. Normally, sampling strategies are designed to generate a representative sample. This means the sample is representative of the population. In other words, the cases in the sample have the variables that are of interest to the researcher in proportions that reflect the population. Sampling is practised in nearly all forms of research, though it is most aligned with variable-centric research and with the use of numeric data and analysis. Sampling from a population comes in two main forms: a non-probability sample (cluster, quota or convenience sampling) or a probability sample (simple random sampling, systematic sampling, stratified sampling). The key difference between a non-probability and probability sample is that in the latter all potential participating cases have an equal chance of being selected. The randomness of probability sampling makes it the better option because it allows the use of more powerful statistical analysis, called inferential statistics.

Science wars: Many of the social sciences are antagonistic. There is inter- and intra-disciplinary rivalry based on theoretical positions, epistemological stances and what is considered good science. Some of this rivalry is based on careerism and is self-serving. However, the diverse epistemological stances have irreducible differences at the level of logic and first principles. This gives rise to science wars. In the 1970s there was intense rivalry between the old guard in the form of positivists of various hues and the radicals – feminists, Marxists, etc. In the 1990s the so-called positivist critique (of mainstream social science) was another science war. These outbreaks of hostilities between academics tend to go out of fashion rather than be resolved.

Social constructivism: Social constructivism is an epistemological position. Social constructivists criticise both positivist and social realist epistemology. They challenge the notion of science as a legitimate concept. They have no faith in science as a project that generates anything resembling universal rules or laws or theory. In this epistemology it is impossible to differentiate truth-claims based in science, or folklore, or common sense, or metaphysics because individuals or actors actively create the social world and all potential measures of that social world. They argue that it is impossible to have a scientific stance, meaning an objective position outside the data and its analysis (if you are a positivist), or to control/filter the subjective effects of power, meaning and bias (if you are a social realist).

Social realism: Social realism is an epistemological position. Social realists believe in an external and measurable social reality, but one that exists through the mediation of our perceptions of it and our actions. Social realists argue that revealing the social world is far more problematic than suggested by positivists. For social realists, doing science is a legitimate goal, but it is understood as a project that is limited by factors that social scientists have great difficulty in controlling for or being objective about. Where positivists strive for objectivity, social realists emphasise subjectivity – perspective – and the appreciation of factors like power, meaning and the need for researcher reflexivity (self-awareness). Any search for truth is always clouded by, among other things, the ways in which researchers and institutions impose bias. Controlling for institutional and researcher bias becomes an important component of socialist realist efforts at doing science, whereas positivists, in their narrow focus on methods, tend to discount these political underpinnings of science. Social realists tend to make explicit the political assumption about epistemology and how it impacts method.

Structuralism and post-structuralism: Structuralism has its origins in linguistic and semiotic analysis. It is a positivist approach that studied the (assumed) underlying laws and generalities of language, rather than what people subjectively thought about language. Structuralism can also be described as being 'decentred', meaning structuralists did not study what individuals or groups thought of the social world, but how their actions were shaped by various rules (of language or of capitalism, for instance). Post-structuralism retained the decentred aspect of structuralism: individual action was not considered important. However, post-structuralism has a social constructivist epistemology, that denied possibilities for science. In essence, the difference between structuralism and post-structuralism is about truth-claims. For its nineteenth-century founders, decentring the focus of research provided the basis for science. For the post-structuralists of the twentieth century, the logic of decentring, of subordinating the individual, provides a further rationale for the abandonment of science as a privileged truth-claim.

Triangulation: Triangulation is the use of more than one method to double- or cross-check the collected and/or partially analysed data from another method.

Validity: Is a way of discussing and assessing the rigour of the research. Validity measures the extent to which the research is accurate, that it measures what was intended, and the extent to which truth-claims can be made. Validity is most readily assessed when the data is a numeric form. Measures of correlation and causality between variables can be used to assess validity. However, all non-numeric data relies on more obviously subjective assessments. These weaker 'tests' that can provide some confidence about validity, including reliability or external validity, internal validity, content or construct validity, face validity or instrumental, peer validity.

Variable-centric, or variable-first research: The researcher begins with some ideas about a few variables and associated values, normally in the form of a proposition or hypothesis. The researcher seeks out an adequate number of cases in order to test the hypothesis. Variable-centric research is closely aligned with hypothesis-testing. Variable-centric research is associated with relatively few variables and many cases. Survey research is the classic example of variable-centric research. The questionnaire contains the questions that are needed to assess the relationship between variables. The researcher uses sampling to find sufficient cases (survey respondents) to test the hypothesis (see Chapter 6).

Variables: Variables are the characteristics or features that are used to describe a case. Variables are always associated with values, in each particular case. Values are the descriptors that make variables measurable. For example, the variable 'Income Level' might have five values, one of which is to be chosen by each survey respondent: (1) less than $5,000, (2) $5,001–$10,000, (3) $10,001–$15,000, (4) $15,001–$20,000, (5) more than $20,000. Experimenters make use of several types of variables: (1) independent variables are the factors that experimenters manipulate to see if they affect the dependent variable; (2) dependent variables are the factors that experimenters measure to see if they are affected by the independent variable; (3) subject variables are the variables that characterise pre-existing differences among study participants.

INDEX

Printed in Great Britain
by Amazon

85245868R00179